Redo Cardiac Surgery in Adults

Venkat R. Machiraju • Hartzell V. Schaff
Lars G. Svensson
Editors

Redo Cardiac Surgery in Adults

Second Edition

Springer

Editors
Venkat R. Machiraju
Department of Cardiothoracic Surgery
University of Pittsburgh Medical Center
Pittsburgh, PA, USA
machvr@upmc.edu

Hartzell V. Schaff
Division of Cardiovascular Surgery
Mayo Clinic
Rochester, MN, USA
schaff@mayo.edu

Lars G. Svensson
Department of Thoracic
and Cardiovascular Surgery
Cleveland Clinic Foundation
Cleveland, OH, USA
svenssl@ccf.org

ISBN 978-1-4939-4154-4 ISBN 978-1-4614-1326-4 (eBook)
DOI 10.1007/978-1-4614-1326-4
Springer New York Dordrecht Heidelberg London

Springer is part of Springer Science+Business Media (www.springer.com)

Preface to the Second Edition

The first edition of Redo Cardiac Surgery in Adults was published in 1996 and was a compilation of the proceedings of the First International Symposium on Redo Cardiac Surgery. During the last 16 years, several changes have occurred, not only in the profiles of the patients requiring redo cardiac surgery, but also in the redo cardiac surgical procedures that are performed. Overall, while the experience of cardiac surgeons has increased, the complexity of the surgical procedures and the comorbid conditions of the patients have also increased. Twenty years ago, redo coronary artery bypass surgery was the most common redo cardiac surgery performed in the adult population. Now, isolated redo coronary artery bypass surgery is virtually gone, and more complex redo valvular surgical procedures along with aortic arch and thoracic aortic procedures are performed routinely. These procedures in turn lead to newer redo cardiac surgical procedures. As younger cardiac surgeons enter the field of cardiac surgery, it will be difficult for them to gain extensive experience in all the redo cardiac surgical procedures during the short period of their training. While experienced surgeons have figured out for themselves how to handle various difficult situations, younger surgeons are always looking for some guidance. There have been several improvements over the years in the management of perioperative complications. Perioperative stroke is addressed quickly with various interventional procedures to limit or obviate any neurological deficit. Similarly, renal failure is managed with early dialysis to prevent mortality and improve survival. The purpose of this book is to give some practical suggestions to surgeons rather than to provide lot of theoretical data to the reader.

The book is divided into a Coronary and General section, which includes coronary artery revascularization procedures and management of the common major perioperative complications, and Mitral and Aortic sections. The authors who contributed the chapters are actively practicing their subspecialty and, as such, they present the current standard of care in managing various surgical problems. Though we cannot discuss rare redo cardiac surgical problems, this book focuses on day-to-day surgical problems that arise during the redo cardiac surgery.

We express our special thanks to Shannon Wyszomierski, Ph.D. for her assistance with the editorial work.

Pittsburgh, PA, USA — Venkat R. Machiraju, MD
Rochester, MN, USA — Hartzell V. Schaff, MD
Cleveland, OH, USA — Lars G. Svensson, MD

Contents

1 **Problems Related to Redo Cardiac Surgery** ... 1
Venkat R. Machiraju

2 **Practical Approaches to the Current "On-Pump" Redo Coronary Artery Bypass Surgery** ... 7
Venkat R. Machiraju

3 **Off-Pump Coronary Artery Bypass Grafting for Repeat Coronary Revascularization** ... 21
Richard J. Myung and John D. Puskas

4 **Management of Perioperative Stroke** ... 29
Amer M. Malik and Lawrence R. Wechsler

5 **Acute Kidney Injury Associated with Cardiac Surgery** ... 37
Mitchell H. Rosner

6 **Pulmonary Factors in Redo Open Heart Surgery** ... 53
David O. Wilson

7 **Transfusion Therapy in Reoperative Cardiac Surgery** ... 57
Anand Padmanabhan and Darrell J. Triulzi

8 **Anesthesia for Redo Cardiac Surgery** ... 63
Cynthia M. Wells and Andrew W. Murray

9 **Options for Advanced Mechanical Support for Cardiogenic Shock Complicating Cardiac Reoperations** ... 67
Christian Bermudez, Kenji Minakata, and Robert L. Kormos

10 **Reoperations for Mitral Valve Disease: Surgical Approaches and Techniques** ... 81
Hartzell V. Schaff and Arman Arghami

11 **Reoperation Following Mitral Valve Repair** ... 89
Rakesh M. Suri and Hartzell V. Schaff

12 **Reoperation for Prosthetic Mitral Valve Endocarditis** ... 99
Kevin L. Greason and Hartzell V. Schaff

13 **Surgical Management of Atrial Fibrillation in Redo Cardiac Operations** ... 109
John M. Stulak and Hartzell V. Schaff

14 **Surgical Management of Tricuspid Valve Disorders** 121
Venkat R. Machiraju

15 **Reoperation for Aortic Valve Disease** 125
Lars G. Svensson

16 **Reoperation Following Homograft Aortic Valve Replacement** 133
Thoralf M. Sundt III

17 **Prosthetic Aortic Valve and Root Endocarditis** 141
Gosta B. Pettersson, Rajesh Ramankutty, Brian Griffin, and Thomas Fraser

18 **Reoperation on the Aortic Arch** 151
Lars G. Svensson

19 **Descending and Thoracoabdominal Aortic Reoperations** 157
Edward Soltesz

20 **Reoperations Following Endovascular Aortic Repair** 171
Eric E. Roselli

21 **Percutaneous Approaches to Valvular Heart Disease After Previous Cardiac Surgery** 195
John M. Stulak and Hartzell V. Schaff

Index 201

Contributors

Arman Arghami, MD Division of Cardiovascular Surgery, Mayo Clinic, Rochester, MN, USA

Christian Bermudez, MD Department of Cardiothoracic Surgery, University of Pittsburgh Medical Center, Pittsburgh, PA, USA

Thomas Fraser, MD Division of Cardiac Infections, Department of Infectious Diseases, Cleveland Clinic, Cleveland, OH, USA

Kevin L. Greason, MD Division of Cardiovascular Surgery, Mayo Clinic, Rochester, MN, USA

Brian Griffin, MD Department of Cardiovascular Medicine, Cleveland Clinic, Cleveland, OH, USA

Robert L. Kormos, MD Department of Cardiothoracic Surgery, University of Pittsburgh Medical Center, Pittsburgh, PA, USA

Venkat R. Machiraju, MD Department of Cardiothoracic Surgery, University of Pittsburgh Medical Center, Pittsburgh, PA, USA

Amer M. Malik, MD Department of Neurology, UPMC Stroke Institute, University of Pittsburgh School of Medicine, Pittsburgh, PA, USA

Kenji Minakata, MD Department of Cardiothoracic Surgery, University of Pittsburgh Medical Center, Pittsburgh, PA, USA

Andrew W. Murray, MBChB Department of Anesthesiology, University of Pittsburgh Medical Center, Pittsburgh, PA, USA

Richard J. Myung, MD Emory University, Wellstar Kennestone Hospital, Marietta, GA, USA

Anand Padmanabhan, MD Department of Pathology, Division of Transfusion Medicine, University of Pittsburgh School of Medicine, Pittsburgh, PA, USA

Gosta B. Pettersson, MD Department of Thoracic and Cardiovascular Surgery, Surgical Director of Lung Transplant Unit, Cleveland Clinic, Cleveland, OH, USA

John D. Puskas, MD Division of Cardiothoracic Surgery, Emory University School of Medicine, Atlanta, GA, USA

Rajesh Ramankutty, MD Department of Thoracic and Cardiovascular Surgery, Surgical Director of Lung Transplant Unit, Cleveland Clinic, Cleveland, OH, USA

Eric E. Roselli, MD Department of Thoracic and Cardiovascular Surgery, Cleveland Clinic, Cleveland, OH, USA

Mitchell H. Rosner, MD Division of Nephrology, University of Virginia Health System, Charlottesville, VA, USA

Hartzell V. Schaff, MD Division of Cardiovascular Surgery, Mayo Clinic, Rochester, MN, USA

Edward Soltesz, MD, MPH Department of Thoracic and Cardiovascular Surgery, Cleveland Clinic, Cleveland, OH, USA

John M. Stulak, MD Division of Cardiovascular Surgery, Mayo Clinic, Rochester, MN, USA

Thoralf M. Sundt III, MD Massachusetts General Hospital, Boston, MA, USA

Rakesh M. Suri, MD, DPhil Division of Cardiovascular Surgery, Mayo Clinic, Rochester, MN, USA

Lars G. Svensson, MD, PhD Department of Thoracic and Cardiovascular Surgery, Cleveland Clinic Foundation, Cleveland, OH, USA

Darrell J. Triulzi, MD Department of Pathology, Division of Transfusion Medicine, University of Pittsburgh School of Medicine, Pittsburgh, PA, USA

Lawrence R. Wechsler, MD Department of Neurology, University of Pittsburgh School of Medicine, Pittsburgh, PA, USA

Cynthia M. Wells, MD Department of Anesthesiology, University of Pittsburgh Medical Center, Pittsburgh, PA, USA

David O. Wilson, MD, MPH Division of Pulmonary, Allergy and Critical Care Medicine, University of Pittsburgh Medical Center, Pittsburgh, PA, USA

Problems Related to Redo Cardiac Surgery

1

Venkat R. Machiraju

Introduction

Redo cardiac surgery has several inherent challenges that can increase mortality and also morbidity to the patient. This chapter will discuss several of the problems associated with technical aspects of redo cardiac surgical procedures. Some aspects will be covered in more depth by other authors in subsequent chapters.

As is true for primary procedures, there are several important patient-related factors that contribute to the risk of operative mortality of redo operations. Older age (>70 years), female sex, diabetes mellitus, chronic obstructive pulmonary emphysema, renal failure or elevated baseline serum creatinine (>2 mg/100 mL), history of stroke, and elevated total body weight are considered as contributing factors for increased risk of mortality during redo cardiac surgery. Additionally, repeat valvular surgery for prosthetic valve endocarditis, a low starting left ventricular ejection fraction (~20%), and urgent operation independently contribute to a higher mortality [1]. Heavy mitral annular and aortic root calcification in elderly makes valvular operation significantly more difficult and challenging. Indeed, the risk of operation is related not only to the comorbid conditions of the patient and the type of operation but also to the number of previous operations. While first-time redo cardiac surgical procedures have an increased risk of mortality for valve-related procedures, generally redo cardiac procedures for coronary artery revascularization alone have been within an acceptable range (3.9%). Second-time redo cardiac surgical procedures, even for coronary artery revascularization, have a notably increased risk of morbidity and mortality.

At the beginning of a redo cardiac surgical procedure, the surgeon can assess the overall potential for morbidity and mortality and give a good understanding to the patient and his or her family of potential complications as well as the likelihood of survival. Preoperative insertion of an intra-aortic balloon for hemodynamic stability or acute myocardial infarction with either right or left ventricular failure from coronary artery occlusion will increase the likelihood of morbidity and mortality. Similarly, patients in cardiogenic shock have a higher surgical risk. It is clear that the preoperative comorbid conditions and the urgency of the need for a surgical procedure dictate the final outcome. In addition, age greater than 80 years is correlated with decreased cognitive function in the postoperative period, which can lead to somnolence and other perioperative complications, such as aspiration pneumonia and gastrointestinal motility disorders. In the end, resource utilization becomes important and, finally, the patient may be transferred to an extended care facility with a tracheostomy, a percutaneous endoscopic gastrostomy (PEG) tube,

V.R. Machiraju, MD (✉)
Department of Cardiothoracic Surgery,
University of Pittsburgh Medical Center,
Pittsburgh, PA, USA
e-mail: machvr@upmc.edu

V.R. Machiraju et al. (eds.), *Redo Cardiac Surgery in Adults*,
DOI 10.1007/978-1-4614-1326-4_1,

and on hemodialysis. This type of discharge from an acute care facility is needed to make a hospital bed available to acutely ill patients, but the 30-day mortality remains very high.

Redo Sternotomy and Institution of Cardiopulmonary Bypass

There is a definite risk of injury to cardiac and vascular structures during redo sternotomy [2]. The incidence of injury is reduced if the pericardium was approximated during the prior surgical procedure. Park and associates from Mayo Clinic reviewed 2,555 cardiac reoperations and found 25% mortality when significant hemorrhagic injury occurred to cardiac structures during sternotomy compared with 6.5% mortality when there was no injury [3]. Institution of bypass prior to sternotomy does not protect the right ventricle from injury. However, with cardiopulmonary bypass, there will be less bleeding and the situation will be more controlled. Exposing the groin vessels without cannulation, using the axillary artery and femoral vein for cardiopulmonary bypass, and initiating bypass through femoral artery and vein have all been recommended to reduce the chance of injury to the structures behind sternum. Even if the femoral vessels are not surgically exposed, it may be prudent to, at least, insert a guide wire percutaneously into femoral vein and artery. This will come in handy in an emergency, as catheters can be threaded over the guide wire quickly.

Generally, the right ventricle becomes adherent to the undersurface of the sternum when the left internal thoracic artery was dissected during the prior surgical procedure. It is important to gently elevate the sternal plate and release the entire right ventricle from the sternum. Small lacerations can be controlled with direct suturing. If injury to the right ventricle occurs before instituting cardiopulmonary bypass, a Foley catheter should be inserted through the rent in the right ventricle and the balloon inflated until the bleeding has decreased. Then, sutures can be applied to close the rent. Immediate heparinization will help to recover blood loss from surgical field into the cardiotomy suction rather than into the cell saver.

Calcified Ascending Aorta

As is true for primary procedures, the aging population requiring redo cardiac surgical procedures will have varying degrees of calcification in the ascending aorta. Atherosclerotic disease in the ascending aorta and arch of the aorta is the primary cause of cerebral emboli during cardiac surgery using cardiopulmonary bypass. This creates a surgical challenge and impacts the decision-making process when planning the surgical procedure. If the aorta is completely calcified and porcelain, it cannot be clamped. The surgeon should make the choice of replacing the entire aorta or performing the procedure using a no-touch technique. If an isolated coronary artery revascularization is necessary, the right and left internal thoracic arteries can be utilized for arterial inflow, as in situ grafts, to avoid manipulation of the aorta. In addition, the Heartstring device (Guidant Corporation, Santa Clara, CA) can be used for proximal anastomosis if there is a softer area in the aorta. An apical-aortic conduit can be used if the primary problem is calcific aortic stenosis [4]. Also, surgical procedures on the mitral valve have been performed without cross-clamping the aorta [5]. Venting the left ventricle will minimize the risk of air embolism risk during this procedure. Awareness of the potential problems will help to minimize surgical risk. Frequently, calcification of the aorta is patchy, and palpation will reveal soft areas for arterial cannulation or application of the aortic cross-clamp. It is useful to lower the aortic pressure by decreasing cardiopulmonary bypass flow transiently before applying an aortic clamp with an atraumatic design. The clamp is placed very low, just above the sinotubular junction, or very high depending upon the external feel. If the aortic calcification is less than 75% of the aortic circumference, the aorta can be safely clamped. Nishi and associates suggest clamping the aorta parallel to the calcification [6].

Coronary Sinus Perfusion

While coronary sinus perfusion protects the myocardium and facilitates the performance of complex surgical procedures, in redo cardiac surgical cases, it is sometimes difficult to thread a retrograde catheter into the coronary sinus because of distortion by the adhesions. Adhesions have to be lysed to the extent that the surgeon can guide the catheter with his fingers into the coronary sinus. Perforation of the coronary sinus generally precludes the use of coronary sinus perfusion. In such cases, antegrade perfusion has to be maintained. In cases with shorter cross-clamp times, the procedure can be managed with cold cardioplegic solution. Because the use of a retrograde catheter can make prolonged surgical procedures safer and the inability to use retrograde perfusion makes the surgical procedure much more difficult, some centers have utilized the experience of an anesthesiologist to insert a retrograde catheter from the neck, using fluoroscopic and echocardiographic guidance. However, occasional attempts to insert these catheters by inexperienced personnel will only waste operating room time and become unsuccessful.

Limited Surgical Dissection

Limited surgical dissection has helped to reduce the morbidity of redo cardiac surgical procedures. When surgeons began doing redo cardiac surgical procedures, it was customary to mobilize the entire heart from the pericardium. This happened because, in an earlier era, the majority of the redo cardiac surgical procedures were coronary artery revascularizations, and it was necessary to mobilize the entire heart when looking for coronary vessels. This extensive surgical dissection increased perioperative bleeding. Redo surgical procedures on the coronary artery are declining, and procedures on the aortic and mitral valves can be performed with minimal surgical dissection and without mobilizing much of the heart. Limiting mediastinal dissection to only those structures for cannulation and exposure may limit morbidity and coagulopathic bleeding. Diffuse capillary bleeding can be managed by correcting coagulopathy and by the use of topical agents, for example, spraying fibrin sealant (Tisseel; Baxter, Deerfield, IL) over the pericardial surface.

Exposure of the Mitral Valve While Limiting Dissection

Adequate visualization of the mitral valve is very important for mitral valve repair or replacement. In deep emphysematous patients, good visualization of mitral valve can be difficult with limited surgical dissection. Dissecting the pleuropericardial attachment from the left chest wall and letting the heart drop into pleural space will help to some extent. An extended transseptal approach or dome approach should help with an easy access to the mitral valve. On occasion, even transecting the aorta and opening the dome of the left atrium have facilitated the exposure of the mitral valve. This was utilized during double valve replacement as the aorta is opened most of the anterior circumference. Retraction with multiple pledgeted sutures on the atrial wall will expose the mitral valve better than a metal retractor. Commissural areas are notorious for a perivalvular leak after prosthetic valve implantation. This is due to lack of good visualization during suture placement. Supra-annular implantation of the mitral prosthesis has decreased perivalvular leaks compared with annular insertion of the prosthesis. During supra-annular implantation, care should be taken not to grab the noncoronary cusp of the aortic valve during suture placement on the anterior mitral annulus.

De-airing of the Heart

De-airing of the heart is one of the important steps to remember before removing the aortic cross clamp and is particularly important when only limited surgical dissection is carried out during redo cardiac surgery, as a sudden ventricular contraction with left ventricular cavity full of air can lead to massive air embolism. The apex of the left ventricle is typically covered with pleuropericardial adhesions and is not easily accessible for de-airing. An echocardiogram during cardiac surgery will help to assess the amount of air in the left-side chambers. Before unclamping the aorta, the air should be evacuated by sticking a needle at the apex of the left ventricle or transseptally or by keeping the aortic root vent on suction. The use of carbon dioxide in the surgical field has also decreased the incidence of air embolism.

Low Cardiac Output Syndrome

Low cardiac output syndrome is one of the main perioperative complications following redo cardiac surgery [7] and is seen in repeat revascularization procedures and in patients with prolonged cardiopulmonary bypass time or prolonged myocardial ischemic time. If the patient has either pulmonary hypertension or mitral valve replacement for ischemic mitral regurgitation, low output syndrome also can occur. Cardiac tamponade is one of the most common causes for postoperative low cardiac output syndrome. This can occur immediately because of postoperative bleeding. However, cardiac tamponade can also be missed if the patient developed an isolated blood clot next to the right atrium, causing external compression of the atrium because of bleeding from the left or right atrial incision. An echocardiogram and chest X-ray should be done immediately to rule out any generalized or local accumulation of blood. Low starting ejection fraction, the presence of ischemic mitral regurgitation, mitral valve replacement, and insertion of a small aortic prosthesis leading to patient prosthetic valve mismatch can also lead to low cardiac output syndrome.

Precautions to avoid low cardiac output syndrome after redo cardiac surgery depend on the nature of the redo procedure. When the entire heart is mobilized for revascularization procedures, all the noncoronary collaterals, which have developed over the years through pericardial adhesions, are disconnected and it becomes necessary to ensure that the patient is adequately revascularized. Complete revascularization should be the primary goal to avoid perioperative complications [8]. Bypassing a small right ventricular branch prevents right ventricular dysfunction. Bypassing the posterior descending or posterolateral branches of the right coronary artery alone may not prevent right ventricular dysfunction unless the proximal coronary artery is open and giving blood to the right ventricle. In patients undergoing valve surgery, if the coronary arteries are normal, there is less chance for myocardial ischemia than in patients undergoing revascularization; however, with prolonged valvular surgery, myocardial preservation can be compromised if the retrograde catheter is not positioned properly. In aortic root surgery, reconnecting the coronary buttons becomes very important. It is necessary to reattach the right coronary button without any kinking or stretching, regardless of how small the coronary artery is.

When low cardiac output syndrome occurs, initial administration of fluid and inotropic therapy should improve the cardiac output. A response to lower doses of inotropes suggests less myocardial damage and probable stunning of myocardium from ischemic arrest. Reversible ischemic changes in the cardiac muscle generally manifest by decreasing the need for chemical agents to improve cardiac output. The need for higher doses of inotropes or pressor agents suggests significant myocardial damage. Both the intra-aortic balloon and recently the new Impella assist device (ABIOMED, Danvers, MA) are helpful to improve the cardiac output. Otherwise, extracorporeal membrane oxygenation (ECMO) needs to be administered until myocardial recovery takes place.

Vasoplegic Syndrome

The incidence of vasoplegic syndrome after cardiopulmonary bypass is 5–15% [9]. Vasoplegic syndrome delays early extubation and also increases the length of stay in the ICU. Vasoplegic syndrome manifests when the patient is markedly hypotensive and requires large doses of vasopressors to maintain adequate blood pressure. This is not only seen in septic conditions but also seen in patients with an extreme degree of hemodilution and also in patients who received milrinone before weaning from cardiopulmonary bypass. Sometimes, in patients with a very low ejection fraction or pulmonary hypertension, milrinone is administered to facilitate easy separation from cardiopulmonary bypass. Such empirical treatments should not be used as they can dilate the vascular bed severely and very large doses of vasopressors will then be required to maintain adequate blood pressure. Along with low systemic blood pressure, the central venous pressure is also low, and administering large quantities of crystalloid solutions further dilute the hemoglobin and increase the need for blood transfusions. The duration of cardiopulmonary bypass, the cardiac temperature during bypass, the volume of cardioplegic solution infused, poor ejection fraction, and preoperative use of angiotensin-converting enzyme (ACE) inhibitors all contribute to vasoplegic syndrome. The use of methylene blue at 1.5 mg/kg to neutralize endogenous nitrous oxide has decreased the requirement for pressor agents while maintaining satisfactory blood pressure.

Emergency Redo Cardiac Surgery

Emergency redo cardiac surgery presents in varying degrees, and the risk of surgery depends on how hemodynamically unstable the patient is [10]. Also, the mortality of emergency redo cardiac surgery depends on the indication for surgery, for example, an acutely thrombosed mechanical valve or a torn cusp of a bioprosthesis. The need for emergency revascularization procedures has decreased over the years because of the advent of various interventional procedures, but there are still occasions when an emergency redo coronary bypass is necessary. At one time, emergency redo coronary artery bypass had a 40–50% mortality rate, but now, in such emergency cases, target vessel revascularization has decreased the overall mortality. For example, in our practice, a patient presented with an acutely thrombosed saphenous vein graft to left anterior descending coronary artery. An off-pump redo bypass surgery was performed through a small left anterior thoracotomy with a reverse saphenous vein from the left axillary artery; the patient went home in 4 days without any problems. Although a redo sternotomy would address other stenotic coronary vessels, it would carry a higher mortality and morbidity. Even in experienced hands, patients who are in cardiogenic shock with pulmonary edema from acute prosthetic valve dysfunction do poorly, and other coexistent risk factors will only increase the likelihood of mortality.

Conclusion

Redo cardiac surgical patients present with various comorbid conditions and can require either simple or very complex surgical procedures. Awareness of all the problems inherent to redo cardiac surgery will facilitate a smoother surgical procedure.

References

1. Christenson JT, Schmziger M, Simmat F. Re operative coronary artery bypass. Risk factors for early mortality and late survival. Eur J Cardiothorac Surg. 1997;1:129–33.
2. Morales D, Williams E, John R. Is resternotomy in cardiac surgery still a problem? Interact Cardiovasc Thorac Surg. 2010;11(3):277–86.
3. Park CB, Suri RM, Burkhart HM, et al. Identifying patients at particular risk of injury during repeat sternotomy: analysis of 2555 cardiac reoperations. J Thorac Cardiovasc Surg. 2010;140(5):1028–35.
4. Crestanello JA, Zehr KJ, Daly RC, Orszulak TA, Schaff HV. Is there a role for the left ventricle apical-aortic conduit for acquired aortic stenosis? J Heart Valve Dis. 2004;13(1):57–62; discussion 62–3.
5. Umakanthan R, Leacche M, Petrocek MR, et al. Safety of minimally invasive mitral valve surgery without aortic cross clamp. Ann Ther Surg. 2008; 85:1544–9.
6. Nishi H, Mitsuno M, Ryomoto M, Miyamoto Y. Comprehensive approach for clamping severely calcified ascending aorta using computed tomography. Interact Cardiovasc Thorac Surg. 2010;10(1):18–20.
7. Rao V, Ivanov J, Weisel RD, Ikonomidis JS, Christakis GT, David TE. Predictors of low cardiac output syndrome after coronary artery bypass. J Thorac Cardiovasc Surg. 1996;112(1):38–51.

8. Maganti MD, Rao V, Borger MA, Ivanov J, David TE. Predictors of low cardiac output syndrome after isolated aortic valve surgery. Circulation. 2005;112(9 Suppl):I448–52.
9. Carrel T, Englberger L, Mohacsi P, Neidhart P, Schmidli J. Low systemic vascular resistance after cardiopulmonary bypass: incidence, etiology, and clinical importance. J Card Surg. 2000;15(5):347–53.
10. Goodwin AT, Ooi A, Kitcat J, Nashef SA. Outcomes in emergency redo cardiac surgery: cost, benefit and risk assessment. Interact Cardiovasc Thorac Surg. 2003;2(3):227–30.

Practical Approaches to the Current "On-Pump" Redo Coronary Artery Bypass Surgery

2

Venkat R. Machiraju

Introduction

The mortality (5–15%) [1] and morbidity are higher for redo coronary artery bypass grafting (CABG) operations than for primary CABG procedures. There are multiple causes for the higher mortality of patients in need of repeat CABG, including left ventricular dysfunction as coronary artery disease (CAD) has progressed and decreased function of multiple organs with advancing age. Several risk stratification models have evolved, over the years, to objectively assess the preoperative risk of patients undergoing cardiac surgery, and a patient can be well-informed about his or her surgical risk prior to the procedure. Whichever risk stratification method is used, risk stratification only gives a general guide to morbidity and mortality, and the individual's outcome depends on whether or not problems occur during the intraoperative course. Advanced age, chronic obstructive lung disease, low serum albumin levels, renal failure, and preoperative hemodialysis for management of renal failure are all predictors of higher morbidity and mortality after cardiac procedures. The timing of surgery (i.e., elective, urgent, and emergent procedures) is also a clear, independent predictor of higher mortality.

Starting in 1967, after the number of primary coronary artery bypass surgeries performed per year increased, the number of redo CABG procedures performed yearly also increased slowly from 2 to 3% to as high as 15% in high-volume centers at the peak period of CABG utilization. Redo CABG was needed in 2.5% of patients within the first 5 years of primary surgery and increased to 17% within 12 years after the first CABG revascularization procedure. Percutaneous catheter interventions and medical therapy have progressed simultaneously and decreased the need for isolated redo coronary bypass. Balloon angioplasty, atherectomy, and stent placement for the management of vein graft atherosclerosis have certainly changed the need for repeat CABG. While most centers performed at least 15% of their revascularization procedures in1990s for recurrent CAD, this volume has significantly decreased in most surgical centers, especially over the last 5 years. Additionally, our appreciation of the benefits of repairing a leaking mitral valve secondary to ischemic CAD or treating calcific aortic stenosis in the elderly has created combined procedures that are more common in the present era than redo CABG alone.

Younger age at the time of the primary revascularization is a good predictor of the need for a second operation during the patient's lifetime. The need for redo CABG also depends very heavily on the type of conduit used for the first operation,

V.R. Machiraju, MD (✉)
Department of Cardiothoracic Surgery,
University of Pittsburgh Medical Center,
Pittsburgh, PA, USA
e-mail: machvr@upmc.edu

V.R. Machiraju et al. (eds.), *Redo Cardiac Surgery in Adults*,
DOI 10.1007/978-1-4614-1326-4_2,

specifically whether an internal thoracic artery (ITA) graft was used or if only vein grafts were used. Using the ITA for bypass grafting was popularized by both Green and Loop [2]. However, before the left ITA became the standard conduit for bypass of the left anterior descending (LAD) coronary artery, several thousand patients had bypass surgery utilizing only saphenous vein grafts. The presence of a well-functioning ITA graft to the LAD has decreased the incidence of redo CABG by at least 50% in a 10-year period. The use of both ITAs as well as the use of other arterial grafts in CABG also diminished the need for repeat revascularization for conduit failures.

Cardiopulmonary bypass time per graft is longer, and incidence of perioperative myocardial infarction is higher for redo CABG than the primary procedure. However, the number of bypass grafts needed in a redo revascularization procedure is generally less than the number of bypass grafts needed during primary revascularization procedures, as some of the grafts from the first operation might be patent. However, there are instances when all the grafts are occluded because of multiple systemic predisposing factors. Single graft or target vessel revascularization procedures have been predominantly performed using off-pump techniques. Most multigraft revascularization procedures are performed on-pump, though some surgeons have initiated off-pump bypass surgery as their primary method of choice even for multiple grafts. If there is hemodynamic instability, cardiopulmonary bypass is still instituted and a beating heart bypass surgery is performed without arresting the heart. Left ITA bypass to the LAD, reverse saphenous vein bypass from descending thoracic aorta to a marginal branch of the circumflex coronary artery, and isolated gastroepiploic artery bypass to distal right coronary artery branches have all been performed off-pump in highly selected cases. The axillary artery is also used as inflow with a reverse saphenous vein to bypass coronary artery branches.

Technical Demands

Successful reentry into the chest, management of patent ITA grafts, establishment of cardiopulmonary bypass, myocardial preservation, prevention of vein graft atheroembolism, and elimination of perioperative hemorrhage are key factors that are under the direct control of the surgeon and improve the final outcome. The occurrence of intraoperative stroke is partly under the control of the surgeon, and onset of renal and pulmonary failure is guided by several factors.

Redo Sternotomy

Safe redo sternotomy is one of the major steps to a good outcome following redo cardiac surgery. Evidence of adhesion of a vein or arterial graft to the back of sternum, history of mediastinal irradiation, presence of an ascending aortic aneurysm, and long-standing mitral or tricuspid valvular disease that causes right heart enlargement are all predisposing factors for catastrophic hemorrhage during sternal reentry. Although in the majority of cases, redo sternotomy can be accomplished without major bleeding, once in a while, an unfortunate incident occurs because the right ventricle, a patent saphenous vein graft or a patent left ITA graft is inadvertently injured. In patients with aortic aneurysms, especially rare aneurysms that are eroding into the sternum, surgeons plan for a safe approach during sternal entry as the diagnosis is evident before the surgery begins. Complications generally occur when the surgeon is least suspicious of such problems and the patient is the most vulnerable at that time.

There are several techniques for safe sternal reentry that are described in the literature, and all of them stress the same singular point. Visualize the structures you are cutting. Lifting the sternal edges or performing mediastinoscopy to lyse the adhesions has been described as giving satisfactory entry into the chest cavity. I have consistently

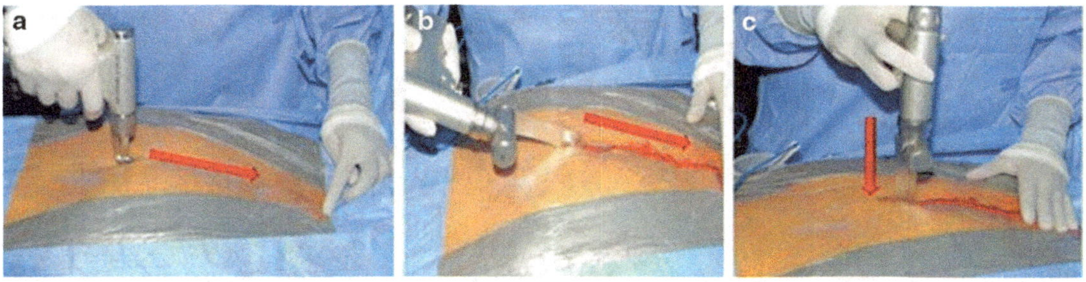

Fig. 2.1 The difference between primary sternotomy (**a**), and safe (**b**) vs. standard (**c**) redo sternotomy techniques (from: Machiraju VR. How to avoid problems in redo coronary artery bypass surgery. J Card Surg. 2004 Jul-Aug;19(4):284–90; Used with permission)

approached the sternum being mindful of the following principles: (1) Safe sternal reentry is one of the key factors for successful outcome. (2) Presume that there may be vital structures adherent to the back of the sternum all the time. (3) The time spent performing a redo sternotomy is not critical but safe entry should be. (4) Visualization of the structures is important to avoid problems with catastrophic bleeding.

Our technique is based on the fact that the direction of the force in primary sternotomy is parallel to the body of the sternum (Fig. 2.1a), and there are no adhesions between the heart and back of the sternum as the intact pericardium shields the cardiac structures. Similarly, even in redo sternotomy, the saw blade is parallel (Fig. 2.1b) instead of perpendicular (Fig. 2.1c), and the sternum is incised up to the posterior table. Because it is the path of least resistance as half of the blade is inside the bone and half outside, in case the hand slips, the saw comes out rather than going into the chest cavity. This safe sternotomy technique is accomplished with a large oscillating saw or a microblade (Fig. 2.1b).

Then, using a spreader, the posterior table of the sternum is incised slowly under direct vision. We leave the sternal wires in place until this stage and then remove them one after another as we incise the posterior table of the sternum. With this technique, we have entered the mediastinal cavity safely without any catastrophic incidents in the last 15 years. We use peripheral cannulation through groin vessels in less than 2% of patients for fear of mediastinal bleeding during sternal reentry and always prefer central cannulation. However, peripheral cannulation techniques are resurging in cardiac surgery.

Patent ITA Grafts

The presence of a well-functioning ITA-to-LAD graft is the most important contributing factor to the patient's long-term survival. Therefore, this graft should be preserved without any damage during redo cardiac surgical procedures. While this is an accepted philosophy among all cardiac surgeons, a patent ITA graft is injured in up to 4% of redo CABG procedures [1]. Though there is universal acceptance of using an ITA-to-LAD graft during the first procedure, there is great variability among surgeons as to how the conduit is attached to the coronary artery. Sometimes, it is too long and a redundant ITA is left inside the mediastinal cavity. Some surgeons bring the ITA in front of the intact pleura, while some surgeons bring it into pericardial cavity between the pleura and the lung parenchyma through a slit incision in the pericardium. Sometimes, a sequential ITA bypass is created to the coronary artery branches

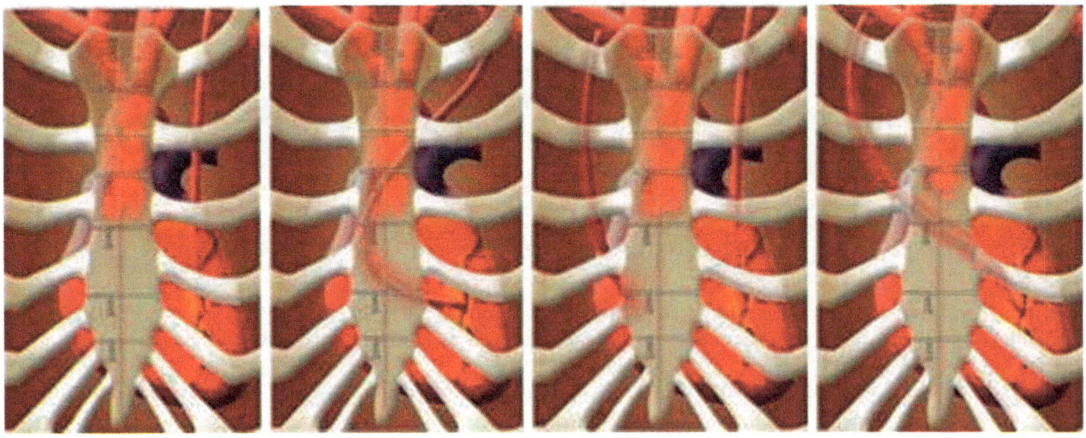

Fig. 2.2 Some of the anatomic possibilities of ITA into coronary artery branches (from: Machiraju used with permission)

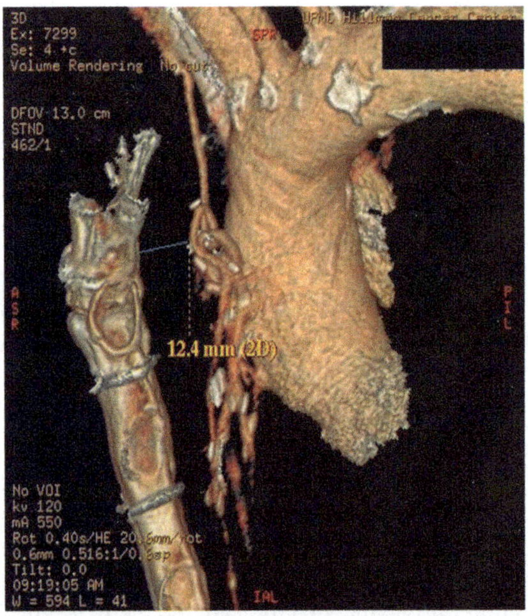

Fig. 2.3 Showing the relationship of a patent right ITA across the midline to the body of the sternum

and, similarly, a skeletonized ITA to a pedicle graft is utilized. Furthermore, now that we have started using both ITAs for primary revascularization, the variations in the arrangement of the two arteries and coronary artery branches have increased (Fig. 2.2). Left ITA to LAD, diagonal and marginal branches, has been used as a pedicle graft. The right ITA has been brought down as a pedicle graft to the right coronary artery and also across the midline to the left-sided coronary artery branches. Even in cases where the right ITA is brought in front of the aorta across the midline, generally it tends to lie down on the aorta and stay much deeper than the back of the sternum (Fig. 2.3). This variability increases the risk for damage of the ITA graft. While the surgeon's prior experience with redo cardiac surgery helps, it is equally true that even the most experienced surgeons have damaged a patent ITA graft. Spending time when dissecting out the ITA is more important for avoiding injury to the structure than the experience of the surgeon.

If the ITA is injured during dissection, immediate hemostasis is important to prevent further blood loss. This is accomplished by ligating, clipping both ends, or successfully resuturing the bleeding site. Some surgeons have placed an intraluminal shunt into the injured ITA to prevent myocardial ischemia. This is more easily said than done because sometimes shunt insertion only causes the tear to get worse and the bleeding to become profuse. The ITA must be satisfactorily mobilized proximal and distal to the tear site before further maneuvers can be performed. If a well-functioning ITA has to be ligated after an injury, an early institution of cardiopulmonary bypass will help to prevent myocardial ischemia. It is prudent to dissect out the right side of the sternum and the heart first rather than the left side, whenever a patent ITA is present perfusing a large region of myocardium. In case, there is an injury to the ITA graft, cardiopulmonary bypass can be instituted quickly avoiding prolonged myocardial ischemia. The right ITA, when available, is the most suitable conduit during redo cardiac surgical procedures to replace an injured left ITA.

There are differing opinions as to whether a patent ITA should be left alone perfusing the myocardium during a redo cardiac surgery or if it should be dissected and clamped so that myocardial temperature can be maintained uniformly with the cardioplegic solution. Smith and associates [3] reviewed 206 patients who had redo cardiac surgery; 118 patients had the ITA dissected and occluded and 88 patients did not have the ITA occluded. In the dissected group, there were seven graft injuries which the authors believe could have been avoided if the ITA had not been dissected. There was no statistical difference in mortality between the groups. It has been my practice, over the years, to dissect out a small portion of the ITA and occlude it during the operation to maintain uniform distribution of cardioplegic solution. There are procedures that require mobilization of a patent ITA, such as revascularizing circumflex coronary artery branches. Also, whenever the chest needs to be opened widely for various procedures, it is necessary to mobilize at least a part of the ITA to avoid stretch injury by the scar tissue. When just replacing an aortic valve, a patent ITA graft can be left alone along with systemic cooling and administration of cold cardioplegic solution.

Institution of Cardiopulmonary Bypass

When instituting cardiopulmonary bypass, the length of the ascending aorta, ascending aortic calcification, and the presence of atherosclerotic and patent vein grafts always create a challenge to finding a suitable place on the aorta for both cannulation and aortic cross-clamping. Carefully separating the superior vena cava and the pulmonary artery on both sides of the aorta is necessary for satisfactory clamping. We have used a Soft-Flow cannula (Edwards Co.) inserted high in the aorta and guided into the beginning of descending thoracic aorta to keep the perfusion site distal to the take of the aortic arch vessels. This, I believe, prevents the "Niagara Falls effect" in front of the arch vessels by avoiding all the turbulence. Direct palpation of the aorta and transesophageal echocardiogram (TEE) give a general idea of the condition of the aorta by which we make a judgment about the site of aortic cannulation. Epiaortic scanning gives further insight into the aorta in doubtful cases. Physical manipulation of the ascending aorta and institution of cardiopulmonary bypass alone can increase the incidence of neurological complications. However, the incidence of intraoperative stroke can be kept at a minimum by perfusing distal to the aortic arch, single aortic clamping, the use of the Soft-Flow aortic cannula, evacuation of all intracardiac air as guided by TEE, and thorough irrigation of the cardiac chambers after excision of the calcified valves. Similarly, fewer neurological complications are observed with axillary artery cannulation as it keeps the site of turbulence away from the take of the arch vessels. Arterial cannula can be inserted over a guide wire as well to minimize manipulation of the aorta.

Myocardial Protection During Redo Cardiac Surgery

The goals of myocardial protection are as follows: (1) The myocardium should be electrically quiescent during the operation. (2) The myocardium should start contracting as soon as the aortic cross-clamp is removed. (3) Minimal inotropic support should be required during separation from cardiopulmonary bypass. (4) Myocardial reperfusion injury in the form of myocardial swelling and decreased contractility should be avoided. Myocardial preservation during cardiac surgery is a balancing act between myocardial ischemia and reperfusion injury. When the myocardium is not protected properly, myocardial stunning and cardiomyocyte necrosis occur depending on the length of ischemia and the time that is needed for the ischemic myocardium to recover during the reperfusion phase. Myocardial damage is attributed to either increase in intracellular calcium, the release of reactive oxygen species or both. These cause loss of the cell's phospholipid layer leading to swelling and loss of cell integrity. After the aortic cross-clamp is removed, cardiac myocyte function may become normal or dysfunctional depending on the level of ischemia, necrosis, or apoptosis.

Although potassium-supplemented (K^+) blood cardioplegia is the hallmark of intraoperative management, myocardial protection varies from surgeon to surgeon and from medical center to medical center. There is no standardized method of cardioplegia administration in the surgical community. There is great variability in the initial and maintenance doses of the plegic solution, solution composition, and route of administration (e.g., antegrade vs. retrograde). Administered cardioplegic solution must reach the myocardium to achieve the goals stated earlier. This may not happen during antegrade induction if there is some aortic insufficiency, severe CAD, or a paucity of collaterals between coronary artery branches. Similarly, cardioplegic solution may give inadequate myocardial protection during retrograde administration if the catheter is not positioned properly in the coronary sinus, if the catheter slips back into the atrium, or if the cardioplegic solution regurgitates back into the atrium due to a very large sinus. It is essential to monitor the coronary sinus pressure and, generally, we tend to keep it between 25 and 40 mmHg. Accidental perforation of coronary sinus and inability to place the retrograde catheter into a small sinus will preclude retrograde administration.

Since TEE is the standard method of monitoring every patient during cardiac surgery, TEE will certainly assist in locating the position of the retrograde catheter when the catheter is positioned at the beginning of the procedure; however, TEE will not help to localize the catheter during the cardiopulmonary bypass period when the heart is arrested and empty. Definitive ways of making sure that the retrograde catheter is properly positioned are by lifting the heart and palpating the balloon catheter in the coronary sinus and opening the right atrium, directly placing the catheter in the coronary sinus, and temporarily occluding the sinus opening with a pledgeted suture until the procedure is completed. Contrary to the popular belief that retrograde delivery of plegia solution does not protect the right ventricle, we have never seen inadequate protection of the right ventricle as long as the posterior descending coronary vein is filled with cardioplegic solution. Generally, we can see that the veins over the right ventricle are filled with bright red blood and that is sufficient for protection. We see right ventricular dysfunction when the left ventricle fails and during aortic surgery when a non-dominant right coronary artery is not properly reattached to the main aorta or to the Dacron graft. We have also revascularized suitable right acute marginal branches and perfused them during the operation. Generally, these grafts flow 15–20 mL of plegia solution per minute, and this is certainly adequate to protect the right ventricle. While a single, ventricular dysfunction (right or left) can be managed relatively easily, biventricular failure certainly requires a ventricular assist device and this is followed by added complications related to the device.

We base our cardioplegia delivery methodology on the following principles: (1) Myocardial edema is bad for functional recovery and so there is no place for crystalloids in the cardioplegic solution. Initiation of cardiopulmonary bypass itself with resulting hemodilution and cytokine release causes some degree of myocardial edema, and adding crystalloid solution to the cardioplegia will further aggravate this process. Therefore, only blood is used as a cardioplegic delivery vehicle. (2) Because oxygen dissociation occurs only at higher temperatures, we keep the plegia temperature around 28°C constantly and have stopped using very cold (4–10°C) plegia. (3) Reperfusion injury occurs only when ischemic periods are created and, so, we deliver continuous retrograde blood cardioplegia through a coronary sinus catheter to avoid myocardial ischemia. Simultaneous antegrade plegia is given through the newly constructed bypass grafts. (4) Since there is significant reduction in the utilization of oxygen, by more than 80% in the quiet arrested heart compared with the normal beating heart, this oxygen demand can be met by giving 100–120 mL of blood continuously instead of larger quantities [4]. (5) Adding adenosine (12 mg) to the induction dose of high dose potassium and magnesium cardioplegic solution generally causes quick cardiac standstill by means of hyperpolarized arrest and limits us from giving larger quantities of cardioplegic solution. By adhering to these principles, even cross-clamping times of 3 h and longer have not resulted in higher rates of inotropic support or intraaortic balloon assistance. During surgical procedures that involve the aortic arch and require circulatory arrest, we administer much colder blood during the portion of the procedure involving the arch and then revert to our standard method once rewarming is started. Systemic temperature is kept at 34–35°C for all patients who do not require circulatory arrest. Blood glucose levels are closely monitored and regulated with insulin therapy. Although there have been several clinical trials of additives to the cardioplegic solution, at present, we only use potassium and magnesium for maintenance of cardiac silence.

Activated neutrophils cause endothelial damage, and the initial insult occurs when contact activation takes place upon initiation of cardiopulmonary bypass. Modalities to filter leukocytes or neutralize the effect of neutrophil-induced toxicity have become a routine part of the clinical practice. Leuko-reduced blood is administered routinely for all patients requiring blood transfusions. Heparin-bonded circuits also decrease the contact activation of neutrophils upon initiation of cardiopulmonary bypass. Several years ago, we adopted administration of 12 mg of adenosine intravenously just before going on cardiopulmonary bypass. Neutrophil activation is mediated by 11b/CD18 members of the integrin family of adhesion receptors, and both adenosine and acadesine inhibit 11b receptor upregulation in a dose-related fashion. Activation of the A1 and A2 adenosine receptors causes significant bradycardia and hypotension, and only activation of the A3 adenosine receptor is helpful to prevent myocardial ischemic injury. While the basis for adenosine treatment is only empirical, it is not cost prohibitive to give a small dose of adenosine after the patient is cannulated and ready to go on cardiopulmonary bypass. As there is no published date, we base our judgment solely on our clinical experience that with adenosine treatment prior to cardiopulmonary bypass, as well at the beginning of cardioplegic induction, even patients with a very low ejection fraction or prolonged cross-clamping come off cardiopulmonary bypass easily.

Clearly, the combined effects of every well-executed technical maneuver during the operation result in good outcomes. It is unlikely that any one step is solely responsible for good or bad functional recovery of the myocardium. While the type of myocardial protection used does not matter much in patients with good left ventricular function requiring a short cross-clamp time, it becomes of paramount importance in patients with poor left ventricular function and a decompensated heart who require a prolonged cross-clamping.

Vein Graft Failure and Prevention of Vein Graft Atheroembolism

Saphenous vein graft failure is one of the main reasons for redo coronary artery bypass surgery. While some vein grafts remain free of disease, others show extensive atheroscelorosis and the underlying mechanisms are intriguing [15]. Injury to intimal layers during the preparation of the vein conduit increases neointimal thickening and smooth muscle proliferation. The most frequent operation in this country still uses the left ITA to bypass the LAD and reverse saphenous vein grafts to bypass the remaining coronary branches. Ten years after CABG surgery, 60–70% of vein grafts are either occluded or show severe stenosis. A diffuse fibromuscular hyperplasia decreases the lumen of vein grafts by 20–30% within the first 12 months. Vein conduits less than 3 mm diameter have a greater chance of failure. A vein with a thick wall at the time of implantation has higher propensity to develop atherosclerotic changes. Patients with hypercoagulable states have higher incidence of graft failure. These patients have either thrombocytosis or hyperfibrinogenemia.

The use of aspirin significantly increases the patency of both vein grafts and arterial grafts, though the patency is not increased by adding warfarin or dipyridamole. High serum lipoproteins are an independent risk factor for developing atheroscelorosis. Clopidogrel (Plavix) has a significant effect on platelet aggregation and decreases the incidence of vein graft closure. It is prescribed primarily by surgeons after off-pump CABG and by cardiologists after stenting a vein graft to treat stenosis.

Saphenous vein valves are a common site for atherosclerosis to occur. Occasionally, there is a congenital valve stenosis, which goes unnoticed at the time of surgery, and only manifests as a stenotic segment seen during angiography performed after surgery. Similarly, there can be vein valve stenosis secondary to phlebitis, which was already present but unsuspected. Although grafts stripped of the venous valves (via a valvulotome) and nonreversed vein grafts are used as in situ grafts for lower extremity revascularization procedures, this is not a common practice for CABG in most centers.

Initial cardioplegia can be given in an antegrade fashion in spite of vein graft stenosis, although retrograde administration for both induction and maintenance has also yielded satisfactory results. Prevention of vein graft atheroembolism using the "no-touch" technique was described by Savage and Cohn [6]. Vein graft atherosclerosis is intraluminal, and any manipulation can result in distal embolization of atherosclerotic material because the material, in general, is very friable and easily dislodged. However, we do not see such loose atherosclerotic material in patients who have received long-term statin therapy [7].

Management of Perioperative Hemorrhage

Maintaining blood in the fluid state necessitates a balance between procoagulant and anticoagulant mechanisms, and shifting the balance can result in either thrombosis or bleeding. Reinfusion of shed blood aspirated from the surgical field by cardiotomy suction can enhance activation of coagulation and inflammation in the systemic circulation. During reinfusion, levels of factor VIIa, markers of thrombin generation, procoagulant microparticles, and activated complement proteins are all increased. Aspiration of shed blood through cardiotomy suction is related to the type of myocardial protection the surgeon uses. Giving intermittent cold cardioplegic solution does not release much blood into the pericardial cavity, so the volume of the cardiotomy suction will be low as well. However, there is chance for reperfusion injury because intermittent ischemia is created and more reactive oxygen species will be liberated when the cross-clamp is released. If continuous tepid cardioplegia is given through a retrograde catheter, there are larger quantities of blood in the pericardial cavity. If this volume is not returned to the pump, there will be significant blood volume loss and bank blood and blood products will need to be transfused, which again causes an inflammatory response.

It has been customary to use an antifibrinolytic agent during cardiopulmonary bypass. It is also clear that the extracorporeal circulation releases the proinflammatory cytokine interleukin (IL)-6 and the anti-inflammatory cytokine IL-10 as is evident in systemic inflammatory response syndrome. While aprotinin, a serine protease inhibitor, decreases the levels of IL-6, it is no longer available for clinical use because of suspected adverse effects on other organs. ε-Aminocaproic acid, a lysine analog that inhibits plasminogen cleavage by tissue plasminogen activator, is commonly used to inhibit fibrinolysis and prevent blood loss. Some surgeons prefer tranexamic acid as an antifibrinolytic agent.

There is an increased incidence of blood transfusions during redo cardiac surgical procedures because of surgical blood loss, prolonged cardiopulmonary bypass time, and low preoperative hemoglobin. Multiple blood transfusions are associated with increased perioperative complications, such as stroke, infection, renal failure, prolonged ventilation and surgical site infections, and increased mortality. However, hematocrit levels lower than 18 during cardiopulmonary bypass are also associated with increased morbidity and mortality because of tissue hypoxia. Postoperatively, patients tolerate hemoglobin levels around 8.0 g/100 mL, and increasing oxygen delivery by giving blood transfusions has not translated into increased oxygen uptake by the tissues in anemic patients. It is also understood that stored red blood cells become depleted of 2,3-diphosphoglycerate (2,3-DPG), which is important for oxygen transfer and several hours are needed for the transfused red blood cells to get replenished with 2,3-DPG. In the practice of most physicians, the threshold to transfuse elderly patients is very low and, as such, older patients tend to get more blood transfusions than younger patients. The need for transfusion of blood products also increases because of increased consumption of the fibrinogen and platelets during cardiopulmonary bypass.

Conduits for Bypass Surgery

ITA, saphenous vein, and radial artery are the most commonly used bypass conduits. These may be available adequately, or the surgeon may have to scramble for alternate conduits like the gastroepiploic artery or the inferior epigastric arteries.

Internal Thoracic Artery

The left ITA is the preferential conduit for redo CABG, provided it was not used during the initial revascularization procedure. Otherwise, the right ITA becomes the next most desirable conduit and should be used whenever possible. There is always some fibrous reaction in this area due to the primary cardiac surgery, and it certainly takes a longer time to dissect out the ITA graft. In my practice, right ITA is used more often as a free graft and is used as a pedicle graft in only 20% of cases. Recycling of previously grafted ITAs can be done in selective cases where there is stenosis at the anastomotic junction or there is an isolated area of narrowing. A patent ITA can be used as an inflow for a T graft with a right ITA or radial artery segment. Many surgeons prefer anastomosing a free ITA graft to the hood of a vein graft or as a T graft, instead of directly attaching it to the aorta. On occasion, when we anastomose to the aorta directly, we make a bigger punch hole in the aorta to avoid anastomotic stricture.

Preparation of Venous Conduits

It is important to avoid conduit injury when preparing venous conduits. Overdistension of the vein and exposure of the vein to lower pH or lower oncotic pressure may cause biochemical or physical injury. Mechanical dilatation of the vein causes excessive distension and injury to the intimal layers and, as such, the pressure should be controlled. In a comparative study, low calcium Plasma-Lyte solution at 37°C resulted in the best venodilatation of all solutions tested to prepare venous grafts.

Vascular smooth muscle cells that proliferate during the first 2 weeks after implantation become the nidus for infiltration of macrophages, which later become foam cells. Intimal thickening itself may be the driving factor for some early graft closures or may promote late atheroscelorosis. Vascular smooth muscle proliferation may be secondary to growth factors derived from either platelets or fibroblasts. Both wall stress and graft injury have been implicated in growth factor production. Additionally, Allen et al. [8] studied the effect of cysteinyl leukotrienes derived from activated leukocytes on saphenous vein grafts and ITA grafts and found that saphenous vein grafts were more sensitive to leukotrienes than the ITA grafts, and this may one of the factors underlying early graft failure in saphenous vein grafts as compared with ITA grafts. As opposed to vein grafts, ITA grafts also have a potent nitric oxide system that protects against vasospasm.

Injury to the saphenous vein endothelium affects the patency of the venous conduit. The endothelium acts as a barrier between blood components and subendothelial muscular layers. Any damage to the endothelium becomes the nidus for vein graft atherosclerosis and graft failure. Surgical manipulation also decreases the antithrombogenic nature of vein graft endothelium and increases vasospasm, thrombogenesis, and occlusive intimal hyperplasia. There is ongoing concern that saphenous vein conduits harvested by endoscopic techniques exhibit more structural and functional damage than those harvested with open surgical techniques. Irrespective of the method used to remove the saphenous vein, the venous endothelium gets damaged when it is subjected to the arterial pressure and a pseudointimal lining develops over time. This is why vein graft atherosclerosis is intraluminal and atheroemboli occur easily with the manipulation of vein grafts.

While the high incidence of vein graft closure after 10 years is clear, there is a debate over replacing angiographically nondiseased vein grafts at the time of redo cardiac surgery. Currently, we believe that this is not necessary and only increases the risk and morbidity [9]. There is no assurance that the newly created vein grafts will last any longer than the grafts they would replace because several factors determine the patency of a new graft. Our preference has been to leave a stenotic vein graft intact and reconstruct a new vein graft beyond the anastomosis of the old graft or to bypass only the diseased segment of the graft. Additionally, it is necessary to leave a stenotic vein graft to the LAD intact while reconstructing with a new ITA graft to avoid malperfusion in this important territory [10].

Radial Artery

In the aged population, as well in diabetic and obese patients, the saphenous vein deteriorates and develops varicosities. The radial artery is the next arterial conduit available after both ITAs have been used. In 1973, Carpentier published the use of the radial artery as a coronary artery bypass conduit but this practice was abandoned in 1976 because of a higher incidence of graft closure. Use of the radial artery in CABG resurged in 1989 after Acar [11] used the radial artery along with vasodilator therapy. The radial artery is a thick-walled muscular artery, which has more elastic lamina than the ITA. Muscular layer response to endothelin I, angiotensin II, norepinephrine, serotonin, and thromboxane-2 results in radial artery spasm. Spasm of the radial artery is the main contributing factor for graft closure and using diltiazem as a vasodilating agent relieves the arterial spasm. Also, using the radial artery to bypass blood vessels that do not have critical stenoses causes competitive blood flow in the native coronary artery and results in graft closure. Currently, use of the radial artery is recommended for coronary artery branches that have >75% stenosis. The radial artery can also develop age-related calcification and is not suitable as a bypass conduit in some elderly patients.

Evidence of sufficient collateral flow in the hand is the most important consideration before radial artery can be taken as a bypass conduit. The modified Allen test is the simplest, most widely available test at bedside and, when inconclusive, digital pulse oximetry, digital plethysmography, and Doppler ultrasonography have been used to assess satisfactory collateral circulation in the hand. Originally, the radial artery was removed by a long forearm incision, which resulted in numbness of the fingers and did not appeal cosmetically to many young patients. Now, the radial artery is removed endoscopically with minimal surgical incisions and higher cosmetic appeal. This is a technically difficult procedure and needs to be performed by practitioners with sufficient training. The radial artery can be removed via pedicle harvesting or using a skeletonization technique. The skeletonized radial artery has higher patency rate as much of the connective tissue around it is removed. However, skeletonization results in leakage of blood from small arterial branches so all the small arterial branches have to be ligated after inflating the artery with vasodilating agents.

Papaverine has been used frequently to dilate the bypass conduits, but is very acidic and causes endothelial cell damage. The effects of papaverine are among the shortest of all available agents, so we use a phenoxybenzamine and verapamil combination in Plasma-Lyte solution and heparin. Because this combination dilates the artery very well, we have also used this solution to dilate

ITAs and have discontinued the use of papaverine. Milronone, another phosphodiesterase inhibitor, also dilates the radial arteries with the effects lasting longer than papaverine.

The radial artery can be used as a T graft from a pedicled ITA or directly from the aorta. The resurgence of use of the radial artery has allowed several surgeons perform primary revascularization procedures using arterial grafts exclusively, thereby limiting the need for redo revascularization procedures. Calcium channel blockers, like diltiazem, increase the patency of radial grafts and, as such, they should be prescribed for up to 1 year after revascularization.

Alternative Conduits

There will always be specific cases where no routine conduits are available and surgeons have to scramble for alternate conduits. In such desperate cases, we have used 4-mm thin-walled polytetrafluoroethylene (Goretex) grafts as an aortocoronary bypass conduit without creating a distal right atrial or superior vena caval anastomosis. We believe that when Permaflow grafts [12] were created, the Goretex graft, which was very big and thick, compromised blood flow into a small coronary artery. Now that the thin-walled Goretex graft, which is used generally for hemodialysis purposes, is available, it can be anastomosed to a coronary artery without impinging on the lumen of the coronary artery.

Indications for Redo Coronary Artery Bypass Surgery

Symptomatic or asymptomatic significant vein graft stenosis to the LAD requires therapeutic intervention. Atherosclerotic lesions in a vein graft to the LAD predict higher rate of death and cardiac events than native vessel disease with the same distribution [13]. Because vein graft atherosclerosis is not necessarily characterized by particular symptoms, vein graft stenosis to the LAD is an indication for reoperation, irrespective of symptoms. In the early 1970s and 1980s, coronary artery primary revascularization was performed with only saphenous vein grafts. Later, the left ITA became the standard conduit to revascularize the LAD. In a few cases, in which the left ITA either did not have sufficient flow or was traumatized during surgical dissection, either the left ITA was used as a free graft or the right ITA was used to revascularize the LAD. Patients who have a functioning left ITA to LAD graft do not gain any increased survival benefit from redo CABG, when the therapeutic intervention is made for non-LAD territory. However, the indication for repeat surgery is based on symptomatology and the presence of valvular disease.

On occasion, we have seen total graft failure following primary CABG requiring repeat surgical intervention. This is seen either very early, within a few months of the initial procedure or as a delayed graft closure. Metabolic conditions, such as uncontrolled diabetes mellitus; polycythemia; local factors, such as poor quality of the saphenous vein or small ITA; or technical conditions, such as poor choice of an anastomotic site in calcified coronary arteries have all contributed to such failure. While it is relatively easy to operate on patients with late graft failure more than 1 year after the procedure, early repeat revascularization, within a few months of the original procedure, is more challenging and difficult when the phlegmon is still present.

Identifying Coronary Artery Branches

It is not easy to dissect out all the coronary artery branches all the time. The LAD may be deeply embedded in the interventricular septum. It is essential to dissect out the part of the LAD that has a larger caliber for graft anastomosis. Once the LAD is identified before it dips underneath the septum, the dissection should be carried out proximally by splitting small portions of the septal muscle until a larger caliber portion of the artery is reached. Secondly, sometimes even the ramus branch or the marginal branches are so deeply embedded in the lateral muscular wall that no trace of the artery is recognized on the surface.

In such cases, the dissection should start proximally near the left atrial appendage downward until the necessary branch is dissected out. Similarly, a suitable portion of the posterolateral branch of the right coronary artery may dip behind the coronary sinus making it difficult for anastomosis.

Combined Surgical Procedures

Patient volumes for isolated redo CABG are decreasing, and the frequency of combined cardiac surgical procedures and repeat revascularization procedures is increasing. The two procedures most commonly combined with redo CABG are aortic valve replacement for age-related calcific aortic stenosis and mitral valve repair or replacement for ischemic mitral regurgitation. Aortotomy for aortic valve replacement may present some challenges if all the saphenous vein grafts that are attached to the ascending aorta are patent. Sometimes, the aortotomy has to be performed between the patent grafts. Percutaneous valve implantation techniques and transapical implantation techniques for aortic prostheses are rapidly advancing; some high-risk surgical patients may be offered alternative approaches for correction of their aortic stenosis.

Ischemic mitral regurgitation is a bigger problem, as it can present as an isolated eccentric jet secondary to posterior papillary muscle outward displacement, a retraction of the P3 segment of the mitral valve secondary to an inferior wall myocardial infarction, or a large central regurgitant jet from annular dilatation and ischemic cardiomyopathy. The cause for mitral regurgitation needs to be properly assessed. Although annuloplasty may correct the mitral regurgitation at the time of surgery, subvalvular surgical procedures, like excising the secondary chordae, approximating the papillary muscles, or posterior leaflet extension, are warranted for long-term satisfactory results.

Conclusions

Redo CABG is a technically challenging operation. In the initial phase of its implementation, the mortality was higher than for primary revascularization procedures for lack of experience in handling the various issues that arise during redo cardiac surgery. As the surgeons performing the procedure have gained experience, the complexity of the patients' comorbid conditions has increased resulting in still higher morbidity and mortality. However, 85% of the patients who survive redo multivessel revascularization live symptom-free for at least 6 years. While isolated, repeat coronary revascularization procedures are on the decline, combined valve and redo CABG procedures are performed regularly in spite of higher morbidity and more perioperative complications. Proper preoperative assessment, skilled intraoperative care, and judicious postoperative management of these highly complex patients should lead to better outcomes.

References

1. Aikens CW, Buckley MJ, Daggett WM, Hilgenberg AD, Vlahakes GJ, Torchiana DF, et al. Reoperative coronary grafting: changing patient profiles: operative indications, techniques and results. Ann Thorac Surg. 1994;58:359–65.
2. Loop FD. The value and conduct of reoperations for coronary atherosclerosis. Semin Thorac Cardiovasc Surg. 1994;6:116–9.
3. Smith RL, Ellman PI, Thompson PW, Girotti ME, Mettler BA, Ailwadi G, et al. Do you need to clamp a patent internal thoracic artery-left anterior descending graft in reoperative cardiac surgery? Ann Thorac Surg. 2009;87:742–7.
4. Buckberg GD, Brazier JR, Nelson RL, Goldstein SM, McConnell DH, Cooper N. Studies of the effects of hypothermia on regional myocardial blood flow and metabolism during cardiopulmonary bypass. I. The adequately perfused beating, fibrillating, and arrested heart. J Thorac Cardiovasc Surg. 1977;73(1):87–94.
5. Lytle BW, McElroy D, McCarthy P. The influence of arterial coronary bypass grafts on the mortality of coronary reoperations. J Thorac Cardiovasc Surg. 1994;107:675–83.
6. Savage EB, Cohn LH. 'No touch' dissection, antegrade-retrograde blood cardioplegia, and single aortic cross-clamp significantly reduce operative mortality of reoperative CABG. Circulation. 1994;90(5 Pt 2):II140–3.
7. Lazar HL. Role of statin therapy in the coronary artery bypass patient. Ann Thorac Surg. 2004;78:730–40.
8. Allen SP, Chester AH, Dashwood MR, Stadjkarimi PJ, Yacoub MH. Preferential vasoconstriction to cysteinyl leukotrienes in the human saphenous vein

compared with the internal mammary artery. Circulation. 1994;90:515–24.
9. Mehta ID, Weinberg J, Jones MF, Tellides G, Kopf GS, Shaw RK, et al. Should angiographically disease-free saphenous vein bypass grafts be replaced at the time of redo coronary artery bypass grafting? Ann Thorac Surg. 1998;65:17–23.
10. Turner FE, Lytle BW, Navia D, Loop FD, Taylor PC, McCarthy PM, et al. Coronary reoperation: results of adding an internal mammary artery graft to a stenotic vein graft. Ann Thorac Surg. 1994;58:1353–5.
11. Acar C, Jebara VA, Portoghese M, Beyssen B, Pagnay JY, Grare P, et al. Revival of radial artery in coronary artery bypass grafting. Ann Thorac Surg. 1992;54:652–60.
12. Weyand M, Kerber S, Schmid C, Rolf N, Scheld HH. Coronary artery bypass grafting with an expanded polytetrafluoroethylene graft. Ann Thorac Surg. 1999;67:1240–5.
13. Lytle BW. The clinical impact of atherosclerotic saphenous vein to coronary artery bypass grafts. Semin Thorac Cardiovasc Surg. 1994;6:81–6.
14. Machiraju VR. How to avoid problems in redo coronary artery bypass surgery. J Card Surg. 2004 Jul-Aug;19(4):284–90.
15. Mills N, Everson CT. Vein graft failure. Curr Opin Cardiol. 1995;10:562–8.

Off-Pump Coronary Artery Bypass Grafting for Repeat Coronary Revascularization

3

Richard J. Myung and John D. Puskas

For decades, cardiopulmonary bypass (CPB) has been used routinely and safely for patients undergoing conventional redo on-pump coronary artery bypass grafting (redo-CABG) surgery. The efficacy and safety of redo-CABG have been well documented across a large spectrum of surgeons and patient populations with mortality rates approaching those of primary CABGs [1]. In many respects, redo-CABG remains the gold standard for repeated coronary revascularization. However, the obligatory aortic manipulation, global myocardial ischemia requiring myocardial protection in advanced coronary disease, and systemic inflammatory response associated with CPB are avoided during redo off-pump coronary artery bypass surgery (redo-OPCAB). To avoid the morbidity attributable to CPB, there has been a resurgence of interest in the application of OPCAB techniques to repeat coronary revascularization.

There is now increasing evidence that OPCAB may provide superior early results, some economic benefit, and equal graft patency. Prospective randomized trials and large retrospective reviews have shown that OPCAB is associated with improved early risk-adjusted morbidity and mortality compared with CABG [2, 3]. In particular, the benefits of OPCAB may be most important to historically high-risk groups, such as women, patients with compromised cardiac function, the elderly, and patients with comorbidities exacerbated by CPB, such as renal insufficiency, pulmonary disease, or cerebrovascular disease. Similarly, improved outcomes may be attributable to OPCAB for secondary endpoints including reoperation for bleeding, renal failure requiring dialysis, prolonged ventilator dependence, prolonged postoperative length of stay, and deep sternal wound infection [4]. Although there are no convincing studies, yet, demonstrating that redo-OPCAB benefits patients, it is easy to surmise that the benefits of OPCAB would translate into this high-risk patient population.

Nonetheless, broad adoption of OPCAB has reached a plateau nationwide, and OPCAB is performed even less frequently following repeat sternotomy. Surgeons participating in the STS database only performed ~20% of isolated primary CABGs using OPCAB techniques in 2009 [5]. While the reason OPCAB has not gained more widespread use is likely multifactorial, there has been reluctance among some surgeons due to reports of worse early and midterm graft patency and a lower degree of complete revascularization [6]. This may be especially true with difficult distal anastomoses in patients with multivessel disease, such as those frequently encountered in the redo setting.

Recently, an improved understanding of OPCAB techniques, including coronary stabiliza-

R.J. Myung, MD (✉)
Assistant Professor of Surgery,
Emory University, Wellstar Kennestone Hospital,
61 Whitcher Street Suite 4100,
Marietta, GA 30060, USA
e-mail: rmyung@emory.edu

J.D. Puskas, MD
Division of Cardiothoracic Surgery,
Emory University School of Medicine,
Atlanta, GA, USA

V.R. Machiraju et al. (eds.), *Redo Cardiac Surgery in Adults*,
DOI 10.1007/978-1-4614-1326-4_3, © Springer Science+Business Media, LLC 2012

tion, distal target visualization, proximal/distal anastomotic devices, and anesthetic/hemodynamic management, has made this highly technical surgery accessible to most surgeons. Ultimately, it is the surgeons' decision whether or not to add OPCAB techniques to their armamentarium for repeat coronary surgery. In many respects, OPCAB surgery for revascularization follows the same principles of OPCAB during primary coronary revascularization: the success of OPCAB depends on the skill of the surgeon and anesthesiologist, their familiarity with advanced OPBCAB techniques for primary revascularization, and appropriate patient selection.

Patient Selection

In general, patients suitable for redo-CABG may also qualify for redo-OPCAB, and there are no absolute contraindications. Ideally, patients well suited for redo-OPCAB are hemodynamically stable with well-preserved left ventricular function and able to withstand fluctuations in hemodynamics as the heart is positioned. Hemodynamic stability is nearly essential in a redo scenario given the additional time required for dissection and performing anastomoses at unfamiliar angles with limited visualization. Factors that facilitate successful redo-OPCAB include large epicardial distal targets, limited adhesions for full mobilization of the heart, targets located on the anterior and inferior walls, and the absence of patent bypass grafts, especially patent mammary grafts.

Redo-OPCAB remains difficult in patients with dilated cardiomyopathies or left ventricular hypertrophy requiring revascularization of the lateral wall due to the limited visibility afforded by the enlarged heart. In addition, the extensive cardiac displacement required for posterior and lateral targets can worsen valvular insufficiency or limit venous return, leading to further hemodynamic instability. Patent left internal mammary artery (LIMA) grafts limit full mobilization of the heart and may be injured during manipulation and displacement of the heart. The surgeon should also measure the degree of risk of sternal reentry as an extremely high-risk patient may require cardiac decompression with CPB prior to safe reentry (Table 3.1).

Table 3.1 Patient selection

Favorable characteristics	Relative contraindications
Stable hemodynamics	Cardiomegaly
Large epicardial targets	Valvular insufficiency
Limited adhesions	High-risk reentry
Anterior and inferior wall distal targets	Lateral wall distal targets
	Patent bypass grafts (patent IMA graft)
	Inexperience with primary OPCAB

Operative Strategy

Many of the techniques for sternal reentry, OPCAB and redo-CABG, have been described in great detail elsewhere and will only be highlighted here as they pertain to redo-OPCAB. In most cases, the patient is positioned in the standard supine position, allowing freedom of movement of the operating table for extreme rotation into all angles. Since the ambient temperature mainly dictates the patient's core temperature without CPB, maintenance of body heat by ancillary methods becomes vital. Routinely using warming blankets or mattresses, minimizing heat loss with the use of warmed fluids, and elevating the room temperature are usually sufficient to maintain the patient's temperature. Monitoring for rapid changes in hemodynamics is essential and consists of an arterial line, pulmonary artery catheter, and, often, transesophageal echocardiography.

The vast majority of redo-OPCAB cases are performed through the previous median sternotomy. Redo-OPCAB has also been safely performed through thoracotomy and minimally invasive direct coronary artery bypass (MIDCAB) approaches that will be discussed later. Entry into a previous median sternotomy allows the best visualization of distal targets, mobilization of the heart from previous adhesions, and easy conversion to CPB, if necessary. It is useful to deflate the lungs and have an assistant retract the sternum anteriorly while the sternum is divided with an oscillating saw, taking care to avoid mediastinal structures that may be adherent to the posterior table of the sternum. Preoperative noncontrast CT scanning provides advance warning when the right ventricle, aorta, or patent grafts are closely adherent to the sternum; in unusual cases, consideration should be given to peripheral cannulation and institution of CPB prior to sternal reentry. After successful entry into the chest, either the right or left internal mammary artery (IMA), if not previously used, can be easily dissected off the posterior table of the sternum using standard techniques. IMA harvest is facilitated by entry into the pleural space following reentry into the sternum with complete mobilization of the heart off the sternum prior to dissection around the IMA. At times, dense adhesions may limit the length of the mammary artery, requiring skeletonization or free grafting to obtain adequate length. Once the IMA is harvested, the retractor is positioned inferiorly in the sternal incision to avoid excessive tension on the innominate vein and aorta, which have not been fully mobilized at this point.

Intrapericardial dissection is undertaken starting from the diaphragm and extending to the right atrium cranially, then out toward the apex. Although somewhat tedious, complete dissection of dense adhesions from a beating heart can be performed safely without excessive bleeding from the epicardium. Additional care should be taken to strictly avoid manipulation of sclerotic vein grafts to minimize the risk of graft embolization. Full mobilization of the heart, aorta, and patent IMA–left anterior descending artery (LAD) graft from surrounding adhesions is often unnecessary, even dangerous at times, and should be tailored to the specific targets that require grafting. Sometimes, surrounding adhesions can help stabilize the area requiring grafting. It is prudent, however, to gain enough access to the ascending aorta and right atrium early in mobilizing the heart to place the patient on CPB quickly, if required. Grafting to the LAD and right coronary artery (RCA) branches can often be completed with minimal dissection of the heart and often requires visualization only of the area surrounding the target. Branches of the circumflex artery require the most complete dissection of the lateral wall, which can be a daunting task in the setting of a patent IMA–LAD graft and dense adhesions. Successful lateral wall grafting is also facilitated by complete dissection of the right lateral border of the heart into the right pleural space since the positioning required to visualize these targets may compromise venous return. Rightward mobilization of the heart to expose the lateral wall also requires complete division of all adhesions between the inferior wall and the diaphragmatic pericardium and extensive division of the pericardium itself from the diaphragm (while preserving the phrenic nerves). Complete dissection of the aorta and pulmonary artery is not required since cross-clamping is unnecessary. Dissection of the ascending aorta can simply be limited to an area for emergent cannulation and placement for proximal grafts. Limiting dissection in this area minimizes the risk for subadventitial dissection and injury to the innominate vein or pulmonary artery.

After the general target area is dissected out completely and the targets are identified, the final sequence of the operation can be planned. Arguably, the closest collaboration between surgeon and anesthesiologist occurs during the construction of distal anastomoses. Communication with an anesthesiologist familiar with off-pump hemodynamics is essential for the success of OPCAB. Needless to say, close attention to hemodynamic parameters at this point can avoid hemodynamic instability during cardiac positioning. In some cases, patients with marginal hemodynamics can be cannulated for pump-supported beating heart surgery, or an intra-aortic balloon pump can be placed to improve hemodynamics. If hemodynamic instability persists, the surgeon should have a low threshold for placing the patient on CPB before cardiogenic shock develops.

The intricacies involving conduit and target selection and graft strategies are beyond the scope of this chapter. However, as a general rule, all anastomoses can be successfully performed with any conduit using OPCAB techniques. The amount of time that the heart is in a nonanatomic position should be minimized, although a "test lift" prior to committing oneself to distal grafting may be useful. Conduit preparation should be performed prior to lifting the heart. Particular attention should be paid to graft length. Conduits in the redo setting often require additional length due to adhesions, the requirement for extremely distal anastomoses, and the presence of old grafts. Additional flexibility can be obtained by direct anastomosis to the distal site of a prior graft by disconnecting the previous atherosclerotic vein graft, graft-to-graft proximal anastomoses, sequential vein grafts, or using additional in situ arterial grafts.

Distal Anastomosis

Prior to distal arteriotomy, the patient is heparinized. A dose of 200 Units/kg with an activated clotting time (ACT) of 300 s provides adequate anticoagulation and prevents unnecessary blood loss, which may be associated with higher levels of anticoagulation. ACT levels are tested and small additional heparin doses (typically 3,000 Units) are given every 30 min. Target vessel stabilization and heart positioning are now performed with several commercially available devices, which combine suction apical positioning and lateral target stabilization devices on flexible arms. The latest iteration of these devices adequately provides stabilization without undue compression of the heart, thereby, producing minimal hemodynamic compromise.

Proximal control of the vessel and patent previous graft is performed with a silastic tape with a blunt needle placed in a double loop circumferentially around the native vessel, proximal to the anastomosis. If necessary, a second snare or soft vascular clamp may be applied around the diseased vein graft, but should not be tightened until after the anastomotic site is opened to prevent distal embolization of atherosclerotic debris from an atherosclerotic vein graft. Only enough tension needs to be applied to restrict flow because the use of a blower–mister facilitates distal visualization even in the presence of a moderate amount of bleeding. In large collateralized targets, either a distal silastic snare (gently applied) or an intracoronary shunt can be used to further enhance visualization.

The sequence of graft construction is often crucial for hemodynamic stability. Generally, easily accessible vessels on the anterior wall should be completed first, as these anastomoses can be performed quickly with very little manipulation of the heart. In addition, collateralized vessels should be completed prior to large collateralizing vessels. For anastomoses that cannot be completed quickly or vessels supplying a large ischemic area, the use of an intercoronary shunt reduces ischemic time and blood loss. In patients with marginal hemodynamics, it may be wise to complete the proximal anastomoses first to provide immediate blood flow to ischemic areas supplied by each target as each distal anastomosis is completed. Similarly, perfusing each graft after completion, as with the perfusion-assisted direct coronary artery bypass (PADCAB) technique, allows for immediate blood flow to individual targets [7].

The LAD is typically the first anastomosis to be performed with an IMA graft, if not previously used. Again, only enough exposure to complete the anastomosis is required and usually placement of a stabilizer is all that is required because the surrounding adhesions facilitate displacement and positioning of the anterior wall. An intracardiac shunt should be used for a large collateralizing LAD supplying an occluded RCA. Anastomoses to diagonal branches can be easily performed in a similar position with little impact on hemodynamics. Additional lysis of adhesions and the application of an apical suction position may be required, depending on the anatomy.

Next, grafts to the distal RCA or its branches are performed. Again, only the posterior wall of the heart requires exposure as placement of the apical suction device along the acute margin of the right ventricle with anteriorly directed lift provides adequate exposure with little hemodynamic insult. Bradycardia caused by proximal stenosis of the RCA can be treated with temporary ventricular pacing wires during completion of the anastomosis. Distal posterior descending artery grafts may require complete dissection of the apex of the heart to place the apex in a more vertical orientation to facilitate visualization.

Finally, grafts along the lateral wall to obtuse marginal branches or left ventricular branch arteries are performed last, sometimes after completing both proximal and distal anastomoses to revascularize other regions of the heart, thereby improving hemodynamic stability during the extreme displacement of the heart often required for visualization of the lateral wall. The apical positioner is used to point the apex of the heart superiorly, in the direction of the surgeon's right shoulder. Marginal hemodynamics after positioning can usually be improved first with small positional changes rather than pharmacologic maneuvers. The Trendelenburg position often improves venous return and is usually sufficient to counteract the reduced venous return from positioning the heart. Full release of the right pericardium and a transverse incision through the right pericardium at the level of the diaphragm laterally toward the phrenic nerve allows the right side of the heart to fall into the adjacent pleural space, thereby improving venous return as well. Elevating the right limb of the sternal retractor on two rolled towels facilitates this maneuver. In addition, a slight relaxation of the rigid arm of the apical suctioning device, while leaving the stabilizer in place, reduces compression of the heart and improves hemodynamics without much detriment to visualization. The ramus intermedius artery is often the most demanding target, especially when it is intramyocardial. Adequate visualization often requires full lysis of adhesions of the lateral wall, pulmonary artery, left atrial appendage, and mobilization of a previous IMA pedicle. It is often easier to enter the left pleural space, completely mobilize the left pericardium down to the level of the phrenic nerve, and dissect the pericardium closer to the area of the target vessel. Unfortunately, there are no easy shortcuts to facilitate this dissection and patience, combined with meticulous technique, is required.

Proximal Anastomosis

Adhesions and limited space surrounding the ascending aorta require some creativity on the part of the surgeon when performing proximal anastomoses. Unlike traditional CABG, OPCAB affords the potential to reduce perioperative strokes caused by manipulation of the aorta. It is imperative to evaluate the ascending aorta with an epiaortic ultrasound as manual palpation to detect atheromatous disease is unreliable due to the degree of adhesions, previous grafts, and felt pledgets frequently present in this area. As is the case in most redo-CABGs, the proximal anastomoses of previous vein grafts are often free of disease and may be the best sites for the creation of new proximal anastomoses. If these sites are unavailable, an additional portion of the ascending aorta must be cleared, with care not to disrupt the innominate vein, pulmonary artery, or dissect in a subadventitial plane.

Often, even the application of a partial occluding vascular clamp is unadvisable. In these situations, proximal anastomotic devices, such as the HEARTSTRING Proximal Seal System (Guidant, Cupertino, CA) or PAS-Port Proximal Anastomosis System (Cardica, Redwood City, CA), can be used to create an anastomosis without application of a clamp. Much of the difficulty of creating proximal anastomoses can be avoided with careful preoperative planning including the use of sequential grafts, in situ pedicled grafts, and graft-to-graft anastomoses. Although long-term patency has yet to be determined, every variation of graft-to-graft anastomosis has been described, including both old and new grafts comprising arterio-arterial, arterio-venous, and veno-venous anastomoses.

Following completion of the grafts, hemodynamic instability, changes in the electrocardiogram, or new wall motion abnormalities may suggest graft compromise. Some surgeons also interrogate each individual graft using transit time flow measurement (VeriQ MediStim, Maple Grove, MN). Finally, protamine is given to reverse anticoagulation, and the remainder of the procedure is completed in standard fashion according to the surgeon's practice.

Application of the previous techniques by an experienced OPCAB surgeon allows performance of ~50% of all redo coronary bypass procedures without use of CPB. It is important that the surgeon is realistic in assessing each patient as a candidate for redo-OPCAB. Elective conversion to conventional CABG is associated with much better outcomes than emergency conversion during hemodynamic collapse, which may be caused by inappropriate attempts to perform redo-OPCAB in patients for whom CPB is necessary. CPB should be available and prepared for immediate institution during every redo-OPCAB case.

Alternative Approaches

Although the vast majority of redo-OPCABs are performed through a previous median sternotomy, alternative approaches through a left thoracotomy may be useful, especially when revascularization of limited target areas is required. Approaches through a thoracotomy may improve outcomes by avoiding the hazards of repeat sternotomy including avoiding injury to underlying structures (especially patent grafts adherent to the sternum), minimizing blood loss, and preventing wound complications. This approach, however, may be contraindicated in patients who cannot tolerate single lung ventilation, have left ventricular hypertrophy, are obese, and require bypass of targets on multiple regions of the heart.

Redo-OPCAB procedures require double-lumen endotracheal intubation. Conduits may be best harvested prior to positioning the patient in the right lateral decubitus position. A muscle-sparing lateral thoracotomy through the fourth, fifth, or sixth interspace is made, depending on the location of the target(s). Through this incision, the entire anterolateral wall can be exposed easily as well as most of the length of the left IMA, if not previously used. The left lung is lowered and the inferior pulmonary ligament is mobilized. Significant adhesions to the lateral wall are uncommon, and the pericardium can usually be lifted free from the underlying myocardium with a longitudinal incision anterior to the phrenic nerve. The coronary targets are identified and each anastomosis created, as described earlier. Often, apical cardiac positioning devices are not required, since traction on the adherent pericardium provides adequate exposure. Care should be taken to provide additional length for each conduit to reach its proximal site along either the subclavian artery or, preferably, the descending thoracic aorta due to its closer proximity. Following completion of the distal anastomosis, the conduit is coursed in a gentle cure anterior to the pulmonary hilum up to the subclavian artery or below the hilum to the descending aorta. The proximal anastomosis is then performed in the usual fashion by placement of a partial occluding side-biting vascular clamp on the descending aorta. Again, the anastomotic devices mentioned earlier can be used when access to the descending aorta is limited. Although long-term outcomes are unknown, this approach has been described in great detail in the literature with excellent early outcomes [8].

Minimally invasive redo-OPCAB techniques continue to evolve. MIDCAB surgery is most useful for anterior wall targets requiring the use of a left IMA. The distal LAD artery may be exposed with a small anterior thoracotomy, and the LAD or diagonal artery may be grafted with a left IMA graft. Robotically assisted or endoscopically assisted IMA harvest with subsequent minithoracotomy has also been described, although its usefulness in the redo setting has yet to be determined.

Outcomes

OPCAB provides at least equivalent outcomes compared with conventional CABG among low-risk patients with regard to hard endpoints, such as mortality, stroke, myocardial infarction, and renal failure, and perhaps has improved outcomes in historically high-risk groups including redo-CABG patients. Despite this, surgeons remain concerned about the completeness of revascularization, long-term graft patency, and excessive mortality in patients converted to CABG from OPCAB [9]. This translates into greater concern regarding the use of OPCAB during redo coronary surgery due to the complex nature of advanced coronary pathology, increasing technical difficulty, and overall greater risk involved. Compounding risks pertaining to redo-OPCAB include greater dissection on a beating heart, a perceived greater threat of atherosclerotic vein embolization, greater hemodynamic instability, and poor outcomes with conversion to CABG. Specifically, incomplete revascularization has been associated with poor long-term outcome. In the redo setting, Di Mauro and colleagues reported a trend toward improved early outcomes of patients undergoing redo-OPCAB; however, this was associated with lower rates of complete revascularization in these patients [10]. It is not known if redo-OPCAB sacrifices long-term outcomes for improved short-term outcomes.

On the other hand, redo-OPCAB offers high-risk patients additional benefits not afforded by traditional CABG. CPB, hypothermic myocardial arrest, problems with myocardial protection, blood loss, and manipulation of the ascending aorta are eliminated or minimized. Unfortunately, there is a paucity of well-controlled comparisons of redo-OPCAB and redo-CABG in the literature, but case reports and retrospective studies suggest improved outcomes with redo-OPCAB [8]. Mishira and colleagues have recently reported results from patients undergoing redo-OPCAB. In this study, 538 patients underwent revascularization during the 10-year study period. Three hundred and thirty-two (61.7%) underwent redo-OPCAB, with 265 (79.8%) patients undergoing bypass through a redo median sternotomy and 67 (20.2%) patients undergoing bypass though thoracotomy. Despite a wide variety of concomitant disease, redo-OPCAB was performed safely with an overall mortality of 3.3%, which was not significantly different from redo-CABG patients [11].

In conclusion, patients requiring repeat coronary artery bypass grafting constitute a high-risk group, who may benefit from redo-OPCAB. However, OPCAB is a more technically challenging procedure than conventional CABG and requires a methodical approach and acquisition of an advanced skill set. This is particularly important when OPCAB techniques are applied to patients who have undergone previous coronary artery bypass surgery.

References

1. Sabik III JF, Blackstone EH, Houghtaling PL, Walts PA, Lytle BW. Is reoperation still a risk factor in coronary artery bypass surgery? Ann Thorac Surg. 2005;80:1719–27.
2. Puskas JD, Cheng D, Knight J, Angelini G, DeCannier D, Diegeler, A, Dullum M, Martin J, Ochi M, Patel N, Sim E, Trehan N, Zamvar V. Off-pump versus conventional coronary artery bypass grafting; a meta-analysis and consensus statement from the 2004 ISMICS Consensus Conference. Innovations. Fall 2005;1(1):3–27.
3. Puskas JD, Edwards FH, Pappas PA, O'Brien S, Peterson ED, Kilgo P, et al. Off-pump techniques benefit men and women and narrow the disparity in mortality after coronary bypass grafting. Ann Thorac Surg. 2007;84(5):1447–54.
4. Puskas JD, Kilgo PD, Lattouf OM, Thourani VH, Cooper WA, Vassiliades TA, et al. Off-pump coronary bypass provides reduced mortality and morbidity and equivalent 10-year survival. Ann Thorac Surg. 2008;86(4):1139–46.
5. Society of Thoracic Surgeons National Adult Cardiac Database: Spring Report 2009. Durham: Duke Clinical Research Institute; 2009.
6. Shroyer AL, Grover FL, Hattler B, Collins JF, McDonald GO, Kozora E, et al. Veterans Affairs Randomized On/Off Bypass (ROOBY) Study Group. On-pump versus off-pump coronary-artery bypass surgery. N Engl J Med. 2009;361(19):1827–37.
7. Cooper WA, Corvera JS, Thourani VH, Puskas JD, Craver JM, Lattouf OM, et al. Perfusion-assisted direct coronary artery bypass provides early reperfusion of ischemic myocardium and facilitates complete revascularization. Ann Thorac Surg. 2003;75(4):1132–9.
8. Mack MJ. Off-pump surgery and alternatives to standard operation in redo coronary surgery. J Card Surg. 2004;19(4):313–9.
9. Khan NE, De Souza A, Mister R, Flather M, Clague J, Davies S, et al. A randomized comparison of off-pump and on-pump multivessel coronary-artery bypass surgery. N Engl J Med. 2004;350(1):21–8.
10. Di Mauro M, Iaco AL, Contini M, Teodari G, Vittolla G, Pano M, et al. Reoperative coronary artery bypass grafting: analysis of early and late outcomes. Ann Thorac Surg. 2005;79:81–7.
11. Mishra YK, Collison SP, Malhotra R, Kohli V, Mehta Y, Trehan N. Ten-year experience with single-vessel and multivessel reoperative off-pump coronary artery bypass grafting. J Thorac Cardiovasc Surg. 2008; 135(3):527–32.

Management of Perioperative Stroke

4

Amer M. Malik and Lawrence R. Wechsler

Introduction

Stroke is currently recognized as the third most common cause of death and the leading cause of adult morbidity in the United States, affecting nearly 795,000 people annually [1]. Perioperative ischemic stroke is an important concern when cardiac surgeries are undertaken. Approximately one million patients worldwide undergo cardiac surgeries annually and coronary artery bypass grafting (CABG) is the most frequent major cardiovascular operation performed. Cardiac surgery is associated with higher perioperative stroke risk compared with general, noncardiac procedures [2–7]. Perioperative ischemic stroke occurs in an estimated 2–6% of CABG surgeries and is often related to the complexity and type of surgery being performed. In patients older than 75 years of age, incidence approaches 9% and is more than twice that of patients 65–74 years old and more than nine times that of patients less than 65 years old [8]. When combined cardiac surgeries (e.g., CABG and valve surgery) are pursued, the incidence of perioperative ischemic stroke tends to be even higher [5, 6].

A.M. Malik, MD, MBA
Department of Neurology, UPMC Stroke Institute, University of Pittsburgh School of Medicine, Pittsburgh, PA, USA

L.R. Wechsler, MD (✉)
Department of Neurology, University of Pittsburgh School of Medicine, Pittsburgh, PA, USA
e-mail: wechslerlr@upmc.edu

Perioperative Stroke Risk

Cardiac surgery involves an intrinsic risk of stroke regardless of the presence of concomitant carotid disease. Timing of surgery is a contributing factor to increased stroke risk. More events are associated with cardiac surgeries performed on an urgent basis rather than those pursued electively [4]. Additionally, intraoperative strokes should be considered differently than postoperative strokes. During the intraoperative period, independent risk factors for stroke are age greater than 70 years, left ventricular ejection fraction less than 40%, prior stroke or transient ischemic attack (TIA), normothermic cardiopulmonary bypass, diabetes mellitus, and peripheral vascular disease [9]. Early postoperative stroke occurs immediately after emergence from anesthesia, and associated risk factors include previous stroke or TIA, aortic atherosclerosis, and duration of cardiopulmonary bypass. Late postoperative stroke involves the development of a neurological deficit remote from first awakening without a neurological deficit. Predictors of delayed stroke include prior stroke or TIA, aortic atherosclerosis, diabetes mellitus, and combined endpoints of atrial fibrillation and low cardiac output. Notably, female gender has been associated with an increased risk of early and delayed postoperative strokes [10]. Air is one of the causative factors for multiple cerebral emboli especially after valvular surgery. However, the use of transesophageal echocardiography as a routine practice during

V.R. Machiraju et al. (eds.), *Redo Cardiac Surgery in Adults*,
DOI 10.1007/978-1-4614-1326-4_4, © Springer Science+Business Media, LLC 2012

cardiac surgery and use of intraoperative carbon dioxide have decreased such incidence.

The mechanisms of stroke related to cardiac surgery also appear to adhere to a time-dependent relationship. In the intraoperative period, macroemboli are the most commonly implicated stroke mechanism, likely resulting from cross-clamping an ascending aortic arch with atherosclerosis [9]. Early postoperative strokes and delayed strokes are associated with emboli and cerebral hypoperfusion, with the former being more common [10].

Coexistent Coronary and Carotid Disease

Carotid endarterectomy (CEA) has been employed as a means of stroke prophylaxis for symptomatic stenosis greater than 70% based on criteria established by the North American Symptomatic Carotid Endarterectomy trial (NASCET) [11]. Evidence from randomized trials also suggests some benefit of CEA for patients with asymptomatic stenosis; however, the magnitude of the benefit is considerably smaller and patients must be selected carefully [12, 13]. In patients with both carotid and coronary disease, CEA has been performed prior to, in conjunction with, or after CABG surgery [14–16]. A staged approach employing CEA prior to CABG is frequently pursued in patients with symptomatic, high-grade carotid lesions whose coronary artery disease is stable. Concurrent CEA is utilized in patients who have unstable angina, high-grade left main lesions and symptomatic high-grade carotid stenoses, bilateral high-grade asymptomatic stenoses, or ipsilateral asymptomatic stenosis and contralateral occlusion [6, 17, 18]. In patients undergoing emergent or urgent CABG who have advanced carotid disease, a reverse-staged approach has been performed. In this option, CEA is delayed for at least 2 weeks because CEA performed immediately after CABG is associated with increased mortality [19]. However, there is a suggestion that CEA in the first week after CABG in neurologically stable patients with minor stroke or TIA is not associated with a higher operative risk vs. late surgery [20].

Recent evidence challenges the belief that prophylactic CEA significantly reduces the incidence of perioperative stroke and suggests that combining CEA and cardiac surgery is unnecessary and ineffective in reducing stroke risk, especially in patients with asymptomatic carotid stenosis [3, 6, 21, 22]. Carotid artery stenting (CAS) and angioplasty are currently being used as alternatives to CEA in preventing stroke in both symptomatic and asymptomatic patients with carotid stenosis [23–29], and a comparison of efficacy of CEA vs. CAS was recently completed in the Carotid Revascularization Endarterectomy vs. Stent Trial (CREST). Among patients with symptomatic or asymptomatic carotid stenosis, the risk of the composite primary outcome of stroke, myocardial infarction, or death did not differ significantly in the CAS group vs. CEA group. During the periprocedural period, CAS was associated with a higher risk of stroke and CEA was associated with a higher risk of myocardial infarction.

Stroke Prevention in Cardiac Surgery

Recommendations on how to best prevent perioperative stroke in patients undergoing cardiac surgery include a few salient management points. A history of TIA or stroke is a strong harbinger of perioperative stroke; therefore, a comprehensive history is a necessity [6, 7, 30]. Significant carotid artery stenosis, even in an asymptomatic patient, has been reported as an independent predictor of stroke risk immediately after CABG [31, 32]. Therefore, aside from careful auscultation for carotid bruits on physical examination, carotid Doppler ultrasonography has been commonly used as a screening tool to determine severe carotid stenosis. This approach has reported detection rates of 5–11% for hemodynamically significant carotid artery stenosis in patients undergoing CABG [33–35]. However, cases are sometimes equivocal with this screening methodology and necessitate further clarification of carotid stenosis severity via catheter carotid angiography and transcranial Doppler [12, 35, 36].

Even when found, however, treatment of the carotid stenosis should follow the guidelines reviewed in the previous section.

Additionally, an intraoperative epiaortic ultrasound or transesophageal echocardiogram should be obtained since aortic atherosclerosis is strongly associated with perioperative stroke risk [4]. These modalities can provide real-time images to assess arterial wall structure, thus permitting plaque and wall characterization and an assessment of the high-risk conditions for cardioembolic stroke [37]. Identification of the location and extent of the atherosclerosis at the time of or prior to the cardiac surgery could modify the surgical approach and alter the site of clamping or aortic cannulation to avoid the calcified plaques [38]. It has been suggested that stroke risk reduction can be achieved with the use of off-pump CABG surgery, avoiding cross-clamping, or using aortic filters [39]. The approach of off-pump CABG is still controversial as recent studies have suggested that off-pump bypass does not produce lower postoperative mortality or stroke rates and has worse composite outcomes and poorer graft patency compared with on-pump CABG surgery [40–43].

Treatment of Perioperative Stroke

Treatment considerations for acute stroke occurring with cardiac surgery are similar to any other acute stroke, except for the special consideration of bleeding risk associated with recent surgery. Knowledge of whether potentially salvageable tissue is present may help guide therapeutic decisions and can be assessed with either computed tomography (CT) or magnetic resonance imaging (MRI) modalities (Figs. 4.1 and 4.2). Intravenous tissue plasminogen activator (t-PA) is currently the only FDA-approved therapy for acute ischemic stroke; however, recent major surgery is an absolute exclusion criterion for intravenous thrombolytic administration because the drug could disrupt hemostasis in the surgical bed and cause significant bleeding.

Patients who have recently had cardiac surgery are thought to be at increased risk for the development of pericardial tamponade, and this situation has been described in the literature [44]. The hypothesis behind this process is believed to be twofold. First, a hypercoagulable state is created from a decrease in t-PA levels

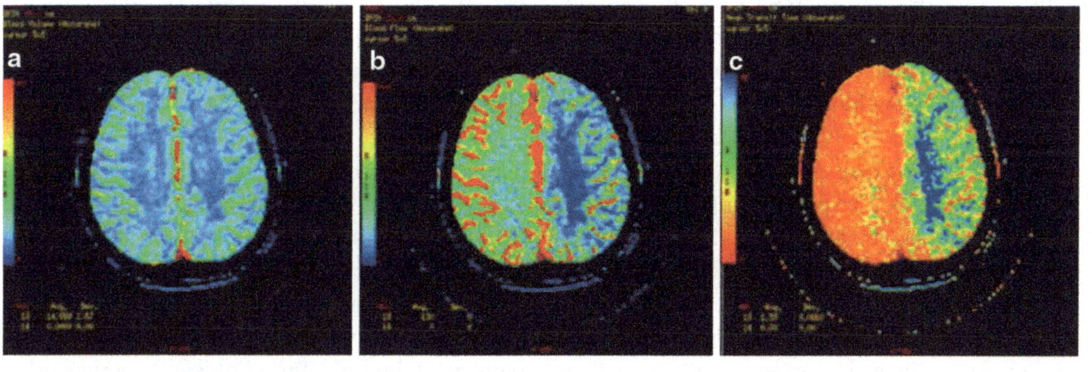

Fig. 4.1 CT brain perfusion scan with sequencing maps for cerebral blood volume (CBV) (**a**), cerebral blood flow (CBF) (**b**), and mean transit time (MTT) (**c**) in a patient with perioperative stroke immediately after a five-vessel CABG. In general, CBV indicates the area of ischemic core, and CBF and MTT indicate the area of ischemic penumbra. These maps indicate a well-preserved CBV without asymmetry but a decreased CBF and increased MTT in brain territory supplied by the left middle cerebral artery. An imaging mismatch is shown indicating that salvageable tissue exists. Concurrent CT angiography of the neck revealed a left internal carotid artery occlusion at the origin. The patient was successfully recanalized with neuroendovascular therapy

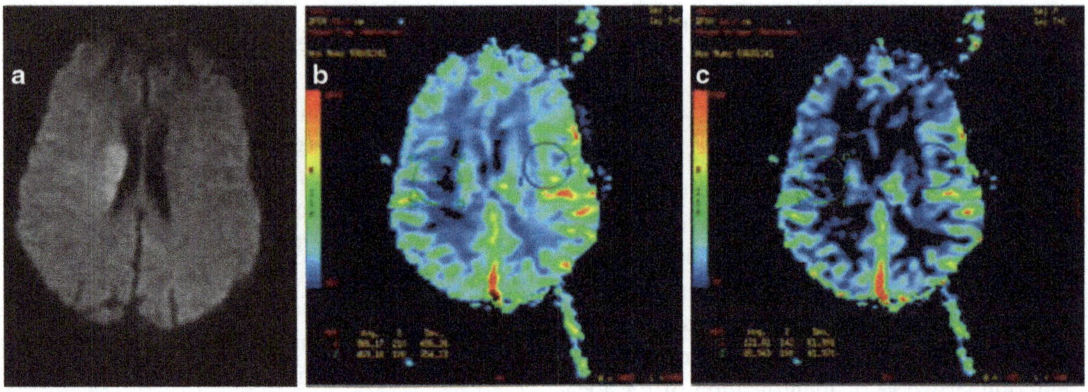

Fig. 4.2 Magnetic resonance diffusion-weighted imaging (DWI) and perfusion-weighted imaging (PWI) in a patient with acute infarction of the right putamen visualized on DWI (**a**) and decreased CBF and CBV visualized on PWI (**b**, **c**), respectively. The area of decreased CBF is much greater than the area of restricted diffusion in the right middle cerebral artery territory, compatible with a large area of ischemic penumbra

and an increase in plasminogen activator inhibitor levels in the postcardiac surgery period after the reverse situation exists perioperatively [45]. Second, platelet dysfunction occurs after CABG and in patients receiving intravenous t-PA for myocardial infarctions, platelet counts less than 100,000 conferred a 7.5-fold increased risk of bleeding [46].

The option that is currently available for reperfusion in instances associated with cardiac surgery is neuroendovascular therapy, an emerging field in ischemic stroke treatment. In general, neuroendovascular therapy is a minimally invasive procedure that utilizes microcatheters and devices, such as balloon angioplasty, stents, and liquid adhesive, and allows the interventionalist to treat the respective problem with the assistance of real-time, bi-plane digital subtraction angiography. Available multimodal neuroendovascular reperfusion therapies include the delivery of intra-arterial pharmacologic thrombolysis, mechanical embolectomy, intravascular stent placement, balloon angioplasty, and manual or continuous aspiration. There are several case reports and case series in the literature identifying successful vessel recanalization after neuroendovascular therapy in cardiac surgery patients [47], and one such case from the University of Pittsburgh School of Medicine is provided as an example (Fig. 4.3).

Recent surgery is generally considered a contraindication to thrombolytic therapy after acute stroke. However, several reports suggest that intervening in patients after cardiac surgery can be accomplished with acceptable risk and promising results [48, 49]. Intravenous t-PA is potentially hazardous because of bleeding into the surgical site, but intra-arterial therapy offers an alternative approach in which less activation of systemic thrombolytic activity should occur. Devices, such as the mechanical embolus removal in cerebral ischemia (MERCI) clot retriever (Concentric Medical, Mountain View, CA) and Penumbra aspiration catheter (Penumbra Inc. USA, Alameda, CA), are now FDA-approved for removal of thrombi from intracranial arteries in patients with acute stroke and represent an attractive option for treatment of acute stroke related to recent cardiac surgery. Moazami et al. reported the results of treatment of 13 patients with stroke 1–12 days following cardiac surgery with either intra-arterial urokinase or t-PA [49]. Seven of the patients achieved thrombolysis in myocardial infarction (TIMI) grade 2 or 3 recanalization. Neurological improvement occurred almost immediately in five patients. A hemothorax requiring chest tube drainage occurred in one patient, and another patient had a small cerebellar hemorrhage without clinical change. Fukuda et al. performed intra-arterial thrombolysis using

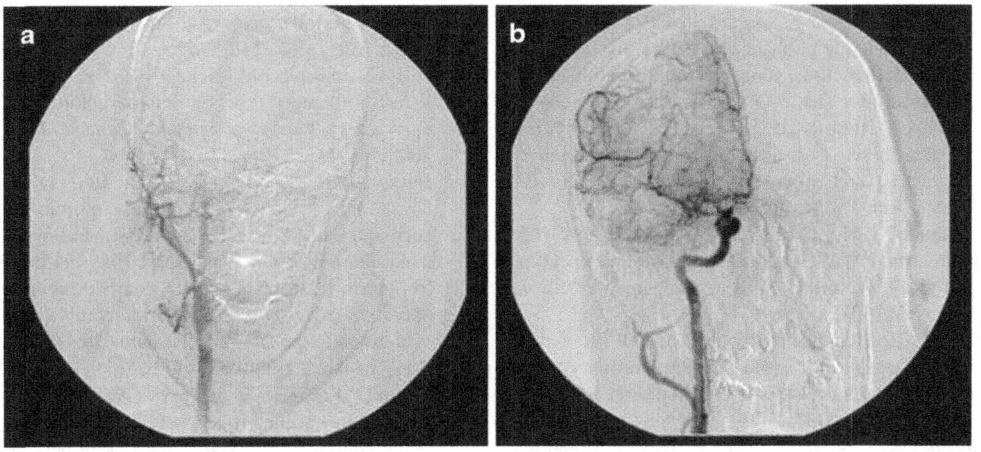

Fig. 4.3 Cerebral digital subtraction angiography in a patient who suffered a perioperative stroke during CABG surgery and was taken for neuroendovascular therapy. Angiography revealed a right proximal middle cerebral artery M1 occlusion (**a**) anterior–posterior view. After intra-arterial thrombolysis and mechanical embolectomy with the MERCI clot retrieval device, the patient experienced successful recanalization with TIMI grade 3 flow (**b**) anterior–posterior view

urokinase on five patients with stroke 2–8 days after cardiac surgery [48]. All patients had at least partial recanalization and neurological improvement occurred in three cases. Only one small hemorrhagic infarct was noted on follow-up CT scans. Katzan et al. reported on six patients receiving intra-arterial thrombolysis after CABG, mitral valve annuloplasty or replacement, aortic valve replacement, or left ventricular assist device surgery. The patients underwent intra-arterial therapy a median of 4.5 days after cardiac surgery, and no clinically significant systemic or intracerebral hemorrhages occurred. At least partial recanalization occurred in four patients, and four patients improved neurologically after their stroke. One patient did expire from massive cerebral edema, although this may have emerged from a lack of collateral flow on the angiogram before the recanalization attempt [50].

These reports suggest that intra-arterial thrombolysis can be performed with good results and acceptable risk in patients with stroke after cardiac procedures. Thrombus removal with endovascular devices may further improve these results. Although hemo-pericardium after intravenous t-PA has been described [44], this complication was not seen in these patients treated with the intra-arterial approach [48–50].

Summary

Acute ischemic stroke is a serious perioperative risk associated with cardiac surgery. Timing plays a key role in the mechanism and development of intraoperative, early postoperative, and late postoperative strokes. Coexistent coronary and carotid disease is an important concern and can be addressed with either CEA or CAS. Prudent surveillance of potentially high-risk patients can help to reduce the incidence of perioperative stroke. Currently, intra-arterial therapy is the only treatment modality available for perioperative stroke and should be pursued when such a situation transpires. If available, emergent consultation and input from a dedicated vascular neurology or stroke physician should be acquired.

References

1. Lloyd-Jones D, Adams RJ, Brown TM, Carnethon M, Dai S, De Simone G, et al. Heart disease and stroke statistics – 2010 update. A report from the American Heart Association. Circulation. 2010 Feb 23;121(7):948–54.
2. Caplan LR. Translating what is known about neurological complications of coronary artery bypass graft surgery into action. Arch Neurol. 2009;66:1062–4.

3. Bond R, Rerkasem K, Shearman CP, Rothwell PM. Time trends in the published risks of stroke and death due to endarterectomy for symptomatic carotid stenosis. Cerebrovasc Dis. 2004;18:37–46.
4. Bucerius J, Gummert JF, Borger MA, Walther T, Doll N, Onnasch JF, et al. Stroke after cardiac surgery: a risk factor analysis of 16,184 consecutive adult patients. Ann Thorac Surg. 2003;75:472–8.
5. McKhann GM, Grega MA, Borowicz Jr LM, Baumgartner WA, Selnes OA. Stroke and encephalopathy after cardiac surgery: an update. Stroke. 2006;37:562–71.
6. Naylor AR, Mehta Z, Rothwell PM, Bell PR. Carotid artery disease and stroke during coronary artery bypass: a critical review of the literature. Eur J Vasc Endovasc Surg. 2002;23:283–94.
7. Nosan DK, Gomez CR, Maves MD. Perioperative stroke in patients undergoing head and neck surgery. Ann Otol Rhinol Laryngol. 1993;102:717–23.
8. Tuman KJ, McCarthy RJ, Najafi H, Ivankovich AD. Differential effects of advanced age on neurologic and cardiac risks of coronary artery operations. J Thorac Cardiovasc Surg. 1992;104:1510–7.
9. Borger MA, Ivanov J, Weisel RD, Rao V, Peniston CM. Stroke during coronary bypass surgery: principal role of cerebral macroemboli. Eur J Cardiothorac Surg. 2001;19:627–32.
10. Hogue Jr CW, Murphy SF, Schechtman KB, Davila-Roman VG. Risk factors for early or delayed stroke after cardiac surgery. Circulation. 1999;100:642–7.
11. North American Symptomatic Carotid Endarterectomy Trial Collaborators. Beneficial effect of carotid endarterectomy in symptomatic patients with high-grade carotid stenosis. N Engl J Med. 1991;325: 445–53.
12. Executive Committee for the Asymptomatic Carotid Atherosclerosis Study. Endarterectomy for asymptomatic carotid artery stenosis. JAMA. 1995;273: 1421–8.
13. Halliday A, Mansfield A, Marro J, Peto C, Peto R, Potter J, et al. Prevention of disabling and fatal strokes by successful carotid endarterectomy in patients without recent neurological symptoms: randomised controlled trial. Lancet. 2004;363:1491–502.
14. Byrne J, Darling III RC, Roddy SP, Mehta M, Paty PS, Kreienberg PB, et al. Combined carotid endarterectomy and coronary artery bypass grafting in patients with asymptomatic high-grade stenoses: an analysis of 758 procedures. J Vasc Surg. 2006;44: 67–72.
15. Kougias P, Kappa JR, Sewell DH, Feit RA, Michalik RE, Imam M, et al. Simultaneous carotid endarterectomy and coronary artery bypass grafting: results in specific patient groups. Ann Vasc Surg. 2007;21: 408–14.
16. Naylor AR. Does the risk of post-CABG stroke merit staged or synchronous reconstruction in patients with symptomatic or asymptomatic carotid disease? J Cardiovasc Surg. 2009;50:71–81.
17. Mackey WC, Khabbaz K, Bojar R, O'Donnell Jr TF. Simultaneous carotid endarterectomy and coronary bypass: perioperative risk and long-term survival. J Vasc Surg. 1996;24:58–64.
18. Hill MD, Shrive FM, Kennedy J, Feasby TE, Ghali WA. Simultaneous carotid endarterectomy and coronary artery bypass surgery in Canada. Neurology. 2005;64:1435–7.
19. Hertzer NR, Loop FD, Beven EG, O'Hara PJ, Krajewski LP. Surgical staging for simultaneous coronary and carotid disease: a study including prospective randomization. J Vasc Surg. 1989;9:455–63.
20. Rerkasem K, Rothwell PM. Systematic review of the operative risks of carotid endarterectomy for recently symptomatic stenosis in relation to the timing of surgery. Stroke. 2009;40:e564–72.
21. Baiou D, Karageorge A, Spyt T, Naylor AR. Patients undergoing cardiac surgery with asymptomatic unilateral carotid stenoses have a low risk of peri-operative stroke. Eur J Vasc Endovasc Surg. 2009;38:556–9.
22. Li Y, Walicki D, Mathiesen C, Jenny D, Li Q, Isayev Y, et al. Strokes after cardiac surgery and relationship to carotid stenosis. Arch Neurol. 2009;66:1091–6.
23. Gray WA, White Jr HJ, Barrett DM, Chandran G, Turner R, Reisman M. Carotid stenting and endarterectomy: a clinical and cost comparison of revascularization strategies. Stroke. 2002;33:1063–70.
24. Kastrup A, Groschel K, Krapf H, Brehm BR, Dichgans J, Schulz JB. Early outcome of carotid angioplasty and stenting with and without cerebral protection devices: a systematic review of the literature. Stroke. 2003;34:813–9.
25. Yadav JS, Wholey MH, Kuntz RE, Fayad P, Katzen BT, Mishkel GJ, et al. Protected carotid-artery stenting versus endarterectomy in high-risk patients. N Engl J Med. 2004;351:1493–501.
26. Sivaguru A, Venables GS, Beard JD, Gaines PA. European carotid angioplasty trial. J Endovasc Surg. 1996;3:16–20.
27. Bonati LH, Ederle J, McCabe DJ, Dobson J, Featherstone RL, Gaines PA, et al. Long-term risk of carotid restenosis in patients randomly assigned to endovascular treatment or endarterectomy in the carotid and vertebral artery transluminal angioplasty study (CAVATAS): long-term follow-up of a randomised trial. Lancet Neurol. 2009;8:908–17.
28. Ederle J, Bonati LH, Dobson J, Featherstone RL, Gaines PA, Beard JD, et al. Endovascular treatment with angioplasty or stenting versus endarterectomy in patients with carotid artery stenosis in the carotid and vertebral artery transluminal angioplasty study (CAVATAS): long-term follow-up of a randomised trial. Lancet Neurol. 2009;8:898–907.
29. Ringleb PA, Hacke W. [stent and surgery for symptomatic carotid stenosis. Space study results]. Nervenarzt. 2007;78:1130–7.
30. Kam PC, Calcroft RM. Peri-operative stroke in general surgical patients. Anaesthesia. 1997;52:879–83.
31. D'Agostino RS, Svensson LG, Neumann DJ, Balkhy HH, Williamson WA, Shahian DM. Screening carotid ultrasonography and risk factors for stroke in coronary artery surgery patients. Ann Thorac Surg. 1996;62:1714–23.

32. Faggioli GL, Curl GR, Ricotta JJ. The role of carotid screening before coronary artery bypass. J Vasc Surg. 1990;12:724–9; discussion 729–31.
33. Berens ES, Kouchoukos NT, Murphy SF, Wareing TH. Preoperative carotid artery screening in elderly patients undergoing cardiac surgery. J Vasc Surg. 1992;15:313–21; discussion 322–3.
34. Anastasiadis K, Karamitsos TD, Velissaris I, Makrygiannakis K, Kiskinis D. Preoperative screening and management of carotid artery disease in patients undergoing cardiac surgery. Perfusion. 2009;24:257–62.
35. Brener BJ, Brief DK, Alpert J, Goldenkranz RJ, Parsonnet V. The risk of stroke in patients with asymptomatic carotid stenosis undergoing cardiac surgery: a follow-up study. J Vasc Surg. 1987;5:269–79.
36. Babikian VL, Feldmann E, Wechsler LR, Newell DW, Gomez CR, Bogdahn U, et al. Transcranial Doppler ultrasonography: year 2000 update. J Neuroimaging. 2000;10:101–15.
37. Ferro JM. Cardioembolic stroke: an update. Lancet Neurol. 2003;2:177–88.
38. Gold JP, Torres KE, Maldarelli W, Zhuravlev I, Condit D, Wasnick J. Improving outcomes in coronary surgery: the impact of echo-directed aortic cannulation and perioperative hemodynamic management in 500 patients. Ann Thorac Surg. 2004;78:1579–85.
39. Abu-Omar Y, Taggart DP. The present status of off-pump coronary artery bypass grafting. Eur J Cardiothorac Surg. 2009;36:312–21.
40. Chu D, Bakaeen FG, Dao TK, Lemaire SA, Coselli JS, Huh J. On-pump versus off-pump coronary artery bypass grafting in a cohort of 63,000 patients. Ann Thorac Surg. 2009;87:1820–6; discussion 1826–7.
41. Fareed KR, Rothwell PM, Mehta Z, Naylor AR. Synchronous carotid endarterectomy and off- pump coronary bypass: an updated, systematic review of early outcomes. Eur J Vasc Endovasc Surg. 2009;37:375–8.
42. Shroyer AL, Grover FL, Hattler B, Collins JF, McDonald GO, Kozora E, et al. On-pump versus off-pump coronary-artery bypass surgery. N Engl J Med. 2009;361:1827–37.
43. Teskin O, Bicer Y, Kaya U, Cicek S. The impact of coronary artery bypass grafting surgical technique on stroke in young and elderly patients. Heart Surg Forum. 2009;12:E17–23.
44. Kasner SE, Villar-Cordova CE, Tong D, Grotta JC. Hemopericardium and cardiac tamponade after thrombolysis for acute ischemic stroke. Neurology. 1998;50:1857–9.
45. Paramo JA, Rifon J, Llorens R, Casares J, Paloma MJ, Rocha E. Intra- and postoperative fibrinolysis in patients undergoing cardiopulmonary bypass surgery. Haemostasis. 1991;21:58–64.
46. Tracy RP, Bovill EG. Fibrinolytic parameters and hemostatic monitoring: identifying and predicting patients at risk for major hemorrhagic events. Am J Cardiol. 1992;69:52A–9.
47. Leker RR, Grigoriadis S, Cohen JE. Endovascular reperfusion therapy for acute ischemic stroke: a meta-analysis. Neurol Res. 2010;32(8):787–791(5). Epub ahead of print.
48. Fukuda I, Imazuru T, Osaka M, Watanabe K, Meguro K, Wada M. Thrombolytic therapy for delayed, in-hospital stroke after cardiac surgery. Ann Thorac Surg. 2003;76:1293–5.
49. Moazami N, Smedira NG, McCarthy PM, Katzan I, Sila CA, Lytle BW, Cosgrove DM III. Safety and efficacy of intraarterial thrombolysis for perioperative stroke after cardiac operation. Ann Thorac Surg. 2001;72:1933–7; discussion 1937–9.
50. Katzan IL, Masaryk TJ, Furlan AJ, Sila CA, Perl II J, Andrefsky JC, et al. Intra-arterial thrombolysis for perioperative stroke after open heart surgery. Neurology. 1999;52:1081–4.

Acute Kidney Injury Associated with Cardiac Surgery

5

Mitchell H. Rosner

Introduction

Acute renal failure (ARF) or acute kidney injury (AKI), depending on the specific definition, occurs in up to 30% of patients undergoing cardiac surgery. ARF that requires dialysis (ARF-D) occurs in approximately 1% of patients undergoing cardiac surgery [1–15]. The development of kidney injury is associated with a high mortality, a more complicated hospital course, and a higher risk of infectious complications [1–15]. Even minimal changes in serum creatinine during the postoperative period are associated with a substantial decrease in survival [16]. Furthermore, the majority of patients who develop ARF-D remain dialysis dependent, leading to significant long-term morbidity and mortality [17]. Despite advances in bypass techniques, intensive care, and delivery of hemodialysis, mortality and morbidity associated with ARF have not markedly changed in the last decade [1–15]. These data highlight the importance of understanding the pathophysiology of ARF associated with cardiac bypass surgery and implementing specific therapies based on this knowledge in well-designed clinical trials.

M.H. Rosner, MD (✉)
Division of Nephrology,
University of Virginia Health System,
Charlottesville, VA, USA
e-mail: mhr9r@virginia.edu

Incidence and Prognosis of ARF After Bypass Surgery

Depending on the definition of ARF, the incidence of ARF varies across studies with a range of 1–30% [1–15]. Conlon et al. described a cohort of 2,843 patients who underwent surgery on cardiopulmonary bypass (CPB) over a 2-year period. ARF (defined as a rise in serum creatinine greater than 1 mg/dL above baseline) occurred in 7.9% of patients and ARF-D occurred in 0.7% [1]. Other studies utilizing a definition of ARF as a rise in serum creatinine ≥50% from baseline demonstrated a rate of ARF as high as 30% [2–15]. Chertow et al. analyzed 42,773 patients who underwent CPB and found an incidence of ARF-D of 1.1% [15]. The incidence of ARF is dependent on the particular type of CPB surgery. Typical coronary artery bypass grafting (CABG) has the lowest incidence of ARF (approximately 2.5%) and ARF-D (approximately 1%), followed by valvular surgery with an incidence of ARF of 2.8% and ARF-D of 1.7%. The highest risk group includes combined CABG/valvular surgery with an incidence of ARF of 4.6% and ARF-D of 3.3% [18, 19].

Mortality associated with the development of ARF is as high as 60% in some studies, but likely averages 15–30% depending on the definition of ARF and the postoperative period studied (hospital discharge or 30-day mortality) [1–15]. In patients who require dialysis, the mortality is uniformly high in all studies and averages 60–70% [1–15]. In the study of Chertow et al., a multivari-

V.R. Machiraju et al. (eds.), *Redo Cardiac Surgery in Adults*,
DOI 10.1007/978-1-4614-1326-4_5, © Springer Science+Business Media, LLC 2012

ate analysis adjusting for comorbid factors identified the occurrence of ARF-D as an independent determinant of the risk for death with an odds ratio of 7.9 [15]. Interestingly, even small increases in serum creatinine are associated with significant mortality. Lassnigg et al. demonstrated that the 30-day mortality of patients who developed a <0.5 mg/dL rise in serum creatinine was 2.77-fold higher than that of patients without a change in serum creatinine, and in patients with a >0.5 mg/dL rise in serum creatinine, 30-day mortality was 18.64-fold higher [16]. These results are qualitatively similar to studies by Thakar et al. in which 31,677 patients who underwent cardiac surgery were analyzed [20]. The development of ARF after CPB also influences long-term mortality, as identified by Loef and colleagues who found that the hazard ratio for death at 100 months after hospital discharge was 1.63 in patients who developed a 25% or greater increase in serum creatinine after surgery [21]. This increase in long-term mortality was independent of whether renal function had recovered by discharge from the hospital. Lok et al. also found that patients who suffered ARF after CPB had a relative risk of death at 1 year of 4.6 as compared with those patients who did not suffer renal injury [22].

Patients who develop ARF-D often remain dialysis dependent. Leacche et al. studied 13,847 patients who underwent CPB procedures [17]. Of those patients who developed ARF-D, 64% required permanent dialysis and the 1-year survival was only 10%. The link between the development of ARF and mortality likely involves numerous factors including some directly related to hemodialysis (hemodynamic instability, catheter-related infections, ventricular ectopy, and visceral ischemia), immune dysregulation associated with ARF, platelet dysfunction, and other less-defined associations. Registry data from Liano et al. have demonstrated that in patients with ARF, infections were the cause of death in 40% [23]. Thakar et al. also demonstrated a high risk of infections in patients who underwent CPB [24]. In patients with ARF-D, the incidence of serious infections, including sepsis, was 58.5% as compared with 3.3% in all patients undergoing CPB [24].

Risk Factors Associated with ARF

Several studies have examined the risk factors associated with the development of ARF after CPB (Table 5.1). The particular type of surgery is quite important, and valvular procedures are associated with a higher risk. In almost all studies, certain risk factors have been repeatedly associated with an increased risk for ARF [2, 4, 6–8, 14, 25–30]. These include female sex, reduced left ventricular function or the presence of congestive heart failure, diabetes mellitus, peripheral vascular disease, preoperative use of an intra-aortic balloon pump (IABP), chronic obstructive pulmonary disease, the need for emergent surgery, and an elevated preoperative serum creatinine. Elevated preoperative serum creatinine is perhaps the most predictive, with the risk of ARF-D approaching 10–20% in patients with a baseline preoperative creatinine 2.0–4.0 mg/dL [25–30]. In patients with a preoperative creatinine greater than 4.0 mg/dL, the risk of ARF-D increases to 25–28% [25–30]. Importantly, almost all the defined risk factors relate to either impaired renal perfusion or decreased renal reserve.

Several other risk factors have been identified but are more controversial and thus, individually likely do not play as prominent a role in determining the risk of ARF. In aggregate, however, these factors may be important and potentially modifiable. These include factors specifically

Table 5.1 Risk factors associated with ARF

Patient-related	Procedure-related
Female sex	Length of CPB
Chronic obstructive pulmonary disease	Cross-clamp time
Diabetes mellitus	Off-pump vs. on-pump
Peripheral vascular disease	Nonpulsatile flow
Renal insufficiency	Hemolysis
Congestive heart failure	Hemodilution
Left ventricular ejection fraction <35%	
Need for emergent surgery	
Cardiogenic shock	
Left main coronary disease	

related to the bypass procedure itself, such as cross-clamp time [31–33], duration of CPB [31–33], pulsatile vs. nonpulsatile bypass flow [34, 35], normothermic vs. hypothermic bypass [36–38], on-pump vs. off-pump CABG [39–45], and redo procedures.

One of the most controversial risk factors is off-pump (OPCAB) vs. traditional on-pump (CABG) coronary bypass surgery. OPCAB obviously removes the bypass circuit but can be associated with greater hemodynamic instability secondary to ventricular compression as the heart is manipulated to access the coronary arteries [42]. This comparison allows separation of the risk factors specifically associated with the bypass procedure itself from other peri-, intra-, and postoperative factors. Early nonrandomized studies suggested that renal tubular injury (as assessed by urinary markers) was lessened in patients who received OPCAB [43, 44]. Subsequent studies have suffered from a lack of randomization, single-site experience, and differences in patient comorbidities and the baseline risk of developing ARF between the OPCAB and CABG groups. Thus, despite several large retrospective series, the answer is still unclear, but the bulk of the data supports a lower risk of ARF in patients undergoing OPCAB, especially for those patients with preexisting renal insufficiency [45–48]. This is further supported by a significant decrease in inflammatory markers in patients undergoing OPCAB as compared with those undergoing CPB [46, 47].

Cardiopulmonary bypass (CPB) is associated with the generation of free hemoglobin and iron through hemolysis that typically occurs during the procedure [48]. Hemolysis may be caused by cardiotomy suction, the duration of perfusion, occlusive roller pumps, turbulent flow in the oxygenator, and blood return through cell savers [48]. This may contribute to oxidative stress and renal tubular injury [49]. In an early study, a low preoperative serum ferritin level (potentially indicative of a reduced ability to bind free iron) was associated with an increased risk for ARF after CPB [50]. However, a larger study could not validate this finding [32].

During CPB, hemodilution is induced to decrease blood viscosity in the hope of improving regional blood flow in the setting of hypoperfusion and hypothermia and limiting the need for blood transfusion [51, 52]. The resulting increase in regional blood flow is thought to offset any risk of decreased oxygen carrying capacity of the blood. However, two recent studies demonstrated that hemodilution (hematocrit <25%) is associated with an increased risk of renal injury as measured by changes in serum creatinine [53, 54]. This may be due to impairment of oxygen delivery to an already hypoxic renal medulla or to alterations in systemic inflammatory mediators caused by regional ischemia.

Predictive Scoring Systems

Several groups have developed clinical scoring systems that help to predict the risk for ARF with CPB [30, 55, 56]. The aim is to select patients at high risk and then to adopt strategies that would offer renal protection. The most recent scoring system analyzed 33,217 patients with a large validation sample. A score was given based on 13 preoperative factors and ranged from 0 to 17 [30] (Table 5.2). In the lowest risk group (score 0–2),

Table 5.2 Cleveland Clinic Foundation Acute Renal Failure scoring system

Risk factor	Points
Female gender	1
Congestive heart failure	2
Left ventricular EF <35%	1
Preoperative use of IABP	2
COPD	1
Insulin requiring diabetes	1
Previous cardiac surgery	1
Emergency surgery	2
Valve surgery only (reference to CABG)	1
CABG + valve (reference to CABG)	2
Other cardiac surgeries	2
Preoperative creatinine 1.2 to <2.1 mg/dL (reference to 1.2)	2
Preoperative creatinine >2.1 (reference to 1.2)	5

Minimum score, 0; Maximum score, 17
Adapted from [30]

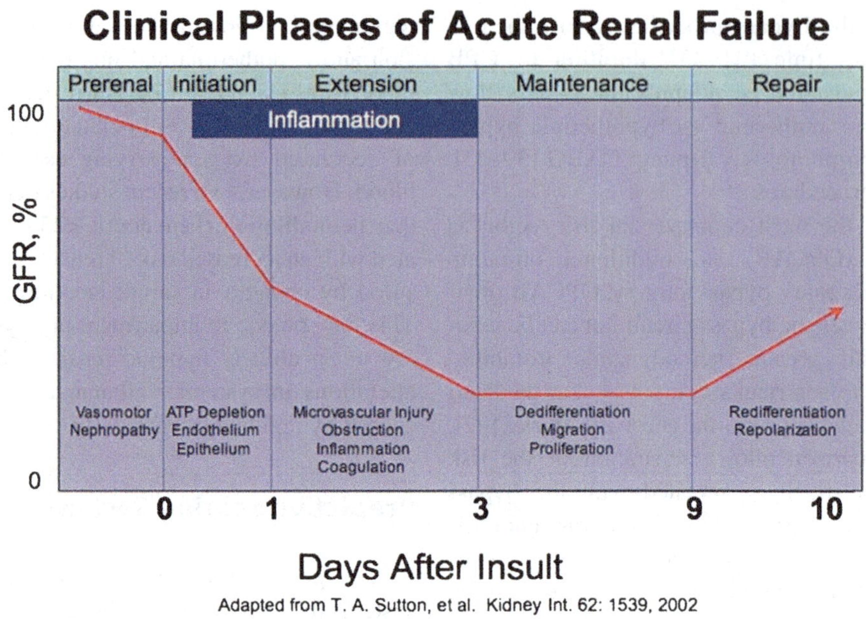

Fig. 5.1 The clinical phases of ARF occur across a continuum of stereotypical pathological changes

the risk of ARF-D was 0.4%, while in the highest risk group (score 9–13), the risk of ARF-D rose to 21.5%. These clinical scoring systems require validation across several medical centers before their routine use can be adopted, but they provide a very useful framework to identify patients who are at risk and may benefit from perioperative or intraoperative renal protective strategies.

Pathogenesis of ARF

No systematic studies of the pathological changes in the kidney have been undertaken in patients with ARF associated with CPB, and it is largely assumed that the pathological lesion is acute tubular necrosis (ATN). This is usually confirmed by the presence of granular casts in the urine of patients who develop ARF. Physiological studies by Moran and Myers substantiated this in 10 patients with protracted severe ARF after CPB [57]. They demonstrated that the transmembrane gradient for glomerular ultrafiltration was significantly diminished, likely from intratubular obstruction and hypertension due to sloughing from injured tubular epithelial cells. They also demonstrated that there was significant transtubular back-leak of glomerular ultrafiltrate across the injured epithelium. These pathological features are likely the downstream result of early events that are depicted in Fig. 5.1 [58–63]. In this schema, ARF begins with an early phase of vasomotor nephropathy in which there are associated alterations in vasoreactivity and renal perfusion leading to prerenal azotemia and eventually cellular ATP depletion and oxidative injury (initiation phase). These processes lead to the activation of bone marrow-derived cells, endothelial cells and renal epithelial cells, and a resulting proinflammatory state. Inflammatory cells adhere to activated endothelium in the peritubular capillaries of the outer medulla, leading to medullary congestion and further hypoxic injury to the S3 segment of the proximal tubule (extension phase). Furthermore, elaboration of inflammatory mediators (as discussed below) leads to additional cellular injury. Tubule cells then begin the process of proliferation (maintenance phase) and redifferentiation. Ultimately, polarity and function are reconstituted (repair phase).

Table 5.3 Pathophysiological factors in ARF

Preoperative	Intraoperative	Postoperative
Lack of renal reserve	Decreased renal perfusion	Systemic inflammation
Renovascular disease	Hypotension	Reduced LV function
Pre-renal azotemia	Lack of pulsatile flow	Vasoactive agents
Recent diuresis	Vasoactive agents	Hemodynamic instability
NPO status	Anesthetic effects	Nephrotoxins
Impaired LV function	Embolic events	Volume depletion
ACEI/ARBs (¿)	CPB-induced inflammation	Sepsis
Nephrotoxins	Nephrotoxins	
IV contrast	Free hemoglobin	
Other medications		
Endotoxemia		
Inflammation		

Clinically, the pathogenesis of ARF associated with CPB can be divided into preoperative, intraoperative, and postoperative events (Table 5.3). The sum of all of these various insults is ultimately reflected in the development of tubular injury that when severe enough is manifested as an increase in serum creatinine often associated with a decreased urine output.

Preoperative Events

As mentioned earlier, patients entering CPB often have received minor or major renal insults. Many patients have had recent myocardial infarctions or severe valvular disease with reduced LV function and reduced renal perfusion. In extreme cases, patients may be in cardiogenic shock and require inotropic support or an IABP. This preexisting renal state may be exacerbated by the use of diuretics, nonsteroidal anti-inflammatory drugs (NSAIDs), angiotensin-converting enzyme inhibitors (ACEIs), or angiotensin receptor blockers (ARBs) that impair the autoregulation of renal blood flow [63]. Furthermore, episodes of preoperative hypotension may lead to sublethal endothelial injury that may impair the production of vasodilatory substances, such as endothelial nitric oxide, and promote vasoconstriction due to the release of endothelin, catecholamines, and angiotensin II, promoting further tubular ischemia and injury [64–66]. Compounding these factors may be a lack of renal functional reserve due to underlying chronic kidney disease, including small and large vessel renovascular disease.

These hemodynamic alterations in the preoperative setting may increase the vulnerability of the kidney (particularly the inner stripe of the outer medulla where metabolic demands are high and the pO_2 is between 10 and 20 mmHg) to any further ischemic or nephrotoxic insult [67, 68].

There may be activation of inflammatory mediators in the preoperative period that also serves to prime the kidney for subsequent injury. Endotoxin levels are elevated in some patients in the preoperative period, despite no evidence of active infection, and these levels have been correlated with postoperative myocardial dysfunction [69–71]. The elevation in preoperative endotoxin levels may reflect the effect of poor cardiac output states contributing to intestinal ischemia and bacterial translocation or may be related to the preoperative care of patients (such as subclinical catheter infections) [72]. Elevated levels of tumor necrosis factor-α (TNFα) have also been shown in patients with preexisting congestive heart failure and may play a role in stimulation of the immune system [73, 74].

Nephrotoxic medications or intravenous contrast given in the immediate preoperative period may lead to overt or occult tubular injury that can interact with other factors to lead to ARF. These nephrotoxic medications include vasoactive (pressor) drugs, NSAIDS, ACEI, ARBs, and antibiotics.

Thus, the preoperative period is a critical time when hemodynamic, nephrotoxic, and inflammatory events can occur that lead to subtle renal injury, which is not necessarily reflected by changes in glomerular filtration rate (GFR). The potential impact of this subtle injury is substantiated by the fact that the preoperative risk scoring systems all rely on factors that ultimately act to reduce renal perfusion, result in lack of renal functional reserve, or set up a proinflammatory milieu.

Intraoperative Events

The intraoperative period is a critical time when patients are exposed to anesthesia and CPB. These events lead to dramatic hemodynamic effects as well as activation of both innate and adaptive immune responses that can initiate or extend renal injury.

Hemodynamic Effects

CPB is associated with significant hemodynamic changes, and the maintenance of cardiovascular stability during CPB requires interplay between the functions of the CPB machine and patient factors, such as systemic vascular resistance, venous compliance, and autoregulatory capacity of various vascular beds. The ultimate goal is to maintain regional perfusion at a level that supports optimal cellular and organ function. Thus, any decrease in renal perfusion during CPB can lead to significant cellular injury, depending on its magnitude and duration.

Oxygen consumption in 1 min (VO_2) is the major determinant of blood flow requirements under normal physiologic conditions and during CPB. Experimentally, CPB flow rates have been determined by calculating VO_2 at different perfusion rates. Perfusion is increased until VO_2 reaches a plateau, after which further increases in CPB flow rates do not lead to increase in oxygen consumption. In general, CPB flow rates of 1.8–2.2 L/min/m^2 are recommended based on this analysis [75, 76]. However, the effect of this CPB flow rate on regional renal blood flow and local oxygen delivery rates is unknown.

In addition to CPB flow rates, perfusion pressure during CPB is also an important determinant of adequate nutrient delivery to vascular beds. Perfusion pressure is determined by the interaction of blood flow and overall arterial resistance. Resistance, in this case, is related to actual friction resistance because of the steady, nonpulsatile nature of CPB, which negates the elastance, inertial, and reflective components of arterial resistance during normal pulsatile flow [77]. Friction resistance is primarily a function of vasomotor tone and blood viscosity (which is further dependent on hematocrit and temperature). Importantly, both variables change during CPB (e.g., blood viscosity increases as hypothermia is induced and vasomotor tone is affected by anesthesia) and lead to associated changes in perfusion pressure. In general, a mean perfusion pressure of 50–70 mmHg is maintained during CPB [77].

It is not known what effect the given hemodynamic goals of a mean perfusion pressure of 50–70 mmHg and CPB flow rates of 1.8–2.4 L/min/m^2 will have on renal perfusion and oxygen delivery. The majority of studies on autoregulation of regional blood flow during CPB have focused on the cerebral circulation and demonstrate preserved cerebral autoregulation of these parameters [78, 79]. Small studies have suggested that mean arterial pressures on CPB greater than 70 mmHg lead to higher intraoperative creatinine clearances but not to changes in postoperative renal function as compared with pressures between 50 and 60 mmHg [80]. Thus, it is likely that renal perfusion and autoregulation are also maintained as long as these hemodynamic goals are met. However, these values are likely near the minimum blood flows that support normal organ function, and any perturbation may lead to ischemia and cellular damage. Furthermore, the effect of these parameters in patients with impaired baseline renal function is not known. In patients

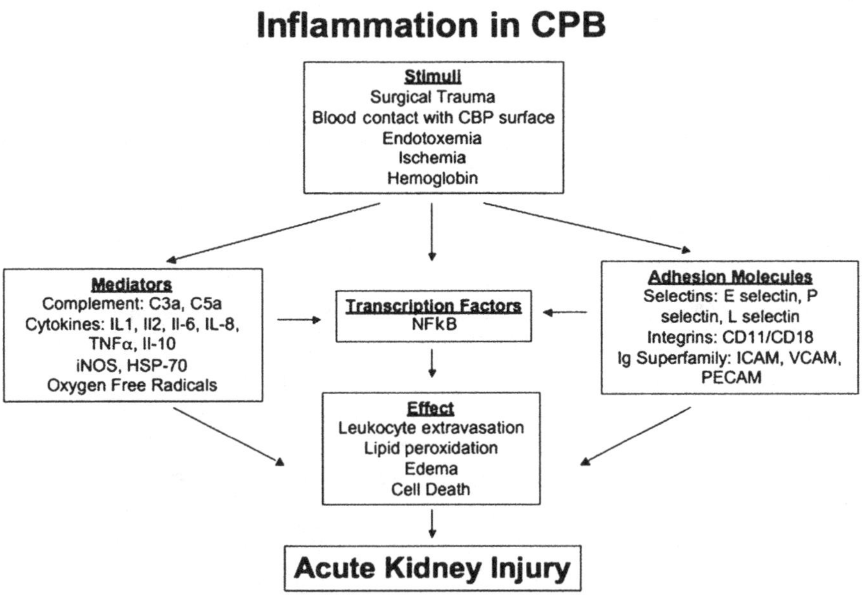

Fig. 5.2 The inflammatory cascade activated by CPB and its role in the production of AKI. Stimuli during the surgical procedure activate a host of inflammatory mediators, adhesion molecules, and proinflammatory transcription factors. These effects lead to cellular injury and ARF

with preexisting hypertension, the relationship between renal blood flow and mean arterial pressure is shifted to the right, so that a higher mean pressure may be required to maintain adequate renal perfusion in these patients [81]. Furthermore, if there is any degree of preexisting ATN, autoregulatory capacity of the kidney may be lost and renal blood flow may become linearly dependent on pressure [82].

Whether alterations of the CPB flow and pressure goals would lead to improved renal outcomes is not known. However, Gold et al. reported that maintenance of higher perfusion pressures, in the range of a mean perfusion pressure of 70 mmHg, was associated with a reduced incidence of cardiac and neurologic complications when compared with patients whose pressures were maintained at 50–60 mmHg [83]. Renal function was not assessed in this study.

Other procedural factors that likely impact renal hemodynamics include hemodilution (oxygen delivery capacity), hypothermia (oxygen consumption), the absence of pulsatile perfusion, and the use of crystalloid vs. colloidal prime solutions. As discussed earlier, with the exception of hemodilution, no deleterious effects on renal function have been found to be associated with alterations in body temperature or in the absence of pulsatile flow.

In total, these hemodynamic changes may lead to regional renal ischemia and cellular injury that could either initiate AKI or extend preexisting renal injury. Furthermore, these hemodynamic changes are potentially modifiable.

Inflammation

CPB provokes a systemic inflammatory response syndrome (SIRS) (Fig. 5.2) [84, 85]. Contact of blood components with the artificial surface of the bypass circuit, ischemia–reperfusion injury, endotoxemia, operative trauma, nonpulsatile blood flow, and preexisting left ventricular dysfunction are all possible causes of SIRS in this setting [86–88]. In its most severe form, a spectrum of injury may be observed that includes one or more of the following clinical manifestations: pulmonary, renal, gut, central nervous system, and myocardial dysfunction; coagulopathy;

vasodilation and increased capillary permeability; hemolysis; pyrexia; and increased susceptibility to infection [89].

During CPB, both neutrophils and vascular endothelium are activated with upregulation of adhesion molecules, such as CD11b and CD41 [89–92]. Platelets also undergo activation, degranulation, and adherence to vascular endothelium [91, 93]. These events led to elaboration of cytotoxic, oxygen-derived free radicals [94], proteases [95], cytokines [96], and chemokines [96, 97]. These inflammatory mediators, such as interleukin (IL)-6, IL-8, and TNFα, increase considerably in the serum during CPB and generally reach peak levels 2–4 h after termination of CPB [84].

CPB is also a potent activator of factor XII (Hageman factor), converting it to factor XIIa [90]. This process initiates the intrinsic coagulation system, the kallikrein system, and the fibrinolytic system [97]. Furthermore, complement proteins are activated through both the classical and alternative pathways [97–99]. Ultimately, this humoral response amplifies the cellular response, leading to neutrophil, endothelial, and monocyte activation and further elaboration of proinflammatory cytokines [59, 97–100]. Finally, diffuse end-organ ischemia likely causes endothelial cells, circulating monocytes, and tissue-fixed macrophages to release cytokines, and oxygen-derived free radicals that further drive the inflammatory response [59, 97–100].

The end result of this generalized inflammatory response induced by CPB within the kidney is not known. Interestingly, animal models of renal ischemia–reperfusion injury have clearly demonstrated the pathological role of interstitial inflammation and the elaboration of proinflammatory cytokines and reactive oxygen species in the production of tubular injury [59, 100–102]. This local inflammatory response in experimental models is identical to that seen on a more global scale during CPB. Thus, it is likely a safe assumption that CPB-induced inflammation has significant deleterious effects on the kidney through similar mechanisms. Despite efforts to produce a CPB system that does not produce contact activation of blood components, this goal has not been realized and CPB still remains a potent proinflammatory stimulus [103, 104].

Other Events Associated with CPB

Macroscopic and microscopic emboli, both gaseous and particulate, are often generated during CPB. These emboli are temporally related to certain intraoperative events, such as aortic cannulation and aortic clamp placement and release [105–108]. One study has demonstrated a significant correlation between the total number of Doppler-detected emboli and postoperative changes in serum creatinine [108]. This suggests that embolic events to the renal circulation may, in part, be responsible for postoperative changes in GFR.

CPB exposes blood to nonphysiological surfaces and shear forces that lead to lysis of red blood cells with release of free hemoglobin into the circulation [109]. In the presence of oxidants, such as hydrogen peroxide and superoxide, free low molecular mass iron is released from the heme moiety into the circulation [110]. This redox active iron is able to participate in organic and inorganic oxygen radical reactions, such as stimulating lipid peroxidation and catalyzing the formation of damaging hydroxyl radicals with subsequent tissue damage [111]. Normally, iron-transporting proteins, such as transferrin and lactoferrin, sequester this free iron and minimize its potential toxicity [112]. However, in some cases, the release of free iron can be so great as to saturate the iron-binding capacity of transferrin. At this point, all iron-binding antioxidant capacity is lost and the serum displays pro-oxidant features [113]. How often this occurs during CPB is not fully known, but it may be as high as 25% of cases [113, 114]. Reperfusion injury during CPB may further exacerbate oxidant stress in the setting of free, circulating iron. However, Tuttle et al. could not find an association between low iron-binding capacity and the risk for ARF after CPB [32]. While desferoxamine has been demonstrated to decrease the occurrence of lipid peroxidation during CPB, there are no studies investigating any protective role of iron chelation in kidney injury [115].

Postoperative Events

The postoperative events that are critical in affecting renal function are similar to traditional causative mechanisms seen in the general intensive care setting. Thus, the use of vasoactive agents, hemodynamic instability, exposure to nephrotoxic medications, volume depletion, and sepsis/SIRS are all critical events that can lead to kidney injury. Another critical factor is postoperative cardiac performance and the need for either inotropic or mechanical support. In the presence of postoperative left ventricular dysfunction, the risk for significant renal injury becomes very high as the vulnerable kidney is subjected to marginal perfusion pressures.

General Measures to Prevent AKI After Cardiac Surgery

Identification of High-Risk Patients

Before cardiac surgery, identifying patients who are at high risk for ARF is critically important. The important risk factors and scoring systems that can be utilized for this identification purpose have been discussed earlier.

Optimization Renal Perfusion and Avoidance of Nephrotoxins

Factors that alter renal blood flow and lead to prerenal azotemia should be identified and corrected. Treatment of volume depletion and congestive heart failure before cardiac surgery will increase cardiac output and renal perfusion. Perioperative hydration, hemodynamic monitoring, and inotropic agents to optimize cardiac output may be necessary. Medications, such as NSAIDS and other nephrotoxic agents, should be discontinued. Whether ACEI and ARBs should be discontinued before surgery is not known and is a source of some debate [116–118]. If radiographic contrast is needed, newer isosmolar contrast agents may be less toxic [119]. In stable patients who have contrast-induced ARF, cardiac surgery should be postponed.

Pharmacological Interventions to Prevent AKI Following Cardiac Surgery

Pharmacological interventions have been attempted with inconsistent results, and currently, there are no drugs with conclusively demonstrated renal protection. The failure of these measures to prevent ARF after cardiac surgery may, in part, be related to a number of factors. First, the pathophysiology of ARF after CPB is more complex than originally considered and simple approaches to target single pathways are unlikely to succeed. Second, late pharmacological intervention is likely to fail. Third, the patient populations that have been studied are often at low risk for renal dysfunction after CPB, thus potentially masking small beneficial effects of therapies. Last, most clinical trials enroll a small number of subjects and are inadequately powered to detect small benefits. Most therapeutic trials in ARF after CPB have been prevention studies in which treatment was initiated before the insult and have shown no significant benefits in the majority of cases.

Drugs That Increase Renal Blood Flow

In low doses (3 μg/kg/min), dopamine stimulates DA-1 and DA-2 dopamine receptors increasing renal blood flow and inhibiting proximal tubule sodium reabsorption. Although dopamine has been used extensively, studies have failed to show its efficacy in ARF following cardiac surgery [120, 121] or ARF associated with other conditions [122]. Thus, there is no role for the use of dopamine in the treatment or prevention of ARF.

Fenoldopam is a selective DA-1 agonist that has been used for the prevention of ARF with variable results. In patients with chronic kidney disease who underwent cardiac angiography, fenoldopam failed to reduce renal dysfunction, 30-day morality, the need for dialysis, or rehospitalization [123]. However, small studies, randomized or uncontrolled, using fenoldopam have demonstrated a reduction of renal dysfunction in patients who underwent cardiac surgery [124–126]. A potential complication is the associated systemic hypotension that occurs after administration of fenoldopam. The beneficial effects of renal vasodilation in this situation may be offset by systemic hypotension that results in an overall net reduction of blood flow to the kidney. This systemic hypotensive effect may be abrogated by local infusion of fenoldopam directly into the renal arteries using a novel vascular delivery system (Benephit™ catheter, AngioDynamics, Latham, NY) [127].

Theophylline, a nonselective adenosine antagonist, is thought to block vasoconstriction induced by A1 adenosine receptors. In a recent clinical trial, theophylline infusion in coronary bypass surgery was ineffective in reducing the incidence of ARF [128].

Drugs That Induce Natriuresis

Atrial natriuretic peptide (ANP) increases natriuresis by increasing GFR and by inhibiting sodium reabsorption by the medullary collecting duct [129]. In a multicenter trial, anaritide, a 25-amino acid synthetic form of ANP, was administered to critically ill patients to treat ATN [130]. The dialysis-free survival was the same whether the patients received anaratide or not. Although a subgroup of patients with oliguria benefited from anaritide in the original study, this observation was not confirmed in a follow-up study [131]. Hypotension was a complicating factor in 46% of the patients who received anaratide [130, 131]. In a recent study, recombinant human ANP (rhANP) was used to treat ARF after cardiac surgery in patients who required inotropic support for heart failure [132]. In patients who received rhANP, there was a significant reduction in the incidence of dialysis at day 21 after the start of treatment. In this trial, ANP was infused at a lower rate (50 ng/kg/min as opposed to 200 ng/kg/min) (thus, lowering the incidence of hypotension) and for a more prolonged period than prior studies. These differences may explain the benefit seen in this study as opposed to earlier ones.

Diuretics may reduce the severity of ARF by preventing tubule obstruction and decreasing oxygen consumption [133]. However, in a double-blind, randomized controlled trial, furosemide treatment was not protective and the incidence of ARF in patients who received furosemide was twice that of the dopamine or placebo group [134]. Similar negative results have been seen in other studies [135, 136].

Mannitol has a variety of effects including the production of an osmotic diuresis with a reduction of tubular obstruction and the capability of scavenging free radicals. Mannitol is often added to the prime solution during CPB with the thought that it may help to maintain urine output during the procedure, minimize tissue edema, and scavenge free radicals [137]. An early study in children who underwent cardiac surgery demonstrated that mannitol was beneficial in the prevention of ARF [138]. However, several other studies have not confirmed these findings, and the potential role of mannitol remains unclear [139–141].

Drugs That Block Inflammation

Inflammation is well documented during CPB and has a prominent role in the pathogenesis of ARF and CPB [63, 97]. It is, thus, an attractive therapeutic target. Pentoxifylline, a phosphodiesterase inhibitor, blocks the activation of neutrophils by TNFα and IL-1 [142] and TNFα release by inflammatory cells [143]. Pentoxifylline reduced cardiac dysfunction and TNFα release in ischemia–reperfusion models [144]. However, pentoxifylline did not affect renal function in elderly patients who underwent cardiac surgery [145]. Dexamethasone also failed to protect against renal dysfunction after cardiac surgery [146]. *N*-acetylcysteine (N-AC) blocks inflammation and oxidant stress in cardiac surgery patients and, thus, may hold promise as a simple, nontoxic protective measure [147, 148]. However, N-AC has not been utilized in a prospective clinical trial that examines renal outcomes.

Other Strategies

The sympathetic nervous system is activated during and after cardiac surgery and may lead to impairment of renal function through a hemodynamic mechanism. Clonidine (an alpha-2 agonist) has been utilized to attenuate these effects, with improvement in hemodynamic stability during CPB [149]. In a small study of 48 normal-risk patients who underwent cardiac surgery, preoperative treatment with clonidine prevented the deterioration of renal function with significantly higher creatinine clearances 24 h after CPB in the clonidine-treated group [150].

Diltiazem has been used in clinical trials to prevent ARF after cardiothoracic surgery. Diltiazem inhibits some of the inflammatory effects of CPB and is often used to prevent vasospasm of radial grafts [151, 152]. Although diltiazem reduced urinary excretion of markers of tubule injury (alpha-glutathione *S*-transferase and *N*-acetyl-β-glucoaminidase) [153], its effectiveness in the prevention of renal dysfunction was inconsistent [154–156].

Summary

CPB surgery is associated with a high risk for AKI. This injury is further associated with substantial morbidity and mortality. The pathogenesis of kidney injury during CPB is complex and involves hemodynamic, inflammatory, and other mechanisms that interact at a cellular level. At present, there are no pharmacological interventions with conclusively demonstrated efficacy in the prevention of renal dysfunction after cardiac surgery. Therapies, such as rhANP, fenoldopam, N-AC, and clonidine, have shown modestly encouraging results in small trials, and their effectiveness needs to be confirmed in larger studies that are appropriately designed to assess renal outcomes.

Ultimately, a successful therapy will utilize strategies that target multiple pathways. This integrated strategy would target hemodynamic, inflammatory, and oxidative pathways and act both at the points of proximal cellular injury and at later downstream events, such as tubular regeneration.

Copyright Acknowledgement This material was previously published in The Clinical Journal of the American Society of Nephrology and is reproduced with the kind permission of the American Society of Nephrology.

References

1. Conlon PJ, Stafford-Smith M, White WD, et al. Acute renal failure following cardiac surgery. Nephrol Dial Transplant. 1999;14:1158–62.
2. Mangano CM, Diamondstone LS, Ramsay JG, Aggarwal A, Herskowitz A, Mangano DT. Renal dysfunction after myocardial revascularization: risk factors, adverse outcomes and hospital resource utilization. Ann Intern Med. 1998;128:194–203.
3. Abel RM, Buckley MJ, Austen WG, Barnett GO, Beck Jr CH, Fischer JE. Etiology, incidence and prognosis of renal failure following cardiac operations. Results of a prospective analysis of 500 consecutive patients. J Thorac Cardiovasc Surg. 1976; 71:323–33.
4. Gailiunas Jr P, Chawla R, Lazarus JM, Cohn L, Merrill JP, Sanders J. Acute renal failure following cardiac operations. J Thorac Cardiovasc Surg. 1980;79:241–3.
5. Ostermann ME, Taube D, Morgan CJ, Evans TW. Acute renal failure following cardiopulmonary bypass: a changing picture. Intensive Care Med. 2000;26:565–71.
6. Andersson LG, Ekroth R, Bratteby LE, et al. Acute renal failure after coronary surgery: a study of incidence and risk factors in 2009 consecutive patients. J Thorac Cardiovasc Surg. 1993;41:237–41.
7. Zanardo G, Michielon P, Paccagnella A, et al. Acute renal failure in the patient undergoing cardiac operation: prevalence, mortality rate, and main risk factors. J Thorac Cardiovasc Surg. 1994;107:1489–95.
8. Mangos GJ, Brown MA, Chan YA, et al. Acute renal failure following cardiac surgery: incidente, outcomes and risk factors. Aust N Z J Med. 1995; 25:284–9.
9. Antunes PE, Prieto D, Ferrao de Oliveira J, Antunes MJ. Renal dysfunction alter myocardial revascularization. Eur J Cardiothorac Surg. 2004;25:597–604.
10. Yeboah ED, Petrie A, Pead JL. Acute renal failure and open heart surgery. Br Med J. 1972;1:415–8.
11. Bhat JG, Gluck MC, Lowenstein J, Baldwin DS. Renal failure after open heart surgery. Ann Int Med. 1976;84:677–82.
12. Hilberman M, Myers BD, Carrie BJ, Derby G, Jamison RL, Stinson EB. Acute renal failure following cardiac surgery. J Thorac Cardiovasc Surg. 1979;77:880–8.
13. Corwin HL, Sprague SM, DeLaria GA, Norusis MJ. Acute renal failure associated with cardiac operations. A case-control study. J Thorac Cardiovasc Surg. 1989;98:1107–12.
14. Schmitt H, Riehl J, Boseilla A, et al. Acute renal failure following cardiac surgery: pre- and perioperative clinical features. Contrib Nephrol. 1991;93: 98–104.
15. Chertow GM, Levy EM, Hammermeister KE, Grover F, Daley J. Independent association between acute renal failure and mortality following cardiac surgery. Am J Med. 1998;104:343–8.
16. Lassnigg A, Schmidlin D, Mouhieddine M, Bachmann LM, et al. Minimal changes of serum creatinine predict prognosis in patients after cardiothoracic surgery: a prospective cohort study. J Am Soc Nephrol. 2004;15:1597–605.
17. Leacche M, Rawn JD, Mihaljevic T, et al. Outcomes in patients with normal serum creatinine and with artificial renal support for acute renal failure developing

after coronary artery bypass grafting. Am J Cardiol. 2004;93:353–6.
18. Abraham VS, Swain JA. Cardiopulmonary bypass and the kidney. In: Kurusz M, Utley JR, Davis RF, editors. Cardiopulmonary bypass: principles and practice. 2nd ed. Philadelphia: Lippincott Williams and Wilkins; 2000. p. 382–91.
19. Grayson AD, Khater M, Jackson M, Fox MA. Valvular heart operation is an independent risk factor for acute renal failure. Ann Thorac Surg. 2003;75: 1829–35.
20. Thakar CV, Worley S, Arrigain S, Yared J-P, Paganini EP. Influence of renal dysfunction on mortality after cardiac surgery: modifying effect of preoperative renal function. Kidney Int. 2005;67:1112–9.
21. Loef BG, Epema AH, Smilde TB, et al. Immediate postoperative renal function deterioration in cardiac surgical patients predicts in-hospital mortality and long-term survival. J Am Soc Nephrol. 2005;16: 195–200.
22. Lok CE, Austin PC, Wanh H, Tu JV. Impact of renal insufficiency on short- and long-term outcomes after cardiac surgery. Am Heart J. 2004;148:430–8.
23. Liano F, Pascual J. Epidemiology of acute renal failure: a prospective, multicenter, community-based study. Madrid Acute Renal Failure Study Group. Kidney Int. 1996;50:811–8.
24. Thakar CV, Yared JP, Worley S, Cotman K, Paganini EP. Renal dysfunction and serious infections after open-heart surgery. Kidney Int. 2003;64:239–46.
25. Chertow GM, Lazarus JM, Christiansen CL, Cook EF, Hammermeister KE, Grover F, et al. Preoperative renal risk stratification. Circulation. 1997;95:878–84.
26. Fortescue EB, Bates DW, Chertow GM. Predicting acute renal failure after coronary bypass surgery: cross-validation of two risk-stratification algorithms. Kidney Int. 2000;57:2594–602.
27. Frost L, Pedersen RS, Lund O, Hansen OK, Hansen HE. Prognosis and risk factors in acute, dialysis-requiring renal failure after open-heart surgery. Scand J Thorac Cardiovasc Surg. 1991;25:161–6.
28. Thakar CV, Liangos O, Yared JP, Nelson D, et al. ARF after open-heart surgery: influence of gender and race. Am J Kidney Dis. 2003;41:742–51.
29. Thakar CV, Liangos O, Yared J-P, Nelson DA, Hariachar S, Paganini EP. Predicting acute renal failure after cardiac surgery: validation and re-definition of a risk stratification algorithm. Hemodial Int. 2003;7:143–7.
30. Thakar CV, Arrigain S, Worley S, Yared J-P, Paganini EP. A clinical score to predict acute renal failure after cardiac surgery. J Am Soc Nephrol. 2005;16:162–8.
31. Slogoff S, Reul GJ, Keats AS, et al. Role of perfusion pressure and flow in major organ dysfunction after cardiopulmonary bypass. Ann Thorac Surg. 1990;50:911–8.
32. Tuttle KR, Worrall NK, Dahlstrom LR, Nandagopal R, Kausz AT, Davis CL. Predictors of ARF after cardiac surgical procedures. Am J Kidney Dis. 2003;41:76–83.
33. Fischer UM, Weissenberger WK, Warters RD, Geissler HJ, Allen SJ, Mehlhorn U. Impact of cardiopulmonary bypass management on postcardiac surgery renal function. Perfusion. 2002;17:401–6.
34. Abramov D, Tamariz M, Serrick CI, et al. The influence of cardiopulmonary bypass flow characteristics on the clinical outcome of 1820 coronary bypass patients. Can J Cardiol. 2003;19:237–43.
35. Urzua J, Troncoso S, Bugedo G, et al. Renal function and cardiopulmonary bypass: effect of perfusion pressure. J Cardiothorac Vasc Anesth. 1992;6:299–303.
36. Provenchere S, Plantefeve G, Hufnagel G, et al. Renal dysfunction after cardiac surgery with normothermic cardiopulmonary bypass: incidence, risk factors and effect on clinical outcome. Anesth Analg. 2003;96:1258–64.
37. The Warm Heart Investigators. Randomized trial of normothermic versus hypothermic coronary artery bypass surgery. Lancet. 1994;343:559–63.
38. Cook DJ. Changing temperature management for cardiopulmonary bypass. Anesth Analg. 1999;88: 1254–71.
39. Magee MJ, Edgerton JR. Beating heart coronary artery bypass: operative strategy and technique. Sem Thorac Cardiovasc Surg. 2003;15:83–91.
40. Loef BG, Epema AH, Navis G, Ebels T, van Oeveren W, Henning RH. Off-pump coronary revascularization attenuates transient renal damage compared with on-pump coronary revascularization. Chest. 2002; 121:1190–4.
41. Ascione R, Lloyd CT, Underwood MJ, et al. On-pump versus off-pump coronary revascularization: evaluation of renal function. Ann Thorac Surg. 1999; 68:493–8.
42. Schwann NM, Horrow JC, Strong MD, Chamchad D, Guerraty A, Wechsler AS. Does off-pump coronary artery bypass reduce the incidence of clinically evident renal dysfunction after multivessel myocardial revascularization? Anesth Analg. 2004;99:959–64.
43. Beauford RB, Saunders CR, Niemeier LA, et al. Is off-pump revascularization better for patients with non-dialysis-dependent renal insufficiency? Heart Surg Forum. 2004;7:E141–6.
44. Gamboso MG, Phillips-Bute B, Landolfo KP, Newman MF, Stafford-Smith M. Off-pump versus on-pump coronary artery bypass surgery and postoperative renal dysfunction. Anesth Analg. 2000;91: 1080–4.
45. Stallwood MI, Grayson AD, Mills K, Scawn ND. Acute renal failure in coronary artery bypass surgery: Independent effect of cardiopulmonary bypass. Ann Thorac Surg. 2004;77:968–72.
46. Fransen E, Maessen J, Dentener M, Senden N, Geskes G, Buurman W. Systemic inflammation present in patients undergoing CABP without extracorporeal circulation. Chest. 1998;113:1290–5.
47. Dybdahl B, Wahba A, Haaverstad R, et al. On-pump versus off-pump coronary artery bypass grafting: more heat-shock protein 70 is released after on-pump surgery. Eur J Cardiothorac Surg. 2004;25:985–92.

48. Wright G. Hemolysis during cardiopulmonary bypass: update. Perfusion. 2001;16:345–51.
49. Baliga R, Ueda N, Waler PD, Shah SV. Oxidant mechanisms in toxic acute renal failure. Am J Kidney Dis. 1997;29:465–77.
50. Davis CL, Kausz AT, Zager RA, Kharasch ED, Cochran RP. Acute renal failure after cardiopulmonary bypass is related to decreased serum ferritin levels. J Am Soc Nephrol. 1999;10: 2396–402.
51. Messmer K. Hemodilution. Surg Clin North Am. 1975;55:659–78.
52. Shah D, Corson J, Karmody A, Leather R. Effects of isovolemic hemodilution on abdominal aortic aneurysmectomy in high risk patients. Ann Vasc Surg. 1986;1:50–4.
53. Swaminathan M, Phillips-Bute BG, Conlon PJ, Smith PK, Newman MF, Stafford-Smith M. The association of lowest hematocrit during cardiopulmonary bypass with acute renal injury after coronary artery bypass surgery. Ann Thorac Surg. 2003; 76:784–92.
54. Karkouti K, Beattie WS, Wijeysundera DN, et al. Hemodilution during cardiopulmonary bypass is an independent risk factor for acute renal failure in adult cardiac surgery. J Thorac Cardiovasc Surg. 2005;129: 391–400.
55. Chertow GM, Lazarus JM, Christiansen CL, et al. Preoperative renal risk stratification. Circulation. 1997;95:878–84.
56. Eriksen BO, Hoff KRS, Solberg S. Prediction of acute renal failure after cardiac surgery: retrospective cross-validation of a clinical algorithm. Nephrol Dial Transplant. 2003;18:77–81.
57. Moran SM, Myers BD. Pathophysiology of protracted acute renal failure in man. J Clin Invest. 1985;76:1440–8.
58. Heinzelmann M, Mercer-Jones MA, Passmore JC. Neutrophils and renal failure. Am J Kidney Dis. 1999;34:384–99.
59. Sheridan AM, Bonventre JV. Cell biology and molecular mechanisms of injury in ischemic acute renal failure. Curr Opin Nephrol Hypertens. 2000;9:427–34.
60. Molitoris BA. Transitioning to therapy in ischemic acute renal failure. J Am Soc Nephrol. 2003;14: 265–7.
61. Sutton TA, Fisher CJ, Molitoris BA. Microvascular endothelial injury and dysfunction during ischemic acute renal failure. Kidney Int. 2002;62:1539–49.
62. Conger JD. Vascular alterations in acute renal failure: roles in initiation and maintenance. In: Molitoris BA, Finn WF, editors. Acute renal failure – a companion to Brenner and Rector's the kidney. Philadelphia: Saunders; 2001. p. 13–29.
63. Okusa MD. The inflammatory cascade in acute ischemic renal failure. Nephron. 2002;90:133–8.
64. Goligorsky MS, Noiri E, Tsukahara H, et al. A pivotal role of nitric oxide in endothelial cell dysfunction. Acta Physiol Scand. 2000;168:33–40.
65. Caramelo C, Espinoza G, Manzarbeitia F, et al. Role of endothelium-related mechanisms in the pathophysiology of renal ischemia/reperfusion in normal rabbits. Circ Res. 1996;79:1031–8.
66. Kohan DE. Endothelins in the kidney: physiology and pathophysiology. Am J Kidney Dis. 1993;22: 493–510.
67. Brezis M, Rosen S. Hypoxia of the renal medulla-its implications for disease. N Engl J Med. 1995;332: 647–55.
68. Chou SY, Porush JG, Faubert PF. Renal medullary circulation: hormonal control. Kidney Int. 1990; 37:1–13.
69. Lequier LL, Nikaidoh H, Leonard SR, et al. Preoperative and postoperative endotoxemia in children with congenital heart disease. Chest. 2000; 117:1706–12.
70. Bennet-Guerrero E, Ayuso L, Hamilton-Davies C, et al. Relationship of preoperative anti-endotoxin core antibodies and adverse outcomes following cardiac surgery. JAMA. 1997;277:646–50.
71. Nilsson L, Kulander L, Nystrom SO, et al. Endotoxins in cardiopulmonary bypass. J Thorac Cardiovasc Surg. 1990;100:777–80.
72. Riddington DW, Venkatesh B, Boivin CM, et al. Intestinal permeability, gastric intramucosal pH, and systemic endotoxemia in patients undergoing cardiopulmonary bypass. JAMA. 1996;275:1007–12.
73. Levine B, Kalman J, Mayer L, et al. Elevated circulating levels of tumor necrosis factor in severe chronic heart failure. N Engl J Med. 1990;323:236–41.
74. Torre-Amione G, Kapadia S, Benedict C, et al. Proinflammatory cytokine levels in patients with depressed left ventricular ejection fraction: a report from the studies of left ventricular dysfunction (SOLVD). J Am Coll Cardiol. 1996;27:1201–6.
75. Parolari A, Alamanni F, Gherli T, et al. Cardiopulmonary bypass and oxygen consumption: oxygen delivery and hemodynamics. Ann Thorac Surg. 1999;67:1320–7.
76. Kirklin JW, Barratt-Boyes BG. Cardiac Surgery. 2nd ed. New York: Churchill Livingstone; 1993. p. 80.
77. Kurusz M, Davis RF, Conti VR. Conduct of cardiopulmonary bypass. In: Gravlee GP, Davis RF, Kurusz M, Utley JR, editors. Cardiopulmonary bypass: principles and practice. Philadelphia: Lippincott Williams and Wilkins; 2000. p. 549–78.
78. Rudy LW, Heymann MA, Edmunds H. Distribution of systemic blood flow during cardiopulmonary bypass. J Appl Physiol. 1973;34:194–200.
79. Harris EA, Seelye ER, Barratt-Boyes BG. On the availability of oxygen to the body during cardiopulmonary bypass in man. Br J Anaesth. 1974; 46:425–31.
80. Urzua J, Troncoso S, Bugedo G, et al. Renal function and cardiopulmonary bypass: effect of perfusion pressure. J Cardiovasc Vasc Anesth. 1992;6:299–303.
81. Palmer BF. Renal dysfunction complicating the treatment of hypertension. N Engl J Med. 2002; 347:1256–61.

82. Kelleher SP, Robinette JB, Conger JD. Sympathetic nervous system in the loss of autoregulation in acute renal failure. Am J Physiol. 1984;246:F379–86.
83. Gold JP, Charlson ME, Williams-Russo P, et al. Improvement of outcomes after coronary artery bypass; a randomized trial comparing intraoperative high versus low mean arterial pressure. J Thorac Cardiovasc Surg. 1995;110:1302–14.
84. Cremer J, Martin M, Redl H, et al. Systemic inflammatory response after cardiac operations. Ann Thorac Surg. 1996;61:1714–20.
85. Taylor K. SIRS – the systemic inflammatory response syndrome after cardiac operations. Ann Thorac Surg. 1996;61:1607–8.
86. Hornick P, Taylor K. Pulsatile and non-pulsatile perfusion: the continuing controversy. J Cardiothorac Vasc Anesth. 1997;11:310–5.
87. Kirklin JK, Blackstone EH, Kirklin JW. Cardiopulmonary bypass: studies on its damaging effects. Blood Purif. 1987;5:168–78.
88. Czerny M, Baumer H, Kilo J, et al. Inflammatory response and myocardial injury following coronary artery bypass grafting with or without cardiopulmonary bypass. Eur J Cardiothorac Surg. 2000;17: 737–42.
89. Fransen E, Maessen J, Dentener M, et al. Systemic inflammation present in patients undergoing CABG without extracorporeal circulation. Chest. 1998;113: 1290–5.
90. Hornick P, Taylor KM. Immune and inflammatory responses after cardiopulmonary bypass. In: Gravlee GP, Davis RF, Kurusz M, Utley JR, editors. Cardiopulmonary bypass: principles and practice. Philadelphia: Lippincott Williams Wilkins; 2000. p. 303–20.
91. Asimakopoulos G, Taylor KM. Effects of cardiopulmonary bypass on leukocyte and endothelial adhesion molecules. Ann Thorac Surg. 1998;66: 2135–44.
92. Galinanes M, Watson C, Trivedi U, et al. Differential patterns of neutrophil adhesion molecules during cardiopulmonary bypass in humans. Circulation. 1996;94 Suppl 2:364–9.
93. Zilla P, Fasol R, Groscurth P, et al. Blood platelets in cardiopulmonary bypass operations. J Thorac Cardiovasc Surg. 1989;97:379–88.
94. Haga Y, Hatori N, Yoshizu H, et al. Granulocyte superoxide anion and elastase release during cardiopulmonary bypass. Artif Organs. 1993;17:837–42.
95. Faymonville ME, Pincemail J, Duchateau J, et al. Myeloperoxidase and elastase as markers of leukocyte activation during cardiopulmonary bypass. J Thorac Cardiovasc Surg. 1991;102:309–17.
96. Frering B, Philip I, Dehous M, et al. Circulating cytokines in patients undergoing normothermic cardiopulmonary bypass. J Thorac Cardiovasc Surg. 1994;108:642–7.
97. Paparella D, Yau TM, Young E. Cardiopulmonary bypass induced inflammation: pathophysiology and treatment. An update. Eur J Cardiothorac Surg. 2002;21:232–44.
98. Musial J, Niewiarowski S, Hershock D, et al. Loss of fibrinogen receptors from the platelet surface during simulated extracorporeal circulation. J Lab Clin Med. 1985;105:514–26.
99. Kirklin JK, Westaby S, Blackstone EH, et al. Complement and the damaging effects of cardiopulmonary bypass. J Thorac Cardiovasc Surg. 1983;86: 845–57.
100. Burne-Taney MJ, Rabb H. The role of adhesion molecules and T cells in ischemic renal injury. Curr Opin Nephrol Hypertens. 2003;12:85–90.
101. Donnahoo KK, Meng X, Ayala A, et al. Early kidney TNF-expression mediates neutrophil infiltration and injury after renal ischemia–reperfusion. Am J Physiol. 1999;277:R922–9.
102. McCoy RN, Hill KE, Ayon MA, et al. Oxidant stress following renal ischemia: changes in the glutathione redox ratio. Kidney Int. 1988;33:812–7.
103. Tennenberg SD, Clardy CW, Bailey WW, et al. Complement activation and lung permeability during cardiopulmonary bypass. Ann Thorac Surg. 1990;50:597–601.
104. Jansen NJ, van-Oeveren W, Gu YJ, et al. Endotoxin release and tumor necrosis factor formation during cardiopulmonary bypass. Ann Thorac Surg. 1992; 54:744–7.
105. Blauth J. Macroemboli and microemboli during cardiopulmonary bypass. Ann Thorac Surg. 1995;59: 1300–3.
106. van der Linden J, Casimir-Ahn H. When do cerebral emboli appear during open heart operations? A transcranial Doppler study. Ann Thorac Surg. 1991;51: 237–41.
107. Barbut D, Hinton RB, Szatrowski TP, et al. Cerebral emboli detected during bypass surgery are associated with clamp removal. Stroke. 1994;25:2398–402.
108. Sreeram GM, Grocott HP, White WD, Newman MF, Stafford-Smith M. Transcranial Doppler emboli count predicts rise in creatinine after coronary artery bypass graft surgery. J Cardiovasc Vasc Anesth. 2004;18:548–51.
109. Moat NE, Evans TE, Quinlan GJ, et al. Chelatable iron and copper can be released from extracorporeally circulated blood during cardiopulmonary bypass. Fed Eur Biochem Soc. 1993;328:103–6.
110. Gutteridge JMC. Iron promoters of the Fenton reaction and lipid peroxidation can be released from hemoglobin by peroxides. Fed Eur Biochem Soc Lett. 1986;201:291–5.
111. Flaherty JT, Weisfeldt ML. Reperfusion injury. Free Radic Biol Med. 1988;5:409–19.
112. Gutteridge JMC, Quinlan GJ. Antioxidant protection against organic and inorganic oxygen radicals by normal human plasma: the important primary role for iron-binding and iron-oxidizing proteins. Biochim Biophys Acta. 1992;1159:248–54.
113. Pepper JR, Mumby S, Gutteridge JMC. Sequential oxidative damage and changes in iron-binding and iron-oxidizing plasma antioxidants during cardiopulmonary bypass surgery. Free Radic Res. 1994; 21:377–85.

114. Pepper JR, Mumby S, Gutteridge JMC. Blood cardioplegia increases plasma iron overload and thiol levels during cardiopulmonary bypass. Ann Thorac Surg. 1995;60:1735–40.
115. Menasche P, Antebi H, Alcindor LG, et al. Iron chelation by deferoxamine inhibits lipid peroxidation during cardiopulmonary bypass in humans. Circulation. 1990;82:IV390–6.
116. Lazar HL. The use of angiotensin-converting enzyme inhibitors in patients undergoing coronary artery bypass graft surgery. Vascul Pharmacol. 2005; 42:119–23.
117. Devbhandari MP, Balasubramanian SK, Codispoti M, et al. Preoperative angiotensin-converting enzyme inhibition can cause severe post CPB vasodilation – current UK opinion. Asian Cardiovasc Thorac Ann. 2004;12:346–9.
118. Kwapisz MM, Muller M, Schindler E, et al. The effect of intravenous quinaprilat on plasma cytokines and hemodynamic variables during cardiac surgery. J Cardiothorac Vasc Anesth. 2004;18: 53–8.
119. Aspelin P, Aubry P, Fransson SG, et al. Nephrotoxicity in High-Risk Patients Study of Iso-Osmolar and Low-Osmolar Non-Ionic Contrast Media Study Investigators. Nephrotoxic effects in high-risk patients undergoing angiography. N Engl J Med. 2003;348:491–9.
120. Woo EB, Tang AT, el-Gamel A, et al. Dopamine therapy for patients at risk of renal dysfunction following cardiac surgery: science or fiction? Eur J Cardiothorac Surg. 2002;22:106–11.
121. Tang AT, El-Gamel A, Keevil B, et al. The effect of 'renal-dose' dopamine on renal tubular function following cardiac surgery: assessed by measuring retinol binding protein (RBP). Eur J Cardiothorac Surg. 1999;15:717–21.
122. Denton MD, Chertow GM, Brady HR. "Renal-dose" dopamine for the treatment of acute renal failure: scientific rationale, experimental studies and clinical trials. Kidney Int. 1996;50:4–14.
123. Stone GW, McCullough PA, Tumlin JA, et al.; for the CONTRAST Investigators. Fenoldopam mesylate for the prevention of contrast-induced nephropathy: a randomized controlled trial. JAMA 2003;290: 2284–91.
124. Ranucci M, Soro G, Barzaghi N, et al. Fenoldopam prophylaxis of postoperative acute renal failure in high-risk cardiac surgery patients. Ann Thorac Surg. 2004;78:1332–7.
125. Caimmi PP, Pagani L, Micalizzi E, et al. Fenoldopam for renal protection in patients undergoing cardiopulmonary bypass. J Cardiothorac Vasc Anesth. 2003;17:491–4.
126. Garwood S, Swamidoss CP, Davis EA, Samson L, Hines RL. A case series of low-dose fenoldopam in seventy cardiac surgical patients at increased risk of renal dysfunction. J Cardiothorac Vasc Anesth. 2003;17:17–21.
127. http://www.angiodynamics.com/products/benephit. Accessed 4/6/2011.
128. Kramer BK, Preuner J, Ebenburger A, et al. Lack of renoprotective effect of theophylline during aortocoronary bypass surgery. Nephrol Dial Transplant. 2002;17:910–5.
129. Light DB, Schwiebert EM, Karlson KH, Stanton BA. Atrial natriuretic peptide inhibits a cation channel in renal inner medullary collecting duct cells. Science. 1989;243:383–5.
130. Allgren RL, Marbury TC, Rahman SN, et al. Anaritide in acute tubular necrosis: Auriculin Anaritide Acute Renal Failure Study Group. N Engl J Med. 1997;336:828–34.
131. Lewis J, Salem MM, Chertow GM, et al. Atrial natriuretic factor in oliguric renal failure. Anaritide Acute Renal Failure Study Group. Am J Kidney Dis. 2000;36:767–74.
132. Sward K, Valsson F, Odencrants P, et al. Recombinant human atrial natriuretic peptide in ischemic acute renal failure. A randomized placebo controlled trial. Crit Care Med. 2004;32:1310–5.
133. Jarnberg PO. Renal protection strategies in the perioperative period. Best Pract Res Clin Anaesthesiol. 2004;18:645–60.
134. Lassnigg A, Donner E, Grubhofer G, et al. Lack of renoprotective effects of dopamine and furosemide during cardiac surgery. J Am Soc Nephrol. 2000; 11:97–104.
135. Lombardi R, Ferreiro A, Servetto C. Renal function after cardiac surgery: adverse effect of furosemide. Ren Fail. 2003;25:775–86.
136. Engelman RM, Gouge TH, Smith SJ, et al. The effect of diuretics on renal hemodynamics during cardiopulmonary bypass. J Surg Res. 1974;16:268–76.
137. Cooper JR, Giesecke NM. Hemodilution and priming solutions. In: Gravlee GP, Davis RF, Kurusz M, Utley JR, editors. Cardiopulmonary bypass: principles and practice. Philadelphia: Lippincott Williams Wilkins; 2000. p. 186–96.
138. Rigden SP, Dillon MJ, Kind PR, et al. The beneficial effect of mannitol on postoperative renal function in children undergoing cardiopulmonary bypass surgery. Clin Nephrol. 1984;21:148–51.
139. Fisher AR, Jones P, Barlow P, et al. The influence of mannitol on renal function during and after open-heart surgery. Perfusion. 1998;13:181–6.
140. Ip-Yam PC, Murphy S, Baines M, Fox MA, Desmond MJ, Innes PA. Renal function and proteinuria after cardiopulmonary bypass: the effects of temperature and mannitol. Anesth Analg. 1994;78:842–7.
141. Carcoana OV, Mathew JP, Davis E, et al. Mannitol and dopamine in patients undergoing cardiopulmonary bypass: a randomized clinical trial. Anesth Analg. 2003;97:1222–9.
142. Sullivan GW, Carper HT, Novick Jr WJ, Mandell GL. Inhibition of the inflammatory action of interleukin-1 and tumor necrosis factor (alpha) on neutrophil function by pentoxifylline. Infect Immun. 1988;56:1722–9.
143. Cagli K, Ulas MM, Ozisik K, et al. The intraoperative effect of pentoxifylline on the inflammatory process and leukocytes in cardiac surgery patients undergoing cardiopulmonary bypass. Perfusion. 2005;20:45–51.

144. Zhang M, Xu YJ, Saini HK, Turan B, Liu PP, Dhalla NS. Pentoxifylline attenuates cardiac dysfunction and reduces TNF-{alpha}level in the ischemic-reperfused heart. Am J Physiol Heart Circ Physiol 2005 Aug;289(2):H832–9.
145. Boldt J, Brosch C, Piper SN, Suttner S, Lehmann A, Werling C. Influence of prophylactic use of pentoxifylline on postoperative organ function in elderly cardiac surgery patients. Crit Care Med. 2001; 29:952–8.
146. Loef BG, Henning RH, Epema AH, et al. Effect of dexamethasone on perioperative renal function impairment during cardiac surgery with cardiopulmonary bypass. Br J Anaesth. 2004;93:793–8.
147. Sucu N, Cinel I, Unlu A, et al. N-acetylcysteine for preventing pump-induced oxidoinflammatory response during cardiopulmonary bypass. Surg Today. 2004;34:237–42.
148. Tossios P, Bloch W, Huebner A, et al. N-acetylcysteine prevents reactive oxygen species-mediated myocardial stress in patients undergoing cardiac surgery: results of a randomized, double-blind, placebo-controlled clinical trial. Thorac Cardiovasc Surg. 2003;126:1513–20.
149. Myles PS, Hunt JO, Holdgaard HO, et al. Clonidine and cardiac surgery: haemodynamic and metabolic effects, myocardial ischaemia and recovery. Anaesth Intensive Care. 1999;27:137–47.
150. Kulka PJ, Tryba M, Zenz M. Preoperative alpha2-adrenergic receptor agonists prevent the deterioration of renal function after cardiac surgery: results of a randomized, controlled trial. Crit Care Med. 1996; 24:947–52.
151. Fansa I, Gol M, Nisanoglu V, et al. Does diltiazem inhibit the inflammatory response in cardiopulmonary bypass? Med Sci Monit. 2003;9:PI30–6.
152. Chanda J, Canver CC. Reversal of preexisting vasospasm in coronary artery conduits. Ann Thorac Surg. 2001;72:476–80.
153. Bergman AS, Odar-Cederlof I, Westman L, et al. Diltiazem infusion for renal protection in cardiac surgical patients with preexisting renal dysfunction. J Cardiothorac Vasc Anesth. 2002;16:294–9.
154. Piper SN, Kumle B, Maleck WH, et al. Diltiazem may preserve renal tubular integrity after cardiac surgery. Can J Anaesth. 2003;50:285–92.
155. Young EW, Diab A, Kirsh MM. Intravenous diltiazem and acute renal failure after cardiac operations. Ann Thorac Surg. 1998;65:1316–9.
156. Amar D, Fleisher M. Diltiazem treatment does not alter renal function after thoracic surgery. Chest. 2001;119:1476–9.

6 Pulmonary Factors in Redo Open Heart Surgery

David O. Wilson

Pulmonary factors are quite relevant for redo cardiac surgery. Postoperative pulmonary complications contribute significantly to overall perioperative morbidity and mortality. This section will review preoperative and postoperative pulmonary considerations in patients undergoing redo cardiac surgery. These factors can be divided into patient-related and procedure-related risks.

In terms of preoperative pulmonary assessment, this discussion will focus on two factors: (1) quality of life/relief of dyspnea in patients with underlying lung disease and pulmonary impairment and (2) preoperative assessment of the risk of prolonged mechanical ventilation. The decision whether to proceed with redo cardiac surgery in patients with significant underlying lung disease, such as chronic obstructive pulmonary disease (COPD), is complicated. In addition to the usual considerations of morbidity and mortality, symptomatic improvement postoperatively is also a concern. In patients with three-vessel coronary artery disease and angina, the decision to proceed with revascularization to reduce cardiac mortality is less challenging. However, in patients with less severe coronary disease and symptomatic, lifestyle-limiting COPD or other lung disease, decision making is more complex. Even with the best-case scenario postoperatively, patients with lifestyle-limiting lung disease may not have symptomatic improvement in dyspnea or quality of life improvement. There are no evidence-based data to guide this decision making, except in the extremes [1], and it is key that patients and families have realistic expectations of what to expect postoperatively.

Patient-related factors relevant to preoperative pulmonary assessment include COPD, restrictive pulmonary impairment, and pulmonary hypertension. COPD has been well studied and is a risk factor for prolonged mechanical ventilation and clinical outcome after cardiac surgery [2]. Restrictive pulmonary impairment, such as related to obesity (with or without obesity hyperventilation syndrome), interstitial lung disease, chest wall deformity, kyphoscoliosis, or respiratory muscle weakness, has been less well characterized, but is of similar importance. Pulmonary function testing and arterial blood gas measurement can address the severity of COPD or restrictive impairment in the appropriate clinical setting. Pulmonary hypertension is especially important in patients with severe underlying lung disease (a poor prognostic factor) and patients undergoing valve surgery. Unfortunately, aside from patients receiving elective surgery who can be persuaded to stop smoking or lose weight, there is usually little that can be done preoperatively to modify the risks of pulmonary complications.

Several studies have examined risk factors for prolonged ventilation in cardiac surgery [2–9]. Some studies have focused on preoperative risk factors and identified groups of patients at greater

D.O. Wilson, MD, MPH (✉)
Division of Pulmonary, Allergy and Critical Care Medicine, University of Pittsburgh Medical Center, Pittsburgh, PA, USA
e-mail: wilsondo@upmc.edu

V.R. Machiraju et al. (eds.), *Redo Cardiac Surgery in Adults*,
DOI 10.1007/978-1-4614-1326-4_6, © Springer Science+Business Media, LLC 2012

risk of prolonged ventilation [3, 4]. One study developed a multivariate prediction model for prolonged ventilation after cardiac surgery, taking into account redo status, and designed a formula to be used to calculate patient-specific risks [9]. The prediction model uses 12 readily available preoperative patient and disease characteristics to predict the need for prolonged ventilation. The characteristics with the greatest weight are aortic surgery, age >75 years, elevated serum creatinine, preoperative ventilation, and previous cardiac surgery (Odds ratios (ORs) 2.4–5.5). The only pulmonary factors in the model are FEV1 < 70% predicted and current smoker, each with an OR of 1.5. Other factors in the model included peripheral vascular disease, ejection fraction <30%, myocardial infarction within 90 days, urgent or emergent surgery, use of cardiopulmonary bypass, and mitral valve surgery. The incidence of prolonged ventilation, defined as >48 h, was ~5% [9].

Another recently published, prospective, observational study assessed predictors of prolonged mechanical ventilation in a cohort of 5,123 cardiac surgical patients [10]. In a logistic regression model, age >65 years, New York Heart Association class 3 or 4, left ventricular ejection fraction (LVEF) >30%, COPD, and chronic renal failure were the only patient-related factors that predicted prolonged mechanical ventilation (ORs 1.296–2.125). Procedure-related factors included redo surgery (OR 2.01), emergency surgery (OR 1.622), red blood cell (RBC) or fresh-frozen plasma (FFP) transfusion greater than 4 U (OR 5.43), and cardiopulmonary bypass time >77 min (OR 2.03). As one can see from the ORs, procedure-related factors were a much more significant risk for prolonged mechanical ventilation than patient-related factors. In addition, COPD was the only pulmonary factor considered.

Another recent study that focused on redo coronary artery bypass grafting (CABG) confirms the significance of procedure-related factors, especially redo status, as risk factors for prolonged mechanical ventilation and, also, perioperative mortality [11]. Compared to first-time CABG and after adjustment for patient-related variables, redo status remained a predictor for prolonged ventilation (OR 1.5) and operative death (OR 2.1). However, after adjusting for patient-related variables, there was no difference in postoperative mid-term survival (1–6 years postoperative) between patients undergoing redo CABG and patients undergoing first-time CABG. The significant predictors of mid-term mortality, based on OR, were all patient-related factors with age > renal failure > reduced LVEF > peripheral vascular disease > congestive heart failure history > respiratory disease [11].

In terms of ventilator weaning and extubation following cardiac surgery, our experience suggests that redo patients may be weaned and extubated using a standard weaning algorithm [12]. As long as the patient met the neurologic, hemodynamic, and pulmonary mechanical and physiologic parameters, extubation was equally successful whether redo or first-time cardiac surgery.

Pulmonary complications are a significant cause of morbidity following cardiac surgery. Chest wall and lung compliance decrease postoperatively, especially within the first 3 days, which may complicate extubation of patients with underlying lung disease and increase the risk for pneumonia by impairing the ability to cough and breathe deeply. Diaphragmatic dysfunction can occur. Atelectasis occurs in up to 70% of patients following cardiac surgery [13]. Acute respiratory distress syndrome (ARDS) complicates cardiopulmonary bypass in ~1% of cases [14]. Postoperative pleural effusions are common and usually develop as a consequence of the surgical procedure. Small, usually left-sided, pleural effusions are common in the early postoperative course following cardiac surgery. They are usually nonspecific, self-limited and require only observation [15]. Postoperative pleural effusions may also occur with postcardiac injury syndrome (Dressler's syndrome) or postoperative heart failure.

A recently published study from Germany suggests that prophylactic nasal continuous positive airway pressure (nCPAP) may be beneficial in preventing postoperative pulmonary complications following cardiac surgery [16]. Five-hundred patients undergoing elective cardiac surgery were randomized into four groups: early extubation control (in the operating room), early extubation nCPAP, late extubation control (in the ICU), and late extubation nCPAP. The control groups received standard postoperative treatment and the study group received at least 6 h of prophylactic nCPAP at 10 cm H_2O. Pulmonary complications including hypoxemia, pneumonia, reintubation rate, and ICU readmission rate were significantly lower in the nCPAP-treated group ($p=0.03$). Thus, nCPAP may be a useful tool to prevent postoperative pulmonary complications in patients recovering from cardiac surgery.

In patients undergoing redo cardiac surgery, preoperative pulmonary assessment allows for refined risk stratification and improved potential for establishing realistic postoperative expectations in patients with pulmonary impairment. Pulmonary complications are a major cause of postoperative morbidity, and newer and evolving concepts for postoperative care, such as prophylactic nCPAP, should be considered in the appropriate clinical setting. In addition, risk factors that can be modified, such as smoking status, or optimized, such as COPD, should be considered.

References

1. Naunheim KS, Wood DE, Krasna MJ, et al. Predictors of operative mortality and cardiopulmonary morbidity in the National Emphysema Treatment Trial. J Thorac Cardiovasc Surg. 2006;131:43–9.
2. Rady M, Ryan T. Preoperative predictors of extubation failure and the effect on clinical outcome after cardiac surgery. Crit Care Med. 1999;27:340–2.
3. Spivack SD, Shimozaki T, Albertini JJ, Deane R. Preoperative prediction of postoperative respiratory outcome. Chest. 1996;109:1222–30.
4. Legare JF, Hirsch GM, Buth KJ, MacDougall C, Sullivan A. Preoperative prediction of prolonged mechanical ventilation following coronary artery bypass grafting. Eur J Cardiothorac Surg. 2001; 20:930–6.
5. Kern H, Redlich U, Hotz H, et al. Risk factors for prolonged ventilation after cardiac surgery using APACHE II, SAPS II, and TISS: comparison of three different models. Intensive Care Med. 2001;27:407–15.
6. Serrano N, Garcia C, Villegas J, et al. Prolonged intubation rates after coronary artery bypass surgery and ICU risk stratification score. Chest. 2005;128: 595–601.
7. Thompson MJ, Elton RA, Mankad PA, et al. Prediction of requirement for, and outcome of, prolonged mechanical ventilation following cardiac surgery. Cardiovasc Surg. 1997;5:376–81.
8. Bezanson JL, Weaver M, Kinney MA, Waldrum M, Weintraub WS. Presurgical risk factors for late extubation in Medicare recipients after cardiac surgery. Nurs Res. 2004;53:46–52.
9. Reddy SLC, Gragson AD, Griffiths EM, Pullan DM, Rushid A. Logistic risk model for prolonged ventilation after adult cardiac surgery. Ann Thorac Surg. 2007;84:528–36.
10. Cislaghi F, Condemi AM, Corona A. Predictors of prolonged mechanical ventilation in a cohort of 5123 cardiac surgical patients. Eur J Anaesthiol. 2009; 26:396–403.
11. Yap CH, Sposato L, Akowuah E, et al. Contemporary results show repeat coronary artery bypass grafting remains a risk factor for operative mortality. Ann Thorac Surg. 2009;87:1386–91.
12. Wilson D, Zapletal J. Weaning after open heart surgery. Am Rev Resp Dis. 1993;147:A873.
13. Sladden RN, Berkowitz DE. Cardiopulmonary bypass and the lung. In: Gravlee GP, Davis RF, Utley IR, editors. Cardiopulmonary bypass. Baltimore: Williams and Wilkins; 1993. p. 468–87.
14. Messent M, Sullivan K, Keogh B, et al. Adult respiratory distress syndrome following cardiopulmonary bypass: incidence and prediction. Anaesthesia. 1992;47:267.
15. Peng MJ, Vargas FS, Cukier A, et al. Postoperative pleural changes after coronary revascularization. Comparison between saphenous vein and internal mammary artery grafting. Chest. 1992;102:327.
16. Zarbock A, Mueller E, Metzer S, Gabriel A, Feindt P, Kindgen-Milles D. Prophylactic nasal continuous positive airway pressure following cardiac surgery protects from postoperative pulmonary complications. Chest. 2009;135:1252–4.

7 Transfusion Therapy in Reoperative Cardiac Surgery

Anand Padmanabhan and Darrell J. Triulzi

Cardiac surgery can be complicated by significant bleeding, particularly in patients with prior cardiothoracic surgery. Redo cardiac procedures can be complicated by adhesions and prolonged cardiopulmonary bypass (CPB), both of which can contribute to excessive bleeding. Approximately 30% of patients undergoing first-time elective coronary artery bypass grafting (CABG) surgery require a blood transfusion [1], and the likelihood of transfusion is even higher in cardiac reoperations (odds ratio 2.32; confidence interval 1.53–2.33) [2]. Thus, the cardiothoracic surgeon and anesthesiologist need to be aware of the symptoms, signs, relevant laboratory tests, pathophysiology, and management strategies for excessive bleeding in the perioperative period of redo cardiac surgery.

Bleeding from a specific anatomic site is typically indicative of surgical bleeding related to blood vessel trauma, while generalized bleeding is typically indicative of systemic coagulopathy. A brisk surgical bleed can rapidly result in generalized coagulopathy if it is not quickly controlled. Symptoms of acute blood loss, such as hypotension, tachycardia, pallor, diaphoresis, oliguria, anuria, acidosis, and altered consciousness, can reflect severe bleeding and should be recognized immediately. Lower preoperative hemoglobin, lower weight, older age, and female sex are independent factors predicting the need for transfusion in CABG surgeries [1]. Other risk factors include preoperative use of antiplatelet or antithrombotic medications, coagulation abnormalities, noncardiac comorbidities, reoperation, and complex or emergent procedures [3]. Frequent intraoperative laboratory testing is highly recommended in high-risk cases and has been greatly facilitated by the availability of a variety of point-of-care testing platforms.

Patients requiring cardiac surgery need to be thoroughly evaluated, with sufficiently time to allow withholding of medications that can interfere with platelet function or the coagulation pathway, such as acetylsalicylic acid, clopidogrel, GpIIb/IIIa inhibitors, and warfarin, before surgery. It is recommended that clopidogrel be discontinued 7 days before the procedure.

In the intraoperative period, prolonged CPB can adversely impact platelet function. This qualitative platelet function defect may cause bleeding despite a physiologically normal platelet count. CPB is also thought to contribute significantly to the hyperfibrinolytic state observed in cardiac surgery [4]. The severalfold increase in plasminogen activator during CPB accelerates conversion of inactive plasminogen to plasmin, which results in clot dissolution. Disseminated intravascular coagulation (DIC), a pathological process of consumptive coagulopathy, can complicate the ability to achieve hemostasis in cardiac surgery. This process of excessive microvascular thrombosis sets the stage for generalized coagulopathy as levels of

A. Padmanabhan, MD • D.J. Triulzi, MD (✉)
Department of Pathology, Division of Transfusion Medicine, University of Pittsburgh School of Medicine, Pittsburgh, PA, USA
e-mail: dtriulzi@itxm.org

V.R. Machiraju et al. (eds.), *Redo Cardiac Surgery in Adults*,
DOI 10.1007/978-1-4614-1326-4_7,

platelets and coagulation factors decrease below hemostatic levels (platelet count <50,000/μL, international normalized ratio (INR) >1.5, and fibrinogen <100 mg/dL).

Another cause of intraoperative bleeding is the use of heparin anticoagulation and its reversal by protamine sulfate during CPB. Multiple studies have examined the issue of activated clotting time (ACT)-guided vs. nonmonitored heparin–protamine dosing and suggest that monitoring does not consistently decrease bleeding or the use of blood products [3]. A randomized prospective trial evaluating use of a whole blood hemostasis system for heparin–protamine administration (Hepcon; Medtronic Blood Management, Englewood, Colorado) showed that compared with the conventional ACT-based dosing group, patients in the Hepcon group had smaller protamine-to-heparin ratios, less chest tube drainage during the immediate postoperative period and needed fewer platelet, fresh frozen plasma (FFP), and cryoprecipitate transfusions [5]. Excessive dosing of protamine, with a resultant increase in the ratio of protamine-to-heparin, impairs platelet function [6]. The Society of Thoracic Surgeons Blood Conservation Guidelines Task Force currently recommends the use of either protamine titration or empiric low-dose regimens (e.g., 50% of total heparin dose) to lower the total protamine dose and lower the protamine-to-heparin ratio [3].

The coagulation pathway can be broadly divided into the extrinsic and intrinsic pathways. The prothrombin time (PT) and INR assess the extrinsic pathway (tissue factor-mediated activation), while the activated partial thromboplastin time (aPTT) is a test of intrinsic pathway (contact activation) function. Preoperatively, all patients should be evaluated for unexplained elevations of PT/INR or aPTT to rule out coagulation factor deficiencies or inhibitors. Serial intraoperative PT/INR, aPTT, and fibrinogen measures should be performed to assess coagulation status and guide transfusion therapy in patients with excessive bleeding. Due to the high doses of heparin used during CPB, intraoperative anticoagulation monitoring using aPTT is not recommended during CPB. For this purpose, the less sensitive ACT test should be used. ACT target levels on CPB should be 300–600 s with an initial ACT >480 s before the initiation of CPB. Thromboelastography (TEG) has been widely utilized for assessment of overall coagulation in a variety of surgical settings. TEG assesses the viscoelastic properties of clot formation and transduces this information into an electrical signal that can be recorded. While TEG-based transfusion algorithms have reduced transfusion in cardiac surgery in some studies [7, 8], there are no clear, validated guidelines for use of this test to assess coagulation status, guide blood component therapy, or predict bleeding risk [9]. A diagnosis of DIC is supported by the clinical presence of diffuse microvascular bleeding with dropping platelet counts, prolonged PT/INR, and decreasing fibrinogen, fibrin split products and D-dimer (if available in the postoperative period).

Numerous tests have been utilized for assessment of platelet function. The bleeding time has generally fallen out of favor and has been replaced by other tests including PFA-100 ("closure time" test; Siemens, Deerfield, IL), Helena Plateletworks (Helena Laboratories Corp., Beaumont, TX), and traditional platelet aggregometry. While each of these tests uses a different hardware and technology, they are similar in that they assess platelet aggregation after stimulation with a variety of platelet agonists. Tests such as VerifyNow (Accumetrics, San Diego, CA) assess platelet function after treatment with aspirin, clopidogrel, and GpIIb/IIIa inhibitors. In most cases, these tests are performed preoperatively for baseline assessment and are not practical to obtain in real time during surgery due mainly to the time required for testing. In patients who require emergency cardiac procedures and are being treated with antiplatelet drugs, such as acetylsalicylic acid or clopidogrel, a 1–2 dose platelet transfusion is recommended prior to surgery.

Management of Bleeding

Typically, red blood cell (RBC) transfusion is considered when >30–40% of the patient's blood volume is lost (>1.5–2 L of blood in a 70-kg patient) [10]. Volume resuscitation should be initially attempted with crystalloids and colloids, unless symptomatic anemia is present. In healthy patients, the effects of oxygen deprivation do not become evident until the hemoglobin concentration falls to 5–6 g/dL. However, a higher hemoglobin threshold should be considered in bleeding cardiac surgery patients who have coronary artery disease and are likely to have associated comorbid cardiorespiratory conditions. There are no consensuses or evidence-based recommendations for the intraoperative transfusion of red cells. Patients are typically maintained at hematocrits between 21 and 24% while on CPB. Cell salvage techniques are often used to minimize the need for allogeneic RBC transfusion [11]. In the postoperative period after successful revascularization, a hemoglobin threshold of 8 g/dL for RBC transfusion does not adversely affect outcomes in patients who undergo primary elective CABG procedures [12]. While the optimal ratio of plasma and platelet units to RBC transfusions is still a matter of debate, it is generally recommended that plasma and platelet transfusions be instituted in situations requiring massive transfusion of RBCs (>10 U/24-h period) to avoid dilutional thrombocytopenia or coagulopathy.

Despite the absence of randomized trials, a count of >50,000/μL normal functioning platelets in a bleeding patient is generally considered adequate for hemostasis. However, in patients with diffuse microvascular bleeding after CPB, the associated qualitative platelet function defect may require platelet transfusion. Evaluation of platelet function in this setting should guide therapy. Plasma transfusions should be used in bleeding patients when the INR is >1.5. Cryoprecipitate (typically available as 6–12 U pools), an excellent source of fibrinogen, should be used to treat hypofibrinogenemia (fibrinogen <100 mg/dL) and DIC. Numerous materials, including mechanical (e.g., porcine/bovine gelatin/collagen), chemical (e.g., polyethylene glycol polymers), and bioactive (e.g., fibrin/thrombin) materials, can be used for local hemostasis. Fibrin sealants, such as Tisseel (Baxter, Westlake Village, CA), are approved for use in cardiac surgery and aid in enhancing coagulation in a localized area [13].

Red Cell Component Selection

Multiple studies support the use of leukoreduced (LR) blood components in cardiac surgery. In patients who underwent cardiac surgery, hospital length of stay declined from 10.1 to 9.5 days with the use of LR blood components and increased to 10.8 days with the reintroduction of non-LR blood components [14]. A meta-analysis of three randomized controlled trials and a more recent prospective randomized controlled trial found decreases in mortality in the short and longer term (1 year) in patients who received LR blood [15–17]. Heart failure was the primary cause of excess mortality in the control group. The mechanisms by which LR blood components prevented adverse outcomes are unclear.

Current anticoagulant preservative storage solutions allow for refrigerated storage of RBCs for up to 42 days. During storage, there is loss of adenosine 5′-triphosphate (ATP), loss of 2,3-bisphosphoglycerate (2,3-DPG), loss of intra-RBC potassium with a concomitant increase in potassium in the storage bag, oxidative damage, and membrane loss. There are also apoptotic changes and RBC shape changes [18]. Given these storage changes, there has been immense interest in the question of whether "old" RBCs are deleterious for patients, or perhaps not as beneficial as "fresh" RBCs. There have been numerous retrospective and some prospective studies that have delved into this topic. A recent comprehensive meta-analysis of the literature on age of transfused RBCs and incidence of complications concluded that it is not possible to clearly determine the relationship between the age of transfused RBCs and outcome on the basis of currently available literature [19]. Prospective, randomized, controlled studies, such as the Age of Blood Evaluation (ABLE) trial, the Age of Red Blood Cells in Premature Infants (ARIPI) study, and the NIH-sponsored Red Cell Storage Duration Study (RECESS), will seek to provide definitive answers to this question.

Recombinant VIIa

Activated factor VII (Factor VIIa; NovoSeven, Novo Nordisk Inc., Princeton, NJ) is a recombinant, activated coagulation factor approved by the FDA for use in patients with congenital hemophilia with inhibitors, in patients with congenital factor VII deficiency, and in patients with acquired hemophilia. Factor VIIa is a potent activator of the extrinsic pathway of coagulation and may be considered in the setting of massive bleeding refractory to aggressive transfusion therapy. Use of factor VIIa is contraindicated in hypercoagulable states, such as DIC. If factor VIIa administration is being considered, there should be vigorous coadministration of blood products; without adequate levels of platelets and coagulation factors, clotting will not occur. Correction of acidosis is also recommended, although there is some controversy whether this affects the ability of factor VIIa to mediate clot formation [20]. The optimal dose of factor VIIa in this setting is unknown but should be the minimum required to achieve hemostasis given the dose-related risk of thrombotic events associated with the use of factor VIIa. A 20–40-μg/kg dose of factor VIIa may aid in achieving hemostasis and can be repeated after 60–90 min. Antifibrinolytic agents, such as aminocaproic acid, tranexamic acid, and aprotinin, inhibit the conversion of plasminogen to plasmin and have been widely used to control bleeding associated with cardiac surgery. While aprotinin appears more effective in decreasing the risk of major hemorrhage than tranexamic acid or aminocaproic acid, it carries a significantly higher mortality risk [21] and is no longer used in this setting. Table 7.1 summarizes the blood component treatment plan for diffuse microvascular hemorrhage in cardiac surgery.

Conclusions

Although blood transfusions are extremely important and often lifesaving in cardiac surgery, cardiothoracic surgeons and anesthesiologists should be aware of the risks of blood transfusion, including transfusion-associated circulatory overload, transfusion-related acute lung injury, and much less common risks, such as transfusion-transmitted infectious diseases, hemolytic transfusion reactions, and anaphylaxis. When severe bleeding is anticipated, as in a patient undergoing redo cardiac surgery, RBC salvage or intraoperative acute normovolemic hemodilution should be considered. Such blood conservation strategies attain even greater importance in patients who have RBC alloantibodies that make obtaining compatible, antigen-negative blood challenging. Blood warmers should be routinely used for transfusion since hypothermia can further exacerbate coagulopathy. Special consideration should also be taken for patient populations that refuse blood transfusion, such as Jehovah's Witnesses, with a clear preoperative plan for the use of nonblood products, such a factor VIIa, desmopressin acetate (DDAVP), and antifibrinolytics in the event of severe bleeding.

Table 7.1 Transfusion therapy in diffuse microvascular hemorrhage

Defect	Laboratory parameters	Treatment
Coagulopathy with factor deficiency	INR > 1.5	Plasma 15–20 mL/kg
Coagulopathy due to fibrinolysis	Fibrinogen <100 mg/dL	Cryoprecipitate 6–12 units; antifibrinolytics
Coagulopathy due to DIC	Fibrinogen <100 mg/dL; INR > 1.5; platelets <50,000/μL	Platelets; plasma; cryoprecipitate
Thrombocytopenia	Platelets <50,000/μL	Platelet transfusion
Platelet dysfunction	Various assays (e.g., prolonged closure time)	Platelet transfusion

References

1. Karkouti K, Cohen MM, McCluskey SA, Sher GD. A multivariable model for predicting the need for blood transfusion in patients undergoing first-time elective coronary bypass graft surgery. Transfusion. 2001;41:1193–203.
2. Alghamdi AA, Davis A, Brister S, et al. Development and validation of transfusion risk understanding scoring tool (TRUST) to stratify cardiac surgery patients according to their blood transfusion needs. Transfusion. 2006;46:1120–9.
3. Ferraris VA, Ferraris SP, Saha SP, et al. Perioperative blood transfusion and blood conservation in cardiac surgery: the society of thoracic surgeons and the society of cardiovascular anesthesiologists clinical practice guideline. Ann Thorac Surg. 2007;83:S27–86.
4. Yavari M, Becker RC. Coagulation and fibrinolytic protein kinetics in cardiopulmonary bypass. J Thromb Thrombolysis. 2009;27:95–104.
5. Despotis GJ, Joist JH, Hogue Jr CW, et al. The impact of heparin concentration and activated clotting time monitoring on blood conservation. A prospective, randomized evaluation in patients undergoing cardiac operation. J Thorac Cardiovasc Surg. 1995;110: 46–54.
6. Mochizuki T, Olson PJ, Szlam F, et al. Protamine reversal of heparin affects platelet aggregation and activated clotting time after cardiopulmonary bypass. Anesth Analg. 1998;87:781–5.
7. Shore-Lesserson L, Manspeizer HE, DePerio M, et al. Thromboelastography-guided transfusion algorithm reduces transfusions in complex cardiac surgery. Anesth Analg. 1999;88:312–9.
8. Royston D, von Kier S. Reduced haemostatic factor transfusion using heparinase-modified thrombelastography during cardiopulmonary bypass. Br J Anaesth. 2001;86:575–8.
9. Samama CM, Ozier Y. Near-patient testing of haemostasis in the operating theatre: an approach to appropriate use of blood in surgery. Vox Sang. 2003; 84:251–5.
10. Murphy MF, Wallington TB, Kelsey P, et al. Guidelines for the clinical use of red cell transfusions. Br J Haematol. 2001;113:24–31.
11. Wang G, Bainbridge D, Martin J, Cheng D. The efficacy of an intraoperative cell saver during cardiac surgery: a meta-analysis of randomized trials. Anesth Analg. 2009;109:320–30.
12. Bracey AW, Radovancevic R, Riggs SA, et al. Lowering the hemoglobin threshold for transfusion in coronary artery bypass procedures: effect on patient outcome. Transfusion. 1999;39:1070–7.
13. Spotnitz WD, Burks S. Hemostats, sealants, and adhesives: components of the surgical toolbox. Transfusion. 2008;48:1502–16.
14. Fung MK, Moore K, Ridenour M, et al. Clinical effects of reverting from leukoreduced to nonleukoreduced blood in cardiac surgery. Transfusion. 2006;46:386–91.
15. Vamvakas EC. WBC-containing allogeneic blood transfusion and mortality: a meta-analysis of randomized controlled trials. Transfusion. 2003;43:963–73.
16. Boshkov LK, Furnary A, Morris C, et al. Prestorage leukoreduction of red cells in elective cardiac surgery: results of a double blind randomized controlled trial. Blood. 2004;104:112a.
17. Boshkov LK, Chien G, VanWinkle G, et al. Prestorage leukoreduction of transfused red cells is associated with significant ongoing 2–12 month survival benefit in cardiac surgery patients. Blood. 2004;104:174a.
18. Zimrin AB, Hess JR. Current issues relating to the transfusion of stored red blood cells. Vox Sanguinis. 2009;96:93–103.
19. Lelubre C, Piagnerelli M, Vincent JL. Association between duration of storage of transfused red blood cells and morbidity and mortality in adult patients: myth or reality? Transfusion. 2009;49:1384–94.
20. Hall K, Forrest P, Sawyer C. The effects of acidosis and hypothermia on blood transfusion requirements following factor VII administration. Anaesth Intensive Care. 2007;35:494–7.
21. Fergusson DA, Hebert PC, Mazer CD, et al. A comparison of aprotinin and lysine analogues in high-risk cardiac surgery. N Engl J Med. 2008;358:2319–31.

8 Anesthesia for Redo Cardiac Surgery

Cynthia M. Wells and Andrew W. Murray

In recent years, an increasing proportion of elderly patients have been referred for repeat cardiac surgery despite the higher morbidity and mortality associated with redo procedures. This patient population requires additional considerations when planning their anesthetic and perioperative care, based on the higher incidence of preexisting conditions in elderly patients as well as the greater surgical risk associated with sternal reentry [1, 2].

The preoperative anesthetic plan for patients undergoing repeat cardiac surgery not only involves a thorough medical history and physical exam, but must also take into consideration factors that enhance perioperative risk. Patients undergoing repeat cardiac surgery are often older, presenting an average of 7–13 years following their original coronary artery bypass grafting or valve procedure [1], and are characterized by an increased incidence of comorbid conditions, such as diabetes mellitus, chronic renal insufficiency, and advanced atherosclerotic disease. Patients with diffuse coronary artery disease and a history of cerebrovascular events are more likely to suffer from postoperative complications, such as myocardial infarction or stroke. A review of the most recent catheterization and echocardiography reports, chest radiogram, and computed tomography (CT) scan reveals important information, such as the patency of prior grafts and the myocardium that they supply, the extent of valve abnormalities, ventricular dysfunction, aortic pathology, and the proximity of vital cardiovascular structures to the posterior sternum.

There are specific preparations necessary for redo cases, in addition to the standard monitors used for cardiac surgery. These preparations include large-bore intravenous access, both above and below the diaphragm, in anticipation of potential blood loss and the need for urgent transfusion and the placement of external defibrillation pads due to the increased risk of arrhythmias during sternotomy and dissection. Cross-matched blood must be available in the operating room and checked prior to incision and the appropriate dose of heparin must be prepared. An arterial line placed before induction of anesthesia allows for precise hemodynamic monitoring. Femoral arterial pressure monitoring should be considered as these cases may have longer cardiopulmonary bypass (CPB) duration with associated underestimation of central blood pressure due to radial arterial spasm. A pulmonary artery catheter will provide valuable information in the majority of patients undergoing redo cardiac surgery, in particular those with underlying ventricular dysfunction, valvular disease, or pulmonary hypertension. The use of transesophageal echocardiography (TEE) as a diagnostic and monitoring tool allows for the continuous assessment of ventricular filling and myocardial and valvular function. In addition, one could consider utilizing cerebral oximetry in high-risk patients.

C.M. Wells, MD • A.W. Murray, MBChB (✉)
Department of Anesthesiology,
University of Pittsburgh Medical Center,
Pittsburgh, PA, USA
e-mail: murrayaw@anes.upmc.edu

V.R. Machiraju et al. (eds.), *Redo Cardiac Surgery in Adults*,
DOI 10.1007/978-1-4614-1326-4_8, © Springer Science+Business Media, LLC 2012

Of greatest concern at the time of sternal reentry is the increased risk of inadvertent trauma to the underlying structures, which may be adherent to the posterior surface of the sternum. Preoperative lateral chest X-ray, CT scan, or magnetic resonance imaging (MRI) may be useful in determining the extent of adherence. Structures at risk include the great vessels, preexisting coronary grafts, and the right ventricle. When damaged, there may be catastrophic hemorrhage or the acute onset of ischemia with rapid decompensation and arrhythmia due to severely compromised myocardial perfusion and function. In the event of such an injury, a mean arterial pressure must be maintained to ensure adequate perfusion to vital organs while minimizing additional blood loss until control is established or the patient is emergently placed on CPB. Occasionally, cannulation via the femoral or axillary artery will precede sternotomy, based on the patient's risk during reentry. Following sternotomy, the surgical dissection time is prolonged secondary to adhesion formation. During exposure, there is the potential for significant bleeding, the development of arrhythmias, and the onset of ischemia due to manipulation of coronary grafts and potential embolization of atheromatous debris into the distal coronary vessels with subsequent transmural myocardial ischemia. Particular vigilance to hemodynamic variations, electrocardiogram (ECG) changes, and new wall motion abnormalities, as seen on TEE, must be maintained during this time.

The challenge and additional risk of performing redo operations continue into the bypass period. There are unique problems related to myocardial preservation that lead to a greater incidence of ventricular dysfunction and postoperative infarction. Right ventricular dysfunction is a significant cause of early morbidity and mortality. This may be due to a prolonged ischemic time, intracoronary embolization, incomplete revascularization, or inadequate myocardial protection despite the use of retrograde cardioplegia to supply territories served by occluded vessels. Treatment of right ventricular failure involves inotropic support, pulmonary vasodilation and, possibly, mechanical ventricular assistance. The presence of impaired left ventricular function preoperatively is an independent risk factor for increased mortality following surgery, or it may have a similar etiology as right-sided dysfunction. Patients with ventricular dysfunction are more likely to require hemodynamic support with vasopressors, inotropic infusions, or mechanical devices, such as an intra-aortic balloon pump, to wean from CPB. Attention must also be given to the potential development of ischemic mitral regurgitation, which may require additional repair.

The postbypass period is often characterized by the continued need for inotropic support and a significant coagulopathy. In addition to the more extensive dissection and longer CPB times associated with redo procedures, the etiology of increased bleeding includes preoperative anticoagulant therapy, CPB-induced platelet dysfunction, hemodilution of clotting factors, hypothermia, and fibrinolysis. The use of antifibrinolytic agents, such as tranexamic acid or e-aminocaproic acid, is recommended to decrease perioperative bleeding with potential dose adjustments for preexisting renal insufficiency. Perioperative bleeding should be treated early to avoid the additional morbidity associated with mediastinal reentry. Clinical signs of coagulopathy, as well as repeat measurements of the collagen-activated platelet count and clotting function with rapid tests, such as a thromboelastogram (TEG), should guide blood product administration. In rare cases, recombinant factor VII may be useful for control coagulopathy but should not be the first-line agent.

Postoperatively, there is a higher incidence of stroke, myocardial infarction, respiratory failure requiring prolonged mechanical ventilation, and renal failure in elderly patients undergoing redo cardiac surgery. However, the short- and long-term outcomes of redo cardiac procedures have improved due to advances in surgical technique, increasing experience, and greater attention to perioperative management. This has led to acceptable risks for elderly patients facing reoperation despite the fact that redo surgery remains a significant risk factor for operative mortality [2]. In addition, different approaches, such as a right thoracotomy for mitral valve surgery or a left thoracotomy for coronary revascularization, may further reduce the risk of sternal reentry in select patients.

References

1. Krane M, Bauernschmitt R, Hiebinger A, et al. Cardiac reoperation in patients aged 80 years and older. Ann Thorac Surg. 2009;87:1379–85.
2. Yap CH, Sposato L, Akowuah E, et al. Contemporary results show repeat coronary artery bypass grafting remains a risk factor for operative mortality. Ann Thorac Surg. 2009;87:1386–91.
3. Kaplan JA, Reich DL, Lake CL, Konstadt SN, editors. Kaplan's cardiac anesthesia. 5th ed. Philadelphia: Elsevier Saunders; 2006.
4. DiNardo JA, Zvara DA. Anesthesia for cardiac surgery. 3rd ed. Malden: Blackwell Publishing; 2008.

Options for Advanced Mechanical Support for Cardiogenic Shock Complicating Cardiac Reoperations

9

Christian Bermudez, Kenji Minakata, and Robert L. Kormos

Mechanical cardiac support has had a fascinating development over the past 4 decades. With the widespread application of cardiopulmonary bypass (CPB) for cardiac interventions, since its first use in 1953 by Dr. Gibbon [1], and the ability to understand the potential and complications of circulatory support, efforts were soon initiated to mechanically replace the heart and to simply support the failing myocardium to allow recovery. Because of the concerns and scrutiny of the initial use of a totally artificial heart (TAH) in 1969 by Dr. Cooley [2], it was not until the mid-1980s, with the first report of the use of a ventricular assist device (VAD) as bridge to transplant by Dr. Portner [3], that mechanical support became a popular method to assist patients with advanced heart failure. Since then, there has been a rapid rise in the number of VADs implanted each year, with more than 800 VAD implantations – including left ventricular assist devices (LVADs), biventricular assist devices (BiVADs), and TAHs – performed for different indications in the United States in 2009 [4]. The experience in patient selection and management of individual centers has contributed to this explosive increase in VAD use but the biggest factor contributing to increased VAD use has likely been the improvements in VAD technology, from the original reports of pulsatile pump use, to the more sophisticated axial flow pumps, and lately centrifugal flow pumps.

The indications for mechanical circulatory support (MCS) include the inability to wean patients safely from CPB (postcardiotomy shock), acute cardiogenic shock syndromes, and various degrees of chronic decompensated heart failure. When chronic decompensated heart failure is the indication for the use of MCS, individual assessment of etiology, patient characteristics, heart transplantation eligibility, and the ability of the native myocardium to overcome the acute event will dictate if the patient is considered a candidate for temporary support to allow myocardial recovery (bridge to recovery), a candidate for heart transplant (bridge to transplant), or a candidate for use of the device as definitive and permanent support (destination therapy). These arbitrary definitions may change, not infrequently, after support initiation depending on the condition and characteristics of the patient.

In cases of acutely decompensated heart failure, the use of a temporary VAD as a bridge to decision is preferred, in most cases, to stabilize the patient, avoiding overutilization of resources and increasing the complexity of the patient management. The etiologies of cardiogenic shock are most commonly acute myocardial infarction (AMI), failure to wean from CPB, acute decompensation of chronic heart failure, acute myocarditis, peripartum cardiomyopathy, and other cardiac disorders, such as valvular disorders and congenital defects. Despite maximal medical therapy with multiple inotropes and vasoactive

C. Bermudez, MD (✉) • K. Minakata, MD
• R.L. Kormos, MD
Department of Cardiothoracic Surgery, University of Pittsburgh Medical Center, Pittsburgh, PA, USA
e-mail: bermudezc@upmc.edu

V.R. Machiraju et al. (eds.), *Redo Cardiac Surgery in Adults*,
DOI 10.1007/978-1-4614-1326-4_9, © Springer Science+Business Media, LLC 2012

medications and intra-aortic balloon pump (IABP) support, the mortality rate remains high for patients with cardiogenic shock [5]. Patients who are marginally stabilized with medical therapy and IABP may be candidates for revascularization or other surgical treatment. In these cases, the interventional or surgical procedure can be performed with MCS on standby. For patients who experience cardiac arrest or who are hemodynamically unstable, the only means of survival is temporary MCS. The primary goal of circulatory assistance with a temporary VAD is to rapidly restore adequate hemodynamics to avoid the development of multiple system organ failure (MSOF). Patients with MSOF due to cardiogenic shock or cardiac arrest have very poor outcomes with long-term implantable LVADs [6].

Assessing the potential for myocardial recovery begins with the initiation of temporary VAD support. Renal, hepatic, pulmonary, and neurologic dysfunctions are frequently assessed to determine severity and reversibility. During support, many patients with MSOF will show improvements that allow consideration of other treatment options, such the use of a long-term device or even a heart transplant, if a donor organ becomes available [7, 8]. Patients with MSOF and a severe irreversible neurologic deficit should not undergo implantation with a long-term device, and consideration to discontinuing VAD support should be given. Assessment of neurologic function is vital before the conversion from a short-term device to a long-term implantable device to avoid use of a costly device in nonviable patients. Recovery and device explant are considered only when renal, hepatic, pulmonary, and neurologic functions are improved. Palliative care with device removal may be necessary for patients without hope for substantial recovery of neurologic function.

The clinical presentation, technologies available, and clinician's expertise will dictate the selection of support in a variety of situations. The mechanical support used in patients with acute decompensated heart failure, including the inability to wean from CPB, cardiogenic shock following an AMI, or acute myocarditis, may differ from the support used in patients with more stable

Table 9.1 Current devices available for mechanical support

Pulsatile	Nonpulsatile
Implantable	*Implantable*
Novacor	DeBakey
HeartMate I XVE	HeartMate II
Thoratec IVAD	Jarvik 2000
CardioWest C-70 TAH	VentrAssist
AbioCor TAH	Others (CorAide, DuraHeart, Evaheart, HeartMate III, HeartWare, Inc.)
Novacor II	
Extracorporeal	*Extracorporeal*
Thoratec PVAD	CentriMag
Abiomed AB 5000 (ventricle)	TandemHeart
Abiomed BVS 5000 (column)	BioMedicus
	Impella

presentations, such as patients with progression of previously stable heart failure in New York Heart Association (NYHA) functional class IIIb or IV. The intended time of support (short term vs. long term), the need for univentricular or biventricular support, and expertise at the individual center are also crucial factors at the time of support selection.

With years of experience, it became clear that noncardiac organ failure is the major cause of death after implantation of MCS. This fatal progression is seen, not infrequently, in patients with acute presentation and advanced cardiogenic shock, with mortality of 50–70% on support regardless of the strategy utilized [9]. The costs and expectations associated with more chronic support have forced the consideration of temporary, less invasive, and less costly support systems in certain acute situations, which gave rise to the bridge-to-bridge concept [10]. The types of support available are described in Table 9.1.

Extracorporeal or paracorporeal devices that allow uni- or biventricular support are generally associated with ease of implantation, and their use is intended for short- or mid-term support. For this reason, these devices are mainly considered for management of acute clinical presentations including postcardiotomy shock, severe hemodynamic deterioration (shock) after MI, acute myocarditis, and in patients with severe ventricular arrhythmias that preclude the use of an LVAD alone. Examples of extra- or paracorporeal devices include the Thoratec PVAD (paracorporeal VAD) (Thoratec, Pleasanton, CA), the Abiomed BVS, and AB 5000 (Abiomed, Danvers, MA), and centrifugal pumps, such as the CentriMag (Levitronix, Waltham, MA). Percutaneous devices worthy of mention for short-term temporary support, especially for management of critical hemodynamic deterioration, include extracorporeal membrane oxygenation (ECMO), the TandemHeart VAD (Cardiac Assist Inc, Pittsburgh, PA), and the Impella cardiac assist device (Abiomed).

Implantable LVADs are used if more prolonged assistance is considered to support the left ventricle as bridge to transplantation or as destination therapy (permanent support). In general, LVADs are used in patients in more stable clinical condition for whom a careful management plan has been discussed. LVAD implantation also requires certain anatomical and physiologic conditions, such as adequate right ventricular function. LVADs have experienced transcendental development with the evolution from first-generation pulsatile pumps to second- and third-generation LVADs (axial and centrifugal flow pumps, respectively) with more sophisticated designs. These include the HeartMate II (Thoratec), Jarvik 2000 (Jarvik Heart Inc., New York, NY), MicroMed/DeBakey VAD (MicroMed Technology Inc., Houston, TX), VentrAssist VAD (Ventracor, New South Wales, Australia), HeartWare (HeartWare Inc, Framingham, MA), Evaheart (Evaheart Medical USA, Pittsburgh, PA), and INCOR (Berlin Heart, Berlin, Germany).

In parallel to the technical evolution of circulatory support devices, multiinstitutional registries (the International Society of Heart and Lung Transplantation (ISHLT) registry and subsequently the Interagency Registry for Mechanically Assisted Circulatory support (INTERMACS)) and large reports from experienced institutions have provided valuable information to categorize different clinical presentations and specific outcomes, facilitating patient and support selection. This combination of improved technology and better patient and support selection has facilitated a rapid improvement in the results of VAD support, which approach those of heart transplantation in specific patient populations [11].

The objective of this review is to analyze the use of mechanical support with specific considerations to reoperative cardiac surgery. It is not the intent of this chapter to neither review all support types available, nor describe in detail the engineering or biocompatibility concepts involved in their design. We will briefly present the support systems most frequently used when patients fail to wean from CPB after redo surgery, along with general concepts for device selection.

Reintervention is one of the most important risk factors for postoperative mortality after coronary bypass, valve repair or replacement, and other cardiac operations [12]. Improvements in surgical techniques and myocardial protection should theoretically minimize the occurrence of these events, but contrarily, the increasing age, comorbidities, and advanced ventricular dysfunction at presentation, in most cases, often after multiple percutaneous interventions, make postoperative ventricular dysfunction an unpleasant but not unexpected complication requiring advanced support in 1–3% of patients [13]. An understanding of the basic strategies and alternatives in postcardiotomy support has become crucial for every cardiac surgeon.

Patients with severe cardiac dysfunction after CPB who have not responded to inotropic and IABP therapy may be considered for more advanced support. Even though the use of IABP therapy has been considered as a first-line treatment in cardiogenic shock, recent reviews and a meta-analysis on the use of IABP therapy for cardiogenic shock accompanying an AMI have shown an absence of a survival benefit at 30 days and an increased rate of stroke and bleeding complications when compared with patients in whom IABP was not used [14]. The use of a more aggressive early circulatory support in patients with severe cardiac dysfunction after CPB may facilitate ventricular unloading increasing the chances of myocardial recovery and survival [15].

After reasonable attempts to correct incomplete or inadequate revascularization or technical problems related to valvular interventions that could be the cause of early postoperative ventricular dysfunction and adequate attempts to wean CPB, circulatory support should not be delayed. The rationale underlying the early use of circulatory support is maintenance of adequate systemic perfusion and prevention of multiorgan failure. Accepted criteria for circulatory support in postcardiotomy shock include a cardiac index less than 2.0 L/min/m^2, systolic blood pressure less than 90 mmHg, and pulmonary capillary wedge pressure greater than 20 mmHg, with evidence of poor organ perfusion, manifested by oliguria and cool extremities, despite adequate inotropic support and use of IABP therapy.

Richenbacher et al. first reported the concept that early hemodynamic stabilization with an LVAD minimizes the risk of hypoperfusion, sequelae, and complications [16]. A less obvious beneficial effect of early support is the left ventricular unloading effect, which decreases myocardial oxygen consumption, reduces left ventricular work, improves myocardial perfusion, and allows recovery of myocardium at risk [17, 18]. Early placement based on predictive models that utilize hemodynamic parameters and levels of inotropic support provide improved rates of weaning and survival to hospital discharge [19].

In addition to the IABP, the most frequently used support systems in postcardiotomy failure include ECMO, pulsatile paracorporeal VADs, such as the Thoratec PVAD, Abiomed BVS 5000, and Abiomed AB 5000, and centrifugal pumps, such as the Levitronix CentriMag. Other technologies, initially designed for percutaneous left ventricular support, have more recently become alternatives for use in postcardiotomy failure including the TandemHeart VAD and Impella microaxial blood pump. Each device is discussed in detail in the following.

Intra-Aortic Balloon Pump

Circulatory support with the IABP has been the mainstay of acute heart failure treatment for over 40 years. Since the first use of the IABP for support of patients with cardiogenic shock in 1968 [20], this device has been the most widely used MCS system with more than 42,000 implantations performed in the United States annually [21]. Initially requiring surgical insertion due to its large size, the introduction of a percutaneous version of the IABP catheter in the early 1980s allowed widespread use. Further improvements, including prefolded balloons and smaller devices, which enable insertion without sheath introducer, have made the IABP one of the preferred systems of cardiologists and cardiothoracic surgeons for the management of left ventricular dysfunction.

The IABP consists of a polyethylene balloon mounted on a double-lumen catheter. The external lumen allows the flux of gas needed for inflation with helium, which has a low density and rapid diffusion coefficient, or carbon dioxide, which has a high solubility in blood and reduces the potential consequences of gas embolization. The central lumen provides access to the guidewire used for percutaneous placement. The IABP catheter is usually inserted into the descending thoracic aorta via the femoral artery and is attached to an external control console. After placement in the proximal descending aorta, the balloon is connected to a drive console that includes a pressurized gas reservoir and a monitor for electrocardiogram (ECG) and pressure wave recording. The drive console allows adjustments in inflation–deflation timing, ideally coordinating inflation with the onset of diastole and deflation just before the onset of systole. This is accomplished using the patient's ECG signal, arterial waveform, or an intrinsic pump rate. The principal effects of the IABP are to increase myocardial oxygen supply and decrease myocardial oxygen demand (left ventricular wall tension) associated with the improvement in diastolic coronary blood flow and the observed reduction in left ventricular afterload. Secondary effects are improvements in cardiac output and ejection fraction and decreases in heart rate and pulmonary capillary wedge pressure [22, 23].

The indications for IABP use have evolved throughout the years. Originally developed to treat cardiogenic shock complicating an AMI, the IABP has now been applied to diverse unstable cardiac conditions, including unstable angina refractory to medical therapy, mechanical complications of AMI, postcardiotomy failure, ischemia-related ventricular arrhythmias, heart failure refractory to medical therapy, and support for high-risk percutaneous coronary intervention and surgical coronary revascularization [24]. The contraindications to IABP use include severe aortic regurgitation, aortic dissection, significant peripheral vascular disease, and contraindications to heparinization. Although different complications of the IABP have been described; the vascular, embolic, and hemorrhagic complications are the most clinically relevant. Limb ischemia ranged from 2 to 5% in some series and careful assessment, and heparinization should be considered if prolonged support is required [25].

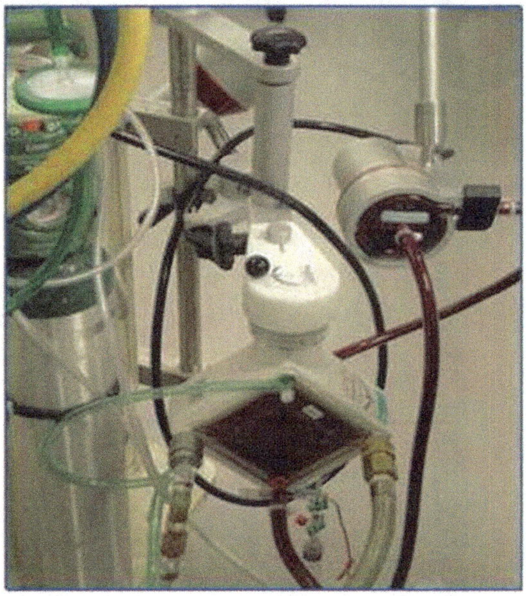

Fig. 9.1 ECMO system combining the use of a centrifugal pump and an oxygenator

Extracorporeal Membrane Oxygenation

ECMO combines a centrifugal or roller pump with an oxygenator (membrane or hollow fiber) (Fig. 9.1). ECMO carries the advantages of providing rapid hemodynamic stabilization and cardiac and respiratory support with up to 6 L/min of nonpulsatile flow even in the presence of severe hypoxemia, which is not infrequent after a prolonged period of CPB. ECMO can be used in central configuration (preferred after prolonged CPB) usually with inflow from the right atrium and outflow in the distal ascending aorta. This is the most frequent approach used for ECMO implantation following unsuccessful weaning from CPB (postcardiotomy failure). Peripheral cannulation (femoral or subclavian artery and femoral vein) is used for acute cardiopulmonary collapse in a nonsurgical environment. Peripheral cannulation is performed percutaneously using the Seldinger technique (femoral vein and femoral artery) with cannula ranging from 17 to 21 Fr for arterial cannulation and 25–29 Fr for venous cannulation, depending on patient's size and characteristics. Occasionally, an 8-mm Dacron graft is anastomosed to the femoral artery for cannula placement to minimize the risk of ischemic complications of the lower extremity [26], but this can be impractical in emergent situations and associated with significant bleeding in the presence of coagulopathy. One of the disadvantages of peripheral cannulation is the inability to effectively decompress the left ventricle if there is an absence of left ventricular function requiring further transseptal drainage of the left atrium or direct surgical implantation of left ventricular, left atrial, or pulmonary arterial drainage. The central cannulation strategy may facilitate ventricular unloading, especially when ventricular contraction is absent or limited, in which case, the peripheral approach may have limited use.

ECMO support has been associated with acceptable outcomes in advanced cardiogenic shock cases, such as those present in acute myocarditis, pulmonary embolism, AMI, and postcardiotomy failure [27–29]. Large institutional reports of ECMO use in postcardiotomy failure [30–32] have shown in-hospital survival rates ranging from 24 to 38%. Despite improvements in pump and oxygenator design, ECMO is still associated with renal (65%), gastrointestinal (18%), bleeding (62%), cerebral (17%), and vascular (16%) complications as well as increased risk of infection, as was evident in a recent, large institutional report [33]. These complications could appear early after ECMO initiation and

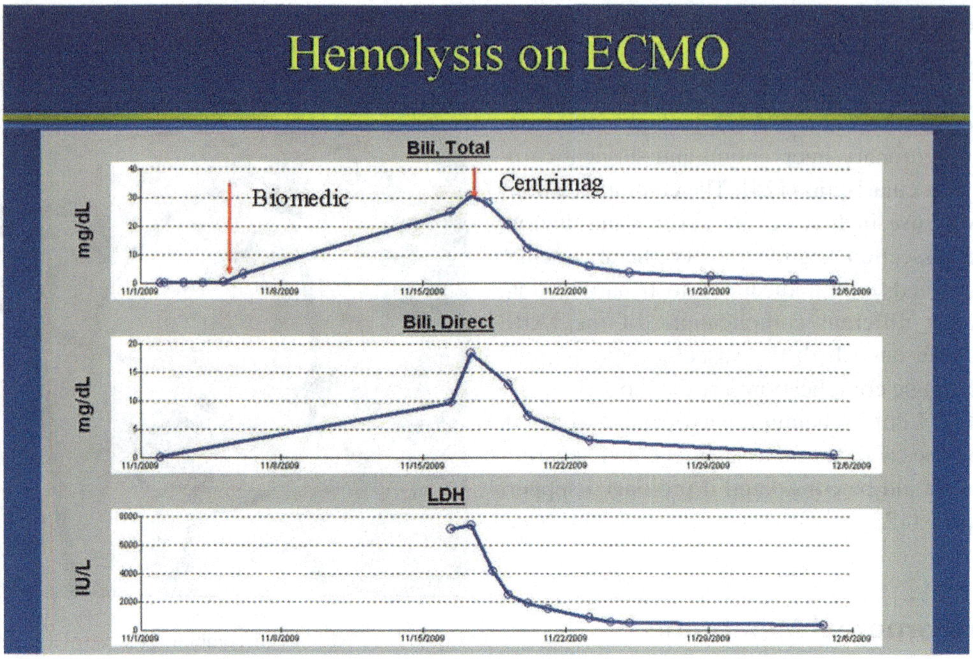

Fig. 9.2 Clinical case of significant hemolysis on ECMO support utilizing first the BioMedicus pump and then the CentriMag. The oxygenator was unchanged

limited the duration of support to 3–7 days in the above-mentioned series.

Despite these potential complications, ECMO is still the most frequently used support in post-cardiotomy shock due to its ability to support hemodynamic and respiratory function, which is frequently affected after prolonged CPB. Our institutional experience (unpublished data) in the postcardiotomy population parallels other series. ECMO use in postcardiotomy shock correlates with a better outcome after coronary bypass failure but a dismal outcome with mortality close to 90–100% in patients with combined coronary bypass surgery and aortic or mitral valve procedures (18 patients from 2003 to 2008), as also reported by Mohr and colleagues [32]. In contrast, the use of ECMO as bridge to decision (recovery or VAD) in cardiogenic shock (non-postcardiotomy) in 42 patients treated at our institution between 2003 and 2008 demonstrated an adequate survival of 57% at 30 days and 53% at 1 year [33], manifesting the influence of the activation of the inflammatory system and organ dysfunction after prolonged CPB rather than inadequate support.

In ECMO, the oxygenator and tubing increase the risk of platelet activation and destruction, which increases the risk of thromboembolic complications. For this reason, strict anticoagulation protocols with activated clotting times (ACTs) ranging from 180 to 220 s are needed and generally require the initiation of heparin hours after CPB with the subsequent risk of significant postoperative bleeding and transfusion requirements. Historically, ECMO systems were mounted with BioMedicus (Medtronic, Minneapolis, MN) centrifugal pumps. Recently, magnetically levitated centrifugal pumps, such as the CentriMag (Levitronix) and Rotaflow (Maquet Corp, Wayne, New Jersey), have facilitated longer support with lower levels of hemolysis and fewer hemorrhagic complications, as seen in our institutional experience (Fig. 9.2).

In situations where left ventricular recovery seems remote or unlikely after CPB, as seen in patients with severe preoperative dysfunction or incomplete revascularization due to inadequate targets, a device more capable of long-term support with the potential to allow patient mobilization and transition the patient to heart transplant should be considered.

Thoratec Paracorporeal Ventricular Assist Device

The Thoratec paracorporeal ventricular assist device (PVAD) is a pneumatically driven pump that can support or substitute for the function of the right or left ventricle and has been considered the workhorse of VADs since its approval as bridge to transplant in 1995 and approval for patients after cardiotomy failure in 1998. The Thoratec PVAD has a 65-mL stroke volume blood pumping chamber made of Thoralon polyurethane and two mechanical valves. With the use of a console or a portable pneumatic driver (such as the Thoratec TLC II), the Thoratec PVAD produces a clinical beat range of 40–110 beats/min and a flow rate of 1.3–7.2 L/min (Fig. 9.3). The PVAD is positioned paracorporeally on the anterior abdominal wall and is suitable for use in smaller patients (body surface area as small as 0.73 m^2). This pulsatile pump allows LVAD, BiVAD, or right ventricular assist device (RVAD) support as needed. The PVAD requires surgical implantation, and the most frequently used cannulation configuration for left ventricular support is in the left ventricular apex, with a 12–15-mm inflow cannula and a 14–18-mm Dacron outflow graft anastomosed to the ascending aorta. Right ventricular support has most frequently drained the right atrium with an 11-mm inflow cannula and a 14–18-mm graft anastomosed to the pulmonary artery. Although left atrial cannulation is easy to insert and remove with minimal dissection or myocardial damage, in practice only right atrial cannulation is used. Direct left ventricular cannulation provides higher VAD flows with a lower risk of thromboembolism especially after AMI and also allows for better decompression of the left ventricle, which may reduce infarct size, improving chances of recovery.

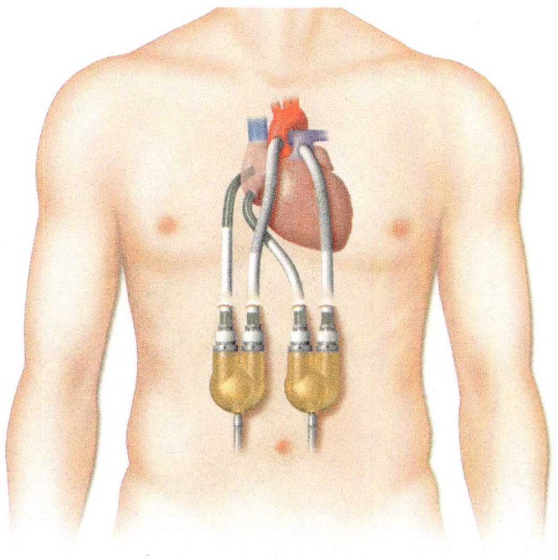

Fig. 9.3 Thoratec PVAD (BiVAD configuration) (reprinted with the permission of Thoratec Corporation)

The use of the PVAD in postcardiotomy patients from the Thoratec registry was associated with survival rates of 44.7% for patients requiring LVAD support (253 patients) and 32.4% for patients requiring BiVAD support. The mean support duration was 21.9 days with 31.2% of the patients requiring BiVAD, 42.8% requiring LVAD, and 13.4% requiring RVAD support [34]. Our institutional experience with the Thoratec PVAD has been extensive with more than 200 PVAD pumps implanted with a survival to transplantation of 74% of cases with LVAD support and 54% of cases with BiVAD support with 17 devices explanted in the total supported population including postcardiotomy support.

Abiomed BVS 5000 and AB 5000 Assist Devices

The BVS 5000 system was the first cardiac assist device approved by the FDA for postcardiotomy support (1992) (Fig. 9.4a).This short-term external pulsatile assist device is capable of providing left, right, or biventricular support. The BVS 5000 system has an upper chamber (atrium) that fills by gravity and a lower pump (ventricle) that

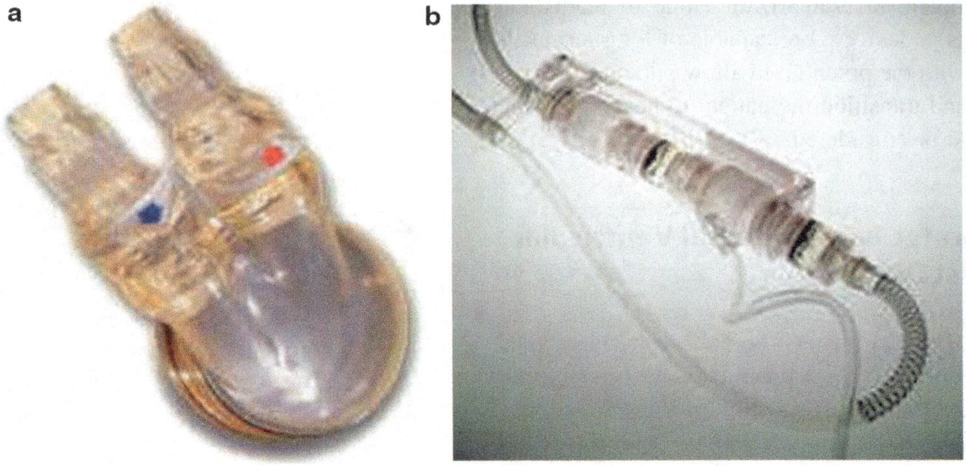

Fig. 9.4 (**a**) Abiomed AB 5000 and (**b**) Abiomed BVS 5000 (used with the permission of Abiomed)

propels the blood out of the pump. Each chamber contains a 100-mL polyurethane bladder. The ventricular pump collapses, via compressed air, ejecting blood to the patient. Inflow cannulas (32–42 Fr) are placed in the right atrium, left atrium, or left ventricle, and outflow cannulas are connected through a 10–12-mm Dacron graft to the pulmonary artery or aorta depending on the type of support required. The cannula design, grafts sizes, and implantation techniques have been adapted to allow consideration of device removal after myocardial recovery.

In the Abiomed Registry, 63% of Abiomed implantations were in postcardiotomy patients with an average age of 56 years. Mean duration of support was 5 days and the longest duration of support was 90 days. Postcardiotomy support resulted in survival in 30%. When the pump was inserted within 3 h of the decision to implant, survival was 60 vs. 20% when insertion was delayed. Success with LVAD support alone was higher than with biventricular support, reflecting the severity of myocardial involvement when BiVAD support is required [35].

The Abiomed AB 5000 is a fully automatic, vacuum-assisted console with a paracorporeal, pneumatically driven, pulsatile pump that allows right, left, or biventricular support (Fig. 9.4b). The pump houses an Angioflex® membrane and two tri-leaflet valves. The pump, connected to cannulas placed in the heart, fills with blood by gravitational force and by vacuum assistance from the drive console. The cannulas and drive console are the same as those used for the BVS 5000. The AB 5000 can provide flow rates of up to 6 L/min. The AB 5000 is utilized in postcardiotomy failure based on data from its predecessor (BVS 5000); the available information suggests improved performance with the AB 5000 if longer support required. In a multicenter, United States registry with 100 patients implanted between 2003 and 2006 for cardiogenic shock following an AMI, 47% required LVAD support, 45% BiVAD, and 8% RVAD with a 30-day survival of 40%. Of these patients, 63% recovered enough left ventricular function to allow removal of the mechanical support. The average time of support-to-recovery was 25 days [36].

Levitronix CentriMag

Levitronix CentriMag is a short-term VAD and extracorporeal system composed of a centrifugal blood pump, an electromagnetic motor, a drive console, an ultrasonic flow probe, and a tubing circuit (Fig. 9.5). The motor generates the magnetic bearing force that levitates the rotor into the pump housing. The magnetic levitation allows the absence of bearings and seals, resulting in

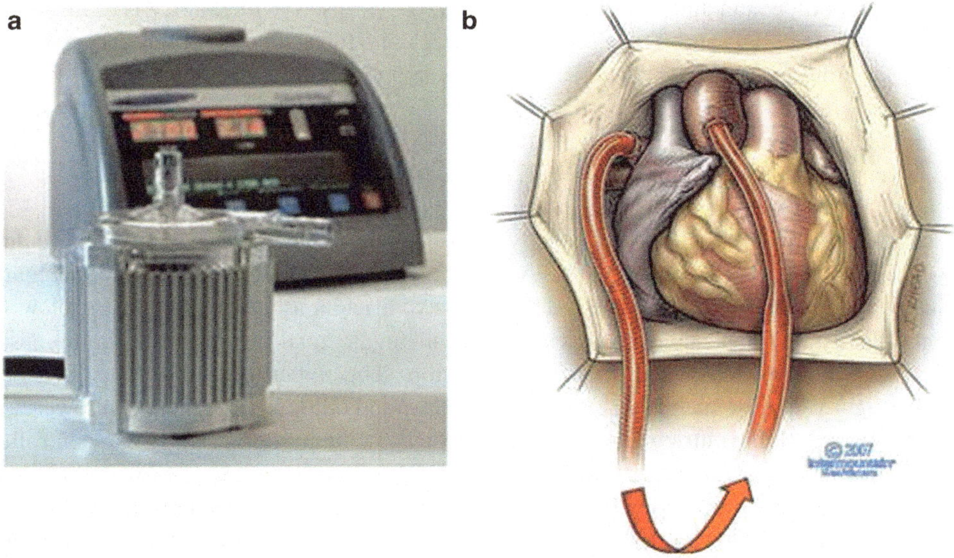

Fig. 9.5 (**a**) CentriMag centrifugal pump with (**b**) cannulation technique for left heart bypass (*left panel*: reprinted with the permission of Thoratec Corporation; *right panel*: used with the permission of Intermountain Healthcare)

minimal friction or heat generation. The device can produce flows up to 10 L/min at a maximum rotational speed of 5,500 rpm under normal physiologic conditions with a priming volume of 31 mL. This magnetic levitation pump is designed to provide high blood flow rates, but with low shear stress on blood components. The small artificial surface area of the CentriMag pump, the absence of device-generated heat, and high blood flow rate minimizes thrombogenicity and may allow for moderate levels anticoagulation during support. Hemolysis has been minimal in the majority of patients supported. The CentriMag pump can be used in an LVAD, RVAD, or BiVAD configuration with cannulation of the left ventricular apex, left atrium, or right atrium for inflow and aorta or pulmonary artery for outflow.

European clinical trials of the CentriMag in postcardiotomy cardiogenic shock have been encouraging with mean support periods of 2 weeks and support for up to 64 days. Overall, 30-day mortality is 50%, which compares favorably with other devices [37]. CentriMag application in other types of acute cardiogenic shock, using the device as bridge to transplant or recovery, is associated with up to 72% survival at 1 month, with some studies demonstrating acceptable outcomes of support for up to 3 months [38]. Our recently reported institutional experience [39] demonstrated a 43% weaning rate from the CentriMag VAD, when used as an RVAD in postcardiotomy shock. Another advantage for CentriMag use in postcardiotomy patients is the ability to connect an oxygenator to the system, transforming the system into ECMO support with oxygenation capabilities. For these reasons, and due to low hemolysis and thromboembolic complication rates, the CentriMag pump has been our preferred support system for isolated right or left ventricular dysfunction postoperatively.

Considerations for Biventricular Support

Although univentricular support is appealing for many reasons, biventricular support is sometimes necessary. However, the addition of an RVAD to an LVAD is not without complications, including (1) technical aspects of crowding the mediastinum with extra cannulae that may prevent sternal closure, (2) additional bleeding sites associated with inflow and outflow attachments to the right heart, and (3) balancing left and right flows. The advantage of adding an RVAD is obvious: total control of the circulation. This is particularly valuable in the setting of profound circulatory collapse or ventricular dysrhythmia [40, 41]. The indication for BiVAD support in the acute setting is also relatively simple: inadequate hemodynamic parameters in the presence of an LVAD alone. Such conditions may arise if there is direct right ventricular dysfunction, such as a right ventricular infarct/ischemia, or secondary conditions affecting the right ventricle, such as massive pulmonary embolism or right ventricular failure due to left ventricular failure. Occasionally (10–20%), the right ventricle may fail following LVAD implantation – specifically when inflow is established from the left ventricle proper – due to distortion of the ventricular septum, geometric disfigurement of the right ventricle, and subsequent dysfunction [42]. Although originally described in association with implantable LVADs in patients with chronic heart failure, this phenomenon has been observed in the short-term device setting as well. Regardless of the cause, management of the right ventricle when an LVAD is implanted is not very different from management without an LVAD. The usual things to consider for right ventricular protection and enhancement of function include (1) ensuring adequate coronary circulation to the right ventricle by grafting stenotic or occluded right coronary artery (RCA) vessels if warranted; (2) dissipating any inadvertent air embolization within the RCA territory by venting the aortic root to remove air as the LVAD is ejecting and wait for the ST segment elevation associated with air emboli to the RCA to normalize; (3) avoiding fluid (crystalloid or colloid products) overload by controlling bleeding; (4) treating reversible pulmonary hypertension by using inhalational or intravenous agents that can augment right ventricular performance and reducing pulmonary artery pressure with agents such as milrinone, epoprostenol, and nitric oxide; (5) avoiding myocardial compression by considering leaving the sternum open to afford enough "play" for the heart to beat without the extra compression caused by sternal approximation. Finally, the RVAD (if used with an LVAD) may only be necessary for a short duration and removal may be an option while leaving the LVAD in place.

TandemHeart

The TandemHeart is a temporary ventricular support system, originally designed for percutaneous left ventricular assistance, driven by a low-speed, centrifugal, dual-chambered, continuous flow pump. The upper pump housing provides the inflow and outflow ports while the lower housing provides communication with the controller and an integral infusion line to provide local cooling and anticoagulation. The pump's impeller rotates at speeds ranging from 3,000 to 7,000 rpm and can generate flow up to 4 L/min. The unique feature of this device is the requirement for placement of the inflow cannula transseptally into the left atrium. The 21-Fr polyurethane inflow cannula has a large end hole and multiple side holes to maintain patency. Cannulation for device implementation is usually performed in the cardiac catheterization laboratory with fluoroscopic guidance. A septal puncture is first performed with Brockenbrough needle passed through a Mullins sheath in the right atrium. A 0.035-in. pigtail guidewire is inserted into the left atrium, and a two-stage (14/21 Fr) dilator is used to dilate the opening in the atrial septum. The inflow cannula is then passed over the wire into the left atrium. Outflow is provided through a 15 or 17-Fr cannula that is placed in the contralateral femoral artery. The pump is placed on the patient's leg near the arterial return cannula. A bedside console provides monitoring and control functions, and it supplies a continuous flow of a heparinized solution to the bearings of the pump. With optimal facilities, equipment, and personnel, support with the TandemHeart can be accomplished within an hour of initial presentation.

The device has been most extensively used for short-term left ventricular support during high-risk percutaneous coronary interventions and treatment of post-infarct cardiogenic shock [43, 44]. Contraindications to TandemHeart support include isolated right ventricular failure, ventricular septal defect (due to the potential for significant right-to-left shunting), and severe peripheral vascular disease. Potential serious device-related complications are persistent patent foramen ovale, limb ischemia, and thromboembolism. In addition, there is the potential for dislodgement of the inflow cannula into the right atrium, which would result in right-to-left shunting and a loss of support.

Reports of TandemHeart use in cardiogenic shock demonstrated acceptable support for days, improving hemodynamic parameters and allowing myocardial recovery or as a bridge to a more permanent device or transplantation with survival rate close to 50% [45]. The presence of vascular complication (14–23%) and bleeding complications from cannulation sites (11–30%) [46, 47] have encouraged TandemHeart use with alternative cannulation strategies, including the central approach (left atrium, ascending aorta), with weaning rates of up to 72% and survival to discharge in 54% of patients, with average support time of 3–4 days, in recent series of postcardiotomy failure [33]. Despite these encouraging results with the use of this and other percutaneous devices to support patients in cardiogenic shock, a recent meta-analysis of controlled trials of these technologies (TandemHeart and Impella) did not show any improvement in survival when compared with IABP therapy despite superior hemodynamic support. The presence of increased risks of bleeding and vascular complications cautions against the use of these percutaneous devices as a first-choice approach in the treatment of cardiogenic shock until more data is available [44, 48].

The Abiomed Impella 5.0 and LD

The Impella 5.0 and Impella LD are intravascular microaxial blood pumps intended to provide short-term mechanical support for acutely reduced left ventricular function in the setting of postcardiotomy heart failure refractory to high-dose inotropic and IABP support. The Impella LD device is inserted across the aortic valve through a 10-mm vascular graft sewn to the ascending aorta, avoiding the use of CPB (Fig. 9.6). The Impella 5.0 is designed for peripheral cannulation through cut down of the femoral artery. The pump diameter of

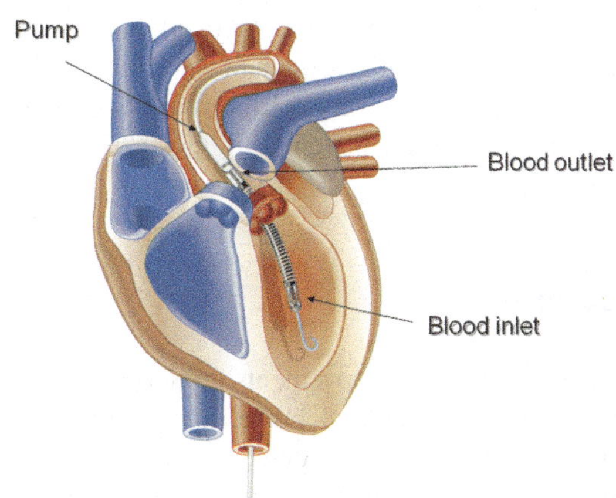

Fig. 9.6 Impella 5.0 (used with the permission of Abiomed)

6.4 mm at the body of the pump and a 7.3-mm at the level of the outflow opening requires adequate vessel size and the absence of peripheral vascular disease if the percutaneous approach is considered. A small electric motor is built into each device, and the 2.8-mm diameter cable leading to the device contains the electrical power supply, which is connected to an external control unit as well as a purge line connected to a purge perfusor, through which heparin is flushed continuously with a pressure of 300–700 mmHg. This 21-Fr microaxial pump is designed to provide between a flow of 3.5–5 L/min at maximal speed (33,000 rpm).

Early postcardiotomy data from three European centers showed the potential of the Impella pump. In patients with residual ventricular function sufficient to generate 1 L/min of flow above the pump flow (3.5–4 L/min), survival was 90%, but survival was only 12% in patients unable to generate 1 L/min of flow due to severe ventricular dysfunction [49]. In the United States, a pilot study designed to be completed in seven centers and originally enrolling 20 patients was not finished after FDA 510(k) approval was obtained for the devices. Unpublished data of 17 patients, supported either centrally or peripherally for postcardiotomy failure, were associated with a 30-day mortality of 12% (two patients) and 6% risk of cerebrovascular events. The average flow was 4.2 L/min and the mean time of support 3.5 days. Other single-center experiences have shown an overall mortality of 50% when used in patients with cardiogenic shock as bridge to transplant or recovery, with up to 66% mortality (two of three patients) in postcardiotomy shock [50].

Summary

Despite all the improvements in surgical techniques and myocardial protection, severe ventricular dysfunction occurs in 1–3% of the patients undergoing cardiac reinterventions. Careful attention to correct incomplete revascularization or inadequate valvular repair/replacement may facilitate ventricular recovery and avoid the need for high doses of inotropic support or advanced mechanical support. When an adequate attempt to remove a patient from CPB fails in the presence of sufficient inotropic support and the use of IABP therapy, early consideration of advanced MCS is necessary. The use of any type of currently available support has its own limitations in these complex situations and per se is associated with mortality in excess of 50%. In reoperative cardiac surgery, the presence of more severe preoperative left ventricular dysfunction, which is frequently seen in redo cardiac surgery patients, and the need for multiple transfusions may increase the degree of pulmonary dysfunction and subsequently cause right ventricular failure. This makes the selection of an adequate support system more complicated for the general cardiac surgeon. Here, we presented a review of the more frequently utilized support systems. In this review, we emphasized systems capable of providing hemodynamic and respiratory support, such as ECMO, and also devices capable of providing left and right ventricular support simultaneously, because severe biventricular dysfunction may be present in ~45% of patients with postcardiotomy shock. The more recent use of percutaneous technologies was briefly mentioned, as these technologies have yielded promising results in a selected group of patients.

The importance of early recognition and management of severe ventricular dysfunction with these advanced support systems may provide better hemodynamic stabilization, prevent multiorgan failure, and allow ventricular unloading, thereby increasing the chances of ventricular recovery. Management in centers with experience in the use of both temporary and more permanent MCS systems is also associated with better outcomes in this high-risk population [51].

References

1. Liotta D, Hall C, Henly W, et al. Prolonged assisted circulation during and after cardiac or aortic surgery. Prolonged partial left ventricular bypass by means of intracorporeal circulation. Am J Cardiol. 1963; 12:399.
2. Cooley DA, Liotta D, Hallman GL, et al. Orthotopic cardiac prothesis for two – staged cardiac replacement. Am J Cardiol. 1969;24(5):723–30.
3. Portner P, Oyer P, McGregor CGA. First human use of an electrically powered implantable ventricular assist system. Artif Organs. 1985;9:36.
4. Interagency Registry for Mechanically assisted circulatory support. http://www.intermacs.org (2011). Accessed 14 Feb 2011.
5. Aggarwal S, Slaughter MS. Acute myocardial infarction complicated by cardiogenic shock: role of mechanical circulatory support. Expert Rev Cardiovasc Ther. 2008;6:1223–35.
6. Kirklin JK, Naftel DC, Kormos RL, Stevenson LW, Pagani FD, Miller MA, et al. Second intermacs annual report: more than 1,000 primary left ventricular assist device implants. J Heart Lung Transplant. 2010; 29:1–10.
7. John R, Liao K, Lietz K, Kamdar F, Colvin-Adams M, Boyle A, et al. Experience with the Levitronix CentriMag circulatory support system as a bridge to decision in patients with refractory acute cardiogenic shock and multisystem organ failure. J Thorac Cardiovasc Surg. 2007;134:351–8.
8. Gregoric ID, Jacob LP, La Francesca S, Bruckner BA, Cohn WE, Loyalka P, et al. The TandemHeart as a bridge to a long-term axial-flow left ventricular assist device (bridge to bridge). Tex Heart Inst J. 2008; 35:125–9.
9. Garatti A, Russo C, Lanfranconi M, et al. Mechanical circulatory support for cardiogenic shock complicating acute myocardial infarction: an experimental and clinical review. ASAIO J. 2007;53:278–87.
10. Pagani F, Lynch W, Swaniker F, et al. Extracorporeal life support to left ventricular assist device bridge to heart transplant: a strategy to optimize survival and resource utilization. Circulation. 1999;100: II206–10.
11. Pagani F et al. Extended mechanical circulatory support with a continuous-flow rotary left ventricular assist device. J Am Coll Cardiol. 2009;54:312–21.

12. Edwards F, Grover F, Shroyer L, et al. The society of thoracic Surgeons cardiac surgery database: current risk assessment. Ann Thorac Surg. 1997;63:903–8.
13. Lee W, Gillinov A, Cameron D, et al. Centrifugal ventricular assist device for support of the failing heart after cardiac surgery. Crit Care Med. 1993; 21:1186–91.
14. Sjauw K, Engström M, Vis M, et al. A systematic review and meta-analysis of intra-aortic balloon pump therapy in ST-elevation myocardial infarction: should we change guidelines? Eur Heart J. 2009;30:459–68.
15. Levin H, Burkoff D, Oz M, et al. Reversal of chronic ventricular dilatation in patients with end-stage cardiomyopathy by prolonged mechanical unloading. Circulation. 1995;91:2717–20.
16. Richenbacher WE, Dash H, Bulck MK, Pierce WS. Utilization of left ventricular assistance in patients with acute myocardial infarction and cardiogenic shock. ASAIO J. 1984;7:32–40.
17. Torre-Amione G et al. Decreased expression of tumor necrosis factor-alpha in failing human myocardium after mechanical circulatory support: a potential mechanism for cardiac recovery. Circulation. 1999; 100:1189–93.
18. Ogletree-Hughes M, Stull L, Sweet W, et al. Mechanical unloading restores beta-adrenergic responsiveness and reverses receptor downregulation in the failing human heart. Circulation. 2001;104:881–6.
19. Samuel L, Holmes E, Thomas M, et al. Management of acute cardiac failure with mechanical assist: experience with the ABIOMED BVS 500. Ann Thorac Surg. 2001;71:S67–72.
20. Kantrowitz A, Tjonneland S, Freed PS, Phillips SJ, Butner AN, Sherman Jr JL. Initial clinical experience with intraaortic balloon pumping in cardiogenic shock. JAMA. 1968;203:113–8.
21. Kozak LJ, Owings MF, Hall MJ: 2005. National Hospital Discharge Survey: 2002 annual summary with detailed diagnosis and procedure data. Vital Health Stat 13:1–199.
22. Sarnoff SJ, Braunwald E, Welch Jr GH, Case RB, Stainsby WN, Macruz R. Hemodynamic determinants of oxygen consumption of the heart with special reference to the tension-time index. Am J Physiol. 1958;192:148–56.
23. Gutterman DD, Cowley Jr AW. Relating cardiac performance with oxygen consumption: historical observations continue to spawn scientific discovery. Am J Physiol Heart Circ Physiol. 2006;291:H2555–6.
24. Cohen M, Urban P, Christenson JT, Joseph DL, Freedman Jr RJ, Miller MF, et al. Intra-aortic balloon counterpulsation in US and non-US centres: results of the benchmark registry. Eur Heart J. 2003;24: 1763–70.
25. Ferguson 3rd JJ, Cohen M, Freedman Jr RJ, Stone GW, Miller MF, Joseph DL, et al. The current practice of intra-aortic balloon counterpulsation: results from the benchmark registry. J Am Coll Cardiol. 2001;38:1456–62.
26. Smith C, Bellomo R, Raman JS, Matalanis G, Rosalion A, Buckmaster J, et al. An extracorporeal membrane oxygenation-based approach to cardiogenic shock in an older population. Ann Thorac Surg. 2001;71:1421–7.
27. Tayara W, Starling R, Yamani M, et al. Improved survival after acute myocardial infarction complicated by cardiogenic shock with circulatory support and transplantation: comparing aggressive intervention with conservative treatment. J Heart Lung Transplant. 2006;25:504–9.
28. Haller I, Kofler A, Lederer W, et al. Acute pulmonary artery embolism during transcatheter embolization: successful resuscitation with veno-arterial extracorporeal membrane oxygenation. Anesth Analg. 2008;107:945–7.
29. Chen J, Ko W, Yu H, et al. Analysis of outcome for patients experiencing myocardial infarction and cardiopulmonary resuscitation refractory to conventional therapies necessitating extracorporeal life support rescue. Crit Care Med. 2006;34:950–7.
30. Smedira N, Moazami N, Golding C, et al. Clinical experience with 202 adults receiving extracorporeal membrane oxygenation for cardiac failure: survival at five years. J Thorac Cardiovasc Surg. 2001;122:92–102.
31. Doll N, Kiaii B, Borger M, et al. Five-year results of 210 consecutive patients treated with extracorporeal membrane oxygenation for refractory postoperative cardiogenic shock. Ann Thorac Surg. 2004;77:151–7.
32. Rastan A, Dege A, Mohr M, et al. Early and late outcomes of 517 consecutive patients treated with extracorporeal membrane oxygenation for refractory postcardiotomy cardiogenic shock. J Thorac Cardiovasc Surg. 2010;139:302–11.
33. Bermudez C, Toyoda Y, Avila F, et al. Use of extracorporeal membrane oxygenation (ECMO) in patients with chronic cardiomyopathy: a word of caution. J Heart Lung Transplant. 2010;29:S179.
34. Hill J, Farrar D, Naka Y, et al. Positive displacement ventricular assist devices. In: Frazier OH, Kirklin JK, editors. ISHLT Monograph Series 1. Elsevier: New York; 2006. p. 53–75.
35. Guyton R, Schonberger J, Everts P, et al. Postcardiotomy shock: clinical evaluation for the BVS 5000 biventricular support system. Ann Thorac Surg. 1993;56:346–56.
36. Anderson M, et al. Mechanical circulatory support improves recovery outcomes in profound cardiogenic shock post AMI. Presented at Transcatheter Therapeutics Oct. 17. Washington; 2006.
37. Shuhaiber J, Jenkins D, Berman M, et al. The Papworth experience with Levitronix CentriMag ventricular assist device. J Heart Lung Transplant. 2008;27:158–64.
38. John R, Liao K, Lietz K, et al. Experience with the Levitronix CentriMag circulatory support system as a bridge to decision in patients with refractory acute cardiogenic shock and multisystem organ failure. J Thorac Cardiovasc Surg. 2007;134:351–8.

39. Bhama J, Kormos R, Toyoda Y, et al. Clinical experience using the Levitronix CentriMag system for temporary right ventricular mechanical circulatory support. J Heart Lung Transplant. 2009;28:971–6.
40. Tsukui H, Teuteberg JJ, Murali S, et al. Biventricular assist device utilization for patients with morbid congestive heart failure: a justifiable strategy. Circulation. 2005;112:165–72.
41. Zhang L, Kapetanakis EI, Cooke RH, et al. Bi-ventricular circulatory support with the Abiomed AB5000 in a patient with idiopathic refractory ventricular fibrillation. Ann Thorac Surg. 2007;83: 298–300.
42. Kormos RL, Gasior T, Antaki J, et al. Evaluation of right ventricular function during clinical left ventricular assistance. ASAIO Trans. 1989;35:547–50.
43. Thiele H, Lauer B, Hambrecht R, et al. Reversal cardiogenic shock by percutaneous left-atrial-to-femoral arterial bypass assistance. Circulation. 2001;104: 2917–22.
44. Thiele H, Sick P, Boudriot E, et al. Randomized comparison of intra-aortic balloon support with a percutaneous left ventricular assist device in patients with revascularized acute myocardial infarction complicated by cardiogenic shock. Eur Heart J. 2005; 26:1276–83.
45. Burkhoff D, O'Neill W, Brunckhorst C, et al. Feasibility study of the TandemHeart percutaneous ventricular assist device for treatment of cardiogenic shock. Catheter Cardiovasc Interv. 2006;68:211–7.
46. Burkhoff D, Cohen H, Brunkhorst C, et al. A randomized multicenter clinical study to evaluate the safety and efficacy of the TandemHeart percutaneous ventricular assist device versus conventional therapy with intra-aortic balloon pumping for treatment of cardiogenic shock. Am Heart J. 2006;152:469.
47. Pitsis A, Visouli A, Burkhoff D, et al. Feasibility study of a temporary percutaneous left ventricular assist device in cardiac surgery. Ann Thoac Surg. 2007;84:1993–9.
48. Cheng J, den Uil C, Hoeks S, et al. Percutaneous left ventricular assist device versus intra-aortic balloon pump counterpulsation for treatment of cardiogenic shock: a meta-analysis of controlled trials. Eur Heart J. 2009;30:2102–8.
49. Siegenthaler M, Brehm K, Strecker T, et al. The impella recover microaxial left ventricular assist device reduces mortality for postcardiotomy failure: a three-center experience. J Thorac Cardiovas Surg. 2004;127:812–22.
50. Garatti A, Colombo T, Russo C, et al. Left ventricular mechanical support with the Impella Recover left direct microaxial blood pump: a single-center experience. Artif Organs. 2006;30:523–8.
51. Goldstein D, Oz M. Mechanical support for postcardiotomy cardiogenic shock. Semin Thorac Cardiovasc Surg. 2000;12:220–8.

Reoperations for Mitral Valve Disease: Surgical Approaches and Techniques

10

Hartzell V. Schaff and Arman Arghami

Introduction

Approximately 10% of all adult cardiac operations involve redo thoracotomy, and clinically significant hemorrhage occurs in up to 8% of patients with a resultant increase in operative morbidity and mortality [1]. Indeed, in some reports, prior cardiac surgery increases the operative risk of mitral valve (MV) surgery almost twofold [2, 3]. Reoperation for MV disease is necessary for a wide variety of problems, such as failure of a previously placed prosthesis, development of a paravalvular leak, endocarditis, or newly diagnosed valve disease in a patient with prior aortic valve replacement or coronary artery bypass. Careful attention to the planning and execution of the operation can minimize surgical risks, and this chapter details those methods that have proved helpful at Mayo Clinic (Rochester, MN) (Fig. 10.1).

H.V. Schaff, MD (✉) • A. Arghami, MD
Division of Cardiovascular Surgery,
Mayo Clinic, Rochester, MN, USA
e-mail: schaff@mayo.edu

Preoperative Preparation

Examination

Several aspects of preoperative clinical examination aid in surgical preparation. For example, patients who require MV reoperation may have clinical signs of associated tricuspid valve regurgitation and right-sided heart failure that can complicate sternal reentry and dissection of the right atrium. Detection of hepatomegaly, especially an enlarged pulsatile liver, suggests tricuspid valve leakage that may need to be corrected during mitral reoperation, and hepatic congestion may also contribute to postoperative coagulopathy. Similarly, patients with marked right ventricular enlargement, especially those with pulmonary artery hypertension, may be at increased risk for myocardial injury during reoperation and peripheral cannulation and institution of cardiopulmonary bypass before dividing the sternum can minimize this risk.

It is also important to carefully assess the adequacy of the femoral vessels and to plan for suitable sites for peripheral cannulation. If there is a question of severe iliofemoral occlusive disease, computerized tomographic angiography (CTA) may be helpful. If there is severe iliofemoral or aortic occlusive disease, preparations should be made for possible cannulation of the axillary artery [4].

V.R. Machiraju et al. (eds.), *Redo Cardiac Surgery in Adults*,
DOI 10.1007/978-1-4614-1326-4_10, © Springer Science+Business Media, LLC 2012

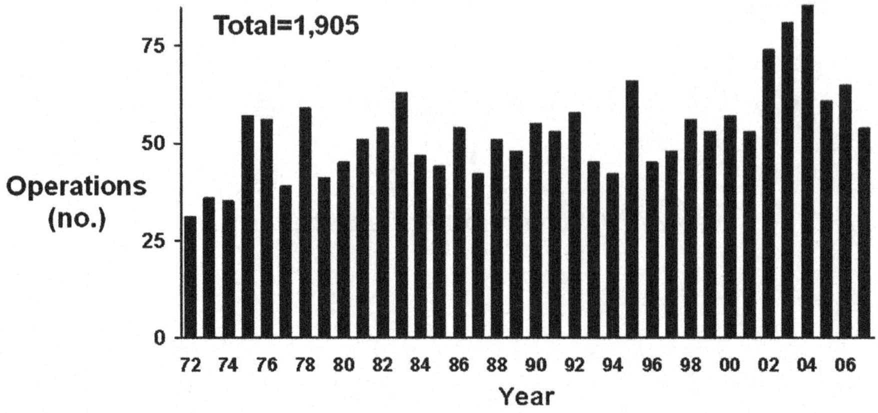

Fig. 10.1 From 1972 through 2007, 1905 patients underwent reoperation for repair or replacement of the mitral valve

Preoperative Imaging

Preoperative chest X-rays are obtained routinely, and lateral views may provide some information on the fullness of the anterior mediastinum and proximity of the heart and great vessels to the sternum. Imaging of the chest with computerized tomographic (CT) scanning is also helpful in providing more detail of the anterior mediastinum and areas of potential injury. Findings that indicate increased risk during sternal reentry include the presence of the right ventricle or aorta <10-mm from the sternum or the presence of a bypass graft crossing the midline <10 mm from the sternum. The usefulness of CT scanning is enhanced by multidetector CT angiography. A retrospective study by Maluenda and associates suggested that preoperative CT scans in patients undergoing cardiac reoperations were associated with shorter perfusion and cross-clamp times, shorter intensive care unit stays, and lower rates of perioperative myocardial infarction [5].

Identification of structures at risk may alter surgical planning. In a small series reported by Aviram et al., operative plans were modified in 6 of 15 patients who underwent repeat coronary revascularization and had preoperative CT scans. These modifications included alternate incisions and cannulation sites as well as changes in plans for myocardial protection [6]. Subsequent reports from the same group suggest a strong trend toward decreased complications in patients who have preoperative multidetector CT scanning [7]. Indeed, Kamdar and associates advocate the routine use of preoperative multidetector CT angiography in patients with prior coronary artery bypass grafting who undergo repeat heart surgery because detection of high-risk findings has a strong association with the adoption of preventive surgical strategies, which they believe has improved surgical outcomes [8].

Preoperative CT imaging is also helpful in determining the presence and extent of calcification of the ascending aorta. Embolic dislodgement of atherosclerotic debris or plaques during surgical manipulation of the aorta is an important cause of perioperative stroke, and in one study, the risk of stroke increased from 1.8% in patients with no aortic disease to 8.6% in patients with documented atherosclerotic disease in the ascending aorta [9].

Cardiac magnetic resonance imaging (MRI) has been used to assess severity of retrosternal adhesions as well as cardiac structure and function. Yoshioka et al. used a technique of tagged cine MRI to assess retrosternal adhesion before redo surgery. With application of a finite element model, determination of strain in the retrosternal area provides a quantitative measure of the severity of adhesion between the sternum and the anterior surface of the heart [10].

In our practice, these additional imaging methods are used liberally but not routinely. For example, we would not obtain such studies in relatively healthy patients undergoing a first MV reoperation who have not had previous coronary artery bypass. However, we would obtain imaging studies in patients having second or third operations, particularly older patients in whom there may be a greater likelihood of atherosclerosis of the ascending aorta and aortic arch.

Hemostasis

Antifibrinolytic drugs, aminocaproic acid or tranexamic acid, are used in all patients undergoing cardiac reoperations at our clinic. These lysine analogs appear equally effective in reducing bleeding and blood transfusions [11], and the use of one agent or the other is determined mainly by cost. At our institution, aminocaproic acid is the most cost-effective. The drug competitively inhibits activation of plasminogen, thereby reducing conversion of plasminogen to plasmin, an enzyme that degrades fibrin clots, fibrinogen and other plasma proteins including the procoagulant factors V and VIII. In high doses, aminocaproic acid also directly inhibits plasmin activity. Our protocol includes a loading dose of 100 mg/kg (e.g., 7 g for a 70-kg patient) that is diluted in 100 mL of normal saline and infused over 30 min. An additional 5 g of aminocaproic acid is added to the priming solution of the cardiopulmonary bypass circuit, and a post-bypass maintenance infusion is used based on the patient's weight and renal function (e.g., 30 mg/kg/h, creatinine <1.6 mg/dL; 20 mg/kg/h, creatinine 1.6–3.2 mg/dL; 10 mg/kg/h, creatinine >3.3 mg/dL; 5 mg/kg/h, creatinine >6.6 mg/dL). The aminocaproic acid infusion should be continued no longer than 2 h into the ICU stay unless a thromboelastogram (TEG) indicates ongoing fibrinolysis.

Antiplatelet therapy is common in patients with cardiac disease, and balance of risk and benefit in patients undergoing reoperation for MV disease is complex. For patients who take only aspirin, we do not routinely advise discontinuation of the medication. Indeed, in patients undergoing primary sternotomy, aspirin use in the perioperative period may reduce adverse cardiac events without increasing the risk of bleeding [12]. Preoperative use of clopidogrel is more problematic. Studies of patients undergoing primary coronary artery bypass operations have documented increased risk of bleeding and need for re-exploration in those who have exposure to clopidogrel 3–5 days preoperatively. Indeed, the manufacturer advises discontinuing the drug for 5 days before elective surgery. Unless there is an urgent indication, reoperation for MV disease should be postponed for at least 5 days after stopping clopidogrel. If such a delay is not practical, preparation should be made for platelet transfusion after cardiopulmonary bypass.

The importance of adequate reversal of warfarin anticoagulation is often overlooked. Patients with MV disease who require anticoagulation can be bridged with unfractionated or fractionated heparin; however, the international normalized ratio (INR) may be slow to return to baseline because of hepatic congestion, and treatment with fresh-frozen plasma or vitamin K will be necessary.

Intraoperative Preparation

Anesthetic management and placement of monitoring lines are similar to primary operations, and transesophageal echocardiography is used in all patients regardless of the surgical approach. An external defibrillator patch is placed to facilitate defibrillation if arrhythmia is provoked during dissection or electrocoagulation and the heart is not fully mobilized. Permanent transvenous pacemakers and defibrillators are reprogramed to avoid interference with the electrocautery. Both groin areas are prepped into the surgical field, and the course of the femoral artery is marked to facilitate subsequent exposure if peripheral cannulation is needed.

Choice of Incision

The choice of incision, resternotomy or right anterolateral thoracotomy, depends on the experience of the surgeon and the need for associated procedures. We prefer a repeat median sternotomy for most patients and believe that this approach is safe and offers the best control of the heart and great vessels. Furthermore, repeat sternotomy allows flexibility if other problems are encountered, such as aortic valve regurgitation, which are underestimated by preoperative examination and echocardiography.

The potential advantages of a lateral thoracotomy for MV reoperation include less dissection and easier avoidance of bypass grafts, particularly those that cross the midline, but there are limitations with a lateral approach in MV reoperations. The lung may be adherent to the right atrium and aorta, and adhesions may prevent safe dissection and isolation of the ascending aorta. Surgeons have managed these problems using peripheral arterial cannulation combined with endoaortic balloon clamping and antegrade cardioplegia [13] or, more commonly, hypothermic ventricular fibrillation during exposure of the valve [14–16]. Indeed, some surgeons use normothermic perfusion and allow the heart to beat during MV reoperation believing this provides the best protection of the myocardium [17, 18]. Avoiding aortic clamping introduces the potential for poor exposure of the MV if there is significant aortic valve regurgitation; also, aortic regurgitation can lead to ventricular distention when the ventricle fibrillates.

Avoiding embolic stroke is a special consideration in the choice of incision for reoperation on the MV. In the experience of Svensson and colleagues, the risk of postoperative stroke was more than twice as high in patients who underwent mitral reoperation via a right thoracotomy compared with patients who had resternotomy (7.5 vs. 2.7%) [19]. Possible mechanisms for this increased risk of neurological dysfunction include embolism from aortic atherosclerosis and retrograde perfusion and incomplete de-airing of the heart. Similarly, Crooke et al. reported that the risk of stroke during MV reoperations was increased fourfold in patients who had retrograde perfusion for cardiopulmonary bypass compared with those who had central aortic cannulation, and they advocate cannulation of the ascending aorta or axillary artery when a lateral thoracotomy is utilized [20].

Resternotomy

Several technical points can increase the safety of resternotomy. First is the decision of whether or not to institute cardiopulmonary bypass prior to dividing the sternum. Extracorporeal circulation and cessation of positive pressure ventilation decompress the heart and lungs, thus minimizing the risk of laceration during resternotomy. This is especially useful when the patient has marked right ventricular and right atrial enlargement and when bypass grafts are near the midline. If cardiopulmonary bypass is not used during initial sternal entry, access for cannulation (femoral or axillary artery, femoral or jugular veins) should be planned (incisions marked) in the event that serious hemorrhage develops.

After the skin incision, the wires are divided and can be left in place to assist in prevention of cardiac injury during sternal opening. For most adult patients, we use an oscillating sagittal saw [21] and initially divide only the anterior table of the sternum. If the divided wires are in place, these are grasped with heavy (Kocher) clamps and pulled upward to further protect substernal structures (Fig. 10.2). Complete division of the sternum begins inferiorly at the xiphisternal junction. Once the inferior-most portion of the sternum is divided, rake retractors are placed on the wound edges, and the assistant retracts upward firmly (Fig. 10.3) but gradually as the adhesions are divided. Particular care should be taken to avoid tearing the innominate vein, which may be encased in scar tissue. This can be especially troublesome if transvenous pacing leads

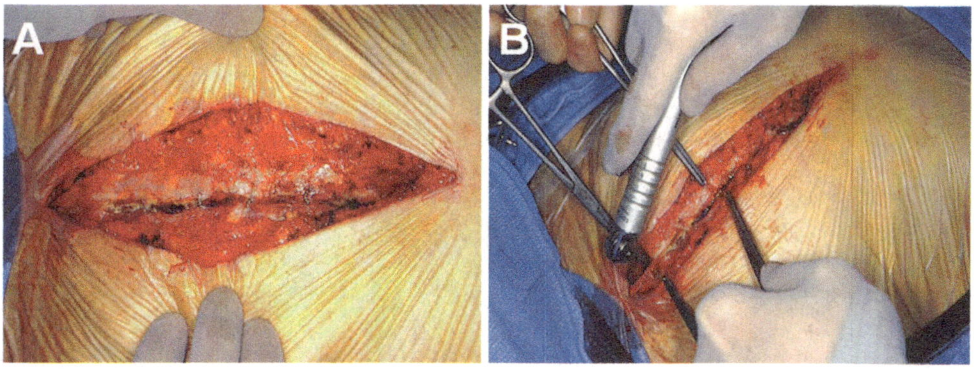

Fig. 10.2 After the skin incision (**a**), wires are divided and pulled upward, and the oscillating saw is used to divide the upper table of the sternum (**b**)

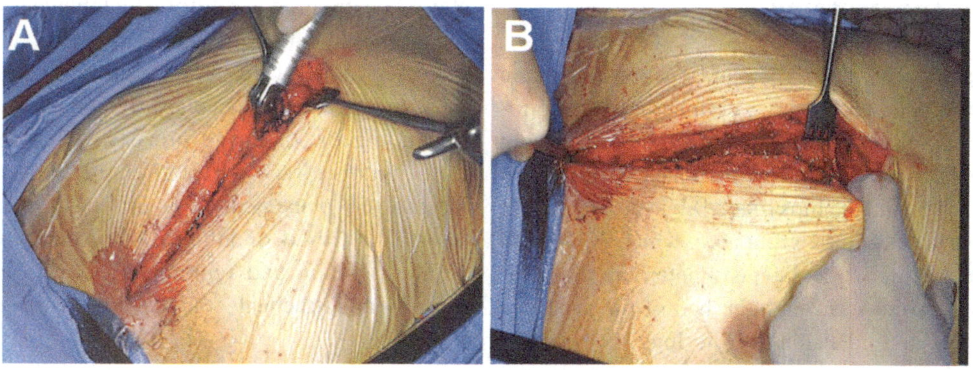

Fig. 10.3 Complete division of the sternum begins at the lower margin (**a**), and upward (anterior) traction on the sternal edges exposes underlying adhesions (**b**) that can be divided under direct vision

have caused phlebitis. O'Brien and colleagues have emphasized the importance of adequate visualization of adhesions, and they recommend dividing only adhesions that are visualized from below and sawing only sternal bone that is freed of adhesions [22].

The first aim of dissection is to isolate the distal ascending aorta to identify an area for cannulation. Next, the right atrium is freed from adhesions to permit venous cannulation. This is done most easily by beginning at the caudal end of the incision. Dissection leftward to free the right ventricle is performed after instituting cardiopulmonary bypass. Once the heart is exposed, a decision is made regarding access to the MV. If the depth of the thorax (anterior–posterior dimension) is normal or not greatly enlarged, and if adhesions are not excessive, then a single venous cannula is used and the MV is approached through a standard incision posterior to the interatrial groove. When adhesions are intense or if the patient has an especially deep chest, it may be easier to cannulate the inferior and superior venae cavae occlusively so that the MV can be exposed through incisions in the right atrium and interatrial septum (Fig. 10.4). With either approach to the MV, exposure is improved by mobilization of the left ventricle so that the apex falls posteriorly. This can be done by dividing pericardial adhesions or by simply opening the left pleural space widely and mobilizing the left ventricular apex extrapericardially.

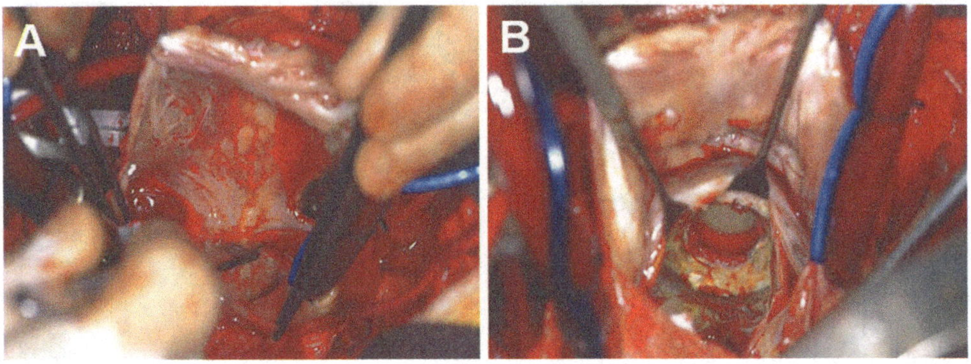

Fig. 10.4 If adhesions make dissection of the standard left atrial incision difficult or if tricuspid repair or replacement is necessary, the MV can be exposed through the atrial septum (**a**, **b**)

Right Thoracotomy

Preparation for anesthesia and operation is made as described previously. A double lumen endotracheal tube allows deflation of the right lung during dissection; the patient is positioned with the left side down, and the hips rotated slightly to the right to give access to the groin area, which is prepped into the field. A right lateral or anterolateral thoracotomy is made through the bed of the fourth or fifth rib, and adhesions of the lung to the chest wall or pericardium are divided using an electrocautery. The pericardium is entered anterior to the phrenic nerve. When possible, the ascending aorta is cannulated for arterial inflow or, alternatively, the right femoral artery is used. Bicaval venous cannulation optimizes exposure, although a single long cannula advanced into the atrium from the femoral vein may be used. Vacuum-assisted drainage can improve venous return when smaller-bore, long cannulas are used [23]. If the aorta can be isolated and clamped, we will maintain normothermia during extracorporeal circulation. If fibrillatory arrest is used for myocardial protection, the patient is cooled to 20–25°C.

The MV is exposed through an incision posterior to the interatrial groove or through the atrial septum if the cavae are cannulated occlusively. After the MV procedure and atrial closure, the patient is rewarmed as necessary, and the heart should be de-aired carefully. The table is tilted in the Trendelenburg position, and a tack vent in the ascending aorta is placed on suction to remove ejected air; echocardiography is helpful in guiding the de-airing process. After discontinuation of extracorporeal circulation, decannulation, and placement of a drainage tube, the incision is closed, and the patient is turned to the supine position and reintubated with a single-lumen endotracheal tube for postoperative ventilation.

Minimally Invasive MV Reoperation

Surgeons who are experienced with minimally invasive approaches have reported satisfactory outcomes with minithoractomy for MV reoperation in selected patients [13, 18]. These minimally invasive techniques utilize small (4–5 cm) inframammary incisions, jugular and femoral venous cannulation, and femoral artery cannulation with or without an endoaortic balloon for aortic occlusion. The same precautions outlined for the right thoracotomy pertain to minimally invasive minithoracotomy, including consideration of the potential complexity of managing aortic valve regurgitation (exposure of the MV, avoiding distention of the left ventricle) and the possible increased risk of stroke [19, 20].

References

1. Follis FM, Pett Jr SB, Miller KB, et al. Catastrophic hemorrhage on sternal reentry: still a dreaded complication? Ann Thorac Surg. 1999;68:2215–9.
2. Edwards FH, Peterson ED, Coombs LP, et al. Prediction of operative mortality after valve replacement surgery. J Am Coll Cardiol. 2001;37:885–92.
3. Rankin RS, Hammill BG, Ferguson TB, et al. Determinants of operative mortality in valvular heart surgery. J Thorac Cardiovasc Surg. 2006;131:547–57.
4. Sabik JF, Nemeh H, Lytle BW, Blackstone EH, Gillinov AM, Rajeswaran J, et al. Cannulation of the axillary artery with a side graft reduces morbidity. Ann Thorac Surg. 2004;77(4):1315–20.
5. Maluenda G, Goldstein MA, Lemesle G, Weissman G, Weigold G, Landsman MJ, et al. Perioperative outcomes in reoperative cardiac surgery guided by cardiac multidetector computed tomographic angiography. Am Heart J. 2010;159(2):301–6.
6. Aviram G, Sharony R, Kramer A, Nesher N, Loberman D, Ben-Gal Y, et al. Modification of surgical planning based on cardiac multidetector computed tomography in reoperative heart surgery. Ann Thorac Surg. 2005;79(2):589–95.
7. Aviram G, Mohr R, Sharony R, Medalion B, Kramer A, Uretzky G. Open heart reoperations after coronary artery bypass grafting: the role of preoperative imaging with multidetector computed tomography. Isr Med Assoc J. 2009;11(8):465–9.
8. Kamdar AR, Meadows TA, Roselli EE, Gorodeski EZ, Curtin RJ, Sabik JF, et al. Multidetector computed tomographic angiography in planning of reoperative cardiothoracic surgery. Ann Thorac Surg. 2008; 85(4):1239–45.
9. van der Linden J, Hadjinikolaou L, Bergman P, Lindblom D. Postoperative stroke in cardiac surgery is related to the location and extent of atherosclerotic disease in the ascending aorta. J Am Coll Cardiol. 2001;38:131–5.
10. Yoshioka I, Saiki Y, Ichinose A, Takase K, Takahashi S, Ohashi T, et al. Tagged cine magnetic resonance imaging with a finite element model can predict the severity of retrosternal adhesions prior to redo cardiac surgery. J Thorac Cardiovasc Surg. 2009;137(4):957–62.
11. Fergusson DA, Hebert PC, Mazer CD, et al. A comparison of aprotinin and lysine analogues in high-risk cardiac surgery. N Engl J Med. 2008;358:2319–31.
12. Oscarsson A, Gupta A, Fredrikson M, Järhult J, Nyström M, Pettersson E, et al. To continue or discontinue aspirin in the perioperative period: a randomized, controlled clinical trial. Br J Anaesth. 2010;104(3): 305–12.
13. Meyer SR, Szeto WY, Augoustides JG, Morris RJ, Vernick WJ, Paschal D, et al. Reoperative mitral valve surgery by the port access minithoracotomy approach is safe and effective. Ann Thorac Surg. 2009; 87(5):1426–30.
14. Tribble CG, Killinger WA, Harman PK, Crosby IK, Nolan SP, Kron IL. Anterolateral thoracotomy as an alternative to repeat median sternotomy for replacement of the mitral valve. Ann Thorac Surg. 1987; 43(4):380–2.
15. Byrne JG, Karavas AN, Adams DH, Aklog L, Aranki SF, Filsoufi F, et al. The preferred approach for mitral valve surgery after CABG: right thoracotomy, hypothermia and avoidance of LIMA-LAD graft. J Heart Valve Dis. 2001;10:584–90.
16. Holman WL, Goldberg SP, Early LJ, McGiffin DC, Kirklin JK, Cho DH, et al. Right thoracotomy for mitral reoperation: analysis of technique and outcome. Ann Thorac Surg. 2000;70:1970–3.
17. Thompson MJ, Behranwala A, Campanella C, Walker WS, Cameron EW. Immediate and long-term results of mitral prosthetic replacement using a right thoracotomy beating heart technique. Eur J Cardiothorac Surg. 2003;24(1):47–51.
18. Seeburger J, Borger MA, Falk V, Passage J, Walther T, Doll N, et al. Minimally invasive mitral valve surgery after previous sternotomy: experience in 181 patients. Ann Thorac Surg. 2009;87(3):709–14.
19. Svensson LG, Gillinov AM, Blackstone EH, Houghtaling PL, Kim KH, Pettersson GB, et al. Does right thoracotomy increase the risk of mitral valve reoperation? J Thorac Cardiovasc Surg. 2007; 134(3):677–82.
20. Crooke GA, Schwartz CF, Ribakove GH, Ursomanno P, Gogoladze G, Culliford AT, et al. Retrograde arterial perfusion, not incision location, significantly increases the risk of stroke in reoperative mitral valve procedures. Ann Thorac Surg. 2010;89(3):723–9.
21. Akl BF, Pett Jr SB, Wernly JA. Use of a sagittal oscillating saw for repeat sternotomy: a safer and simpler technique. Ann Thorac Surg. 1984;38(6):646–7.
22. O'Brien MF, Harrocks S, Clarke A, Garlick B, Barnett AG. How to do safe sternal reentry and the risk factors of redo cardiac surgery: a 21-year review with zero major cardiac injury. J Card Surg. 2002;1:4–13.
23. Nyawo B, Botha P, Pillay T, Clark SC, Tocewicz K, Forty J, et al. Clinical experience with assisted venous drainage cardiopulmonary bypass in elective cardiac reoperations. Heart Surg Forum. 2008; 11(1):E21–3.

11 Reoperation Following Mitral Valve Repair

Rakesh M. Suri and Hartzell V. Schaff

Introduction

The management of mitral valve regurgitation (MR) has evolved significantly over the past 2 decades. During that time, there has been a change in the pathology and, consequently, the pathophysiology of patients referred for operative treatment. In current practice in the Western world, consequent to the decline in the frequency of postinflammatory valvopathy, most patients presenting for mitral valve (MV) surgery have degenerative valve disease. Two factors have been influential in broadening the indications for performing MV repair. First, patients are identified earlier and followed more regularly to prevent the deleterious consequences of chronic persistent MR on left ventricular (LV) size and function. Second, the outcome of surgical management has improved, and the long-term durability of primary and reoperative valve repair has been clearly established.

MV repair is the standard of care for the correction of significant MR due to degenerative valve disease [1–4], and studies have demonstrated superior survival and equivalent, if not better, durability as compared with valve replacement. But, late reoperation on the repaired MV may be necessary, and the linearized rate of reoperation ranges from 0.5 to 1.5% per year [4]. There is a natural hesitance to perform a second mitral repair because of concern that patients with failed initial repair might have poor tissue quality, limiting the durability of re-repair. Also, there has been speculation that secondary MV repair might have greater risk than valve replacement. This chapter reviews operative methods and outcomes of reoperation on the MV after initial repair.

R.M. Suri, MD, DPhil (✉) • H.V. Schaff, MD
Division of Cardiovascular Surgery, Mayo Clinic, Rochester, MN, USA
e-mail: suri.rakesh@mayo.edu

Indications for Surgery

Detailed longitudinal studies and improved techniques of two-dimensional and Doppler echocardiography have allowed clinicians to identify evidence-based "trigger points" to recommend MV surgery in patients with significant MR [5–7]. Accurate echocardiographic delineation of both the anatomic cause and the severity of MR permits stratification of patients and the selection of an optimal treatment strategy based upon well-defined outcomes. These have been reflected in the American College of Cardiology/American Heart Association Guidelines for the Management of Patients with Valvular Heart Disease [8, 9]. Current class I indications for MV surgery for chronic severe MR include the presence of symptoms without severe LV dysfunction (severe LV dysfunction is characterized by LV ejection fraction [LVEF] > 30% and left ventricular end-systolic dimension [LVESD] < 55 mm) and the absence of symptoms with mild-to-moderate LV dysfunction (LVEF

V.R. Machiraju et al. (eds.), *Redo Cardiac Surgery in Adults*,
DOI 10.1007/978-1-4614-1326-4_11, © Springer Science+Business Media, LLC 2012

30–60% and LVESD > 40 mm). Moreover, mitral repair (vs. mitral replacement) is recommended in patients with chronic severe MR, whenever possible, and the guidelines suggest that patients should be appropriately referred to ensure that the option of surgical mitral repair is made available to them. Class IIA indications for MV surgery (preferably repair) in degenerative mitral disease include the presence of chronic severe MR in asymptomatic patients with a normal LVEF (>60%) if the patient (a) is sent to a center where the likelihood of a successful mitral repair is greater than 90%, (b) has new onset atrial fibrillation, or (c) has documented pulmonary hypertension. Finally, patients with moderate-to-severe symptoms and severe LV dysfunction along with an anatomic abnormality of the mitral apparatus amenable to valvuloplasty should also undergo repair.

Integration of these guidelines into the management of patients with recurrent MR after initial valve repair requires judgment. First, the risk of a second procedure will, in most patients, be increased compared with initial operation. Guidelines for management of asymptomatic patients are predicated on very low operation mortality (<1%) as well as a high likelihood of valve repair vs. replacement. In clinical practice, patients with recurrent severe MR are followed closely with echocardiographic assessment of LV size and function every 6–12 months. Intervention would be advised if symptoms develop or if there is objective progression of LV dilation or decreased systolic function. When reoperation is necessary, both the surgeon and the patient may feel that valve replacement is the best strategy to avoid a third operation.

Surgical Methods

The approach to the MV during reoperation is dictated by the experience of the surgeon and the need for additional procedures. In most patients, we proceed with repeat median sternotomy; alternatively, a right anterolateral thoracotomy may be used (see Chap. 9) [28, 29]. Once the heart is exposed, a decision is made regarding access to the MV. If the depth of the thorax (anterior–posterior dimension) is normal or not greatly enlarged and if adhesions are not excessive, then a single venous cannula is used with plans to expose the MV via a standard incision posterior to the interatrial groove. In patients with a deep chest and when adhesions limit dissection, it may be prudent to cannulate the inferior and superior vena cava occlusively, so that the MV can be exposed through incisions in the right atrium and interatrial septum. With either approach to the MV, exposure is improved by mobilization of the LV so that the apex falls posteriorly. This can be done by dividing pericardial adhesions or by simply opening the left pleural space widely and mobilizing the LV apex extrapericardially.

Once the valve is exposed, the leaflets and annulus should be inspected carefully to determine the cause of failure of the initial repair; filling the ventricle with saline facilitates assessment. The decision to re-repair the valve or proceed with replacement depends on several factors, such as adequacy of exposure, identification of the cause of recurrent MR, quality of the tissues, and expectations of the patient. There are multiple causes for recurrent valve leakage. Some patients will exhibit new pathology, such as another ruptured chord. In others, recurrent MR will be due to failure of the initial repair owing to disruption of the prior leaflet repair or dehiscence of the annuloplasty ring. We have encountered patients with leaflet perforation due to suture dehiscence at the annulus following a quadrangular excision, and we have seen others with perforation of the anterior leaflet caused by annuloplasty sutures for full rings placed too low in the leaflet tissue rather than in the annulus. These perforations are easily repaired, directly with pledget-reinforced suture or by autologous pericardial patch.

For recurrent or residual prolapsing segments of the posterior leaflet, we use triangular leaflet resection (Figs. 11.1 and 11.2) or leaflet plication, as first described by McGoon [10]. Anterior leaflet pathology is usually corrected by resuspension using 4–0 Gore-Tex neochordae; some surgeons

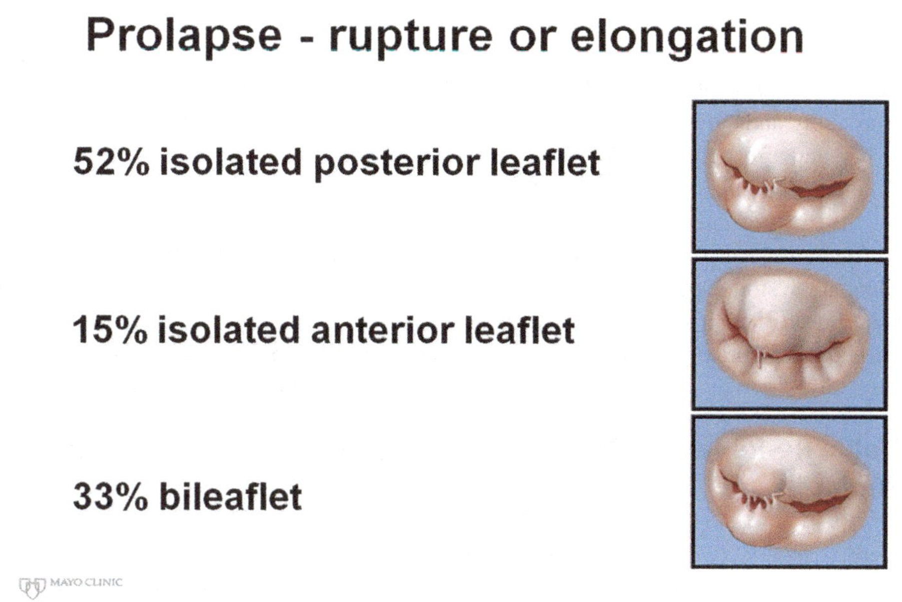

Fig. 11.1 All patients in the Mayo repair series had mitral leaflet prolapse due to chordal rupture or elongation. Fifty-two percent of patients had isolated posterior leaflet prolapse, 15% had isolated anterior leaflet (AL) prolapse, and 33% had bileaflet disease. By permission of Mayo Foundation for Medical Education and Research. All rights reserved

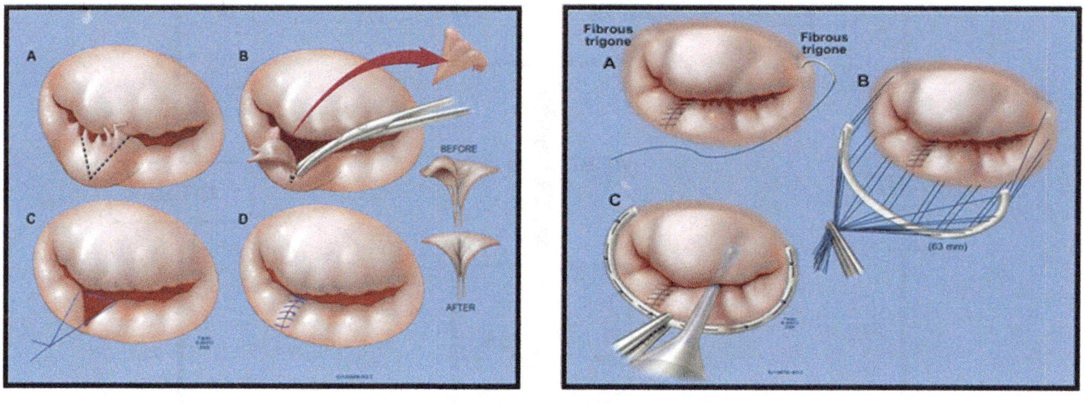

Fig. 11.2 Primary repair of posterior leaflet prolapse consists of triangular resection of the prolapsing segment followed by two-layer running Prolene reconstruction. This eliminates the prolapsing segment and restores normal leaflet coaptation. All repairs are supported by a standard length 63 mm annuloplasty band. By permission of Mayo Foundation for Medical Education and Research. All rights reserved

use artificial chords liberally for posterior leaflet repair. During initial valve repair, we favor a 63-mm posterior annuloplasty band anchored between the right and left fibrous trigones. In patients who undergo reoperation, the initial repair often included a ring or partial ring annuloplasty, and the surgeon will have to determine whether the annuloplasty is sufficiently tight to provide adequate systolic apposition of the anterior and posterior leaflets; if not, the annuloplasty can be revised by resuture or replacement.

Mitral Valve Re-Repair vs. Mitral Valve Replacement

As stated previously, there may be reluctance to attempt re-repair at the time of reoperation, and the surgeon often simply proceeds with prosthetic replacement. Certainly, this is best strategy for some patients, but valve repair has definite advantages over replacement. With successful valve repair, patients who maintain sinus rhythm resume full activities without the need for chronic anticoagulation. In addition to reducing morbidity, valve repair improves patient survival compared with prosthetic replacement. For example, in our experience with 1,411 patients who underwent MV repair (1,173 patients, 83%) or MV replacement (238 patients, 17%) between January 1, 1980 and December 31, 1999, valve repair was an important predictor of late survival, independent of age, preoperative functional class, and the presence or absence of coronary artery disease [4]. Furthermore, patients who have MR corrected by repair have more complete remodeling compared with patients having MV replacement [11].

Our experience suggests that the beneficial effects of repair vs. replacement are also achieved after reoperation [12]. Between January 1, 1970 and January 1, 2005, a total of 145 patients underwent mitral reoperation for recurrent MR at Mayo Clinic, Rochester Minnesota. One hundred and seven patients had their first MV repair at our institution (5% of 2,122 patients having primary MV repair for degenerative leaflet prolapse during the study period), and 38 had their first operation elsewhere (Fig. 11.3). At reoperation, 64 patients (44%) had MV re-repair, and 81 patients

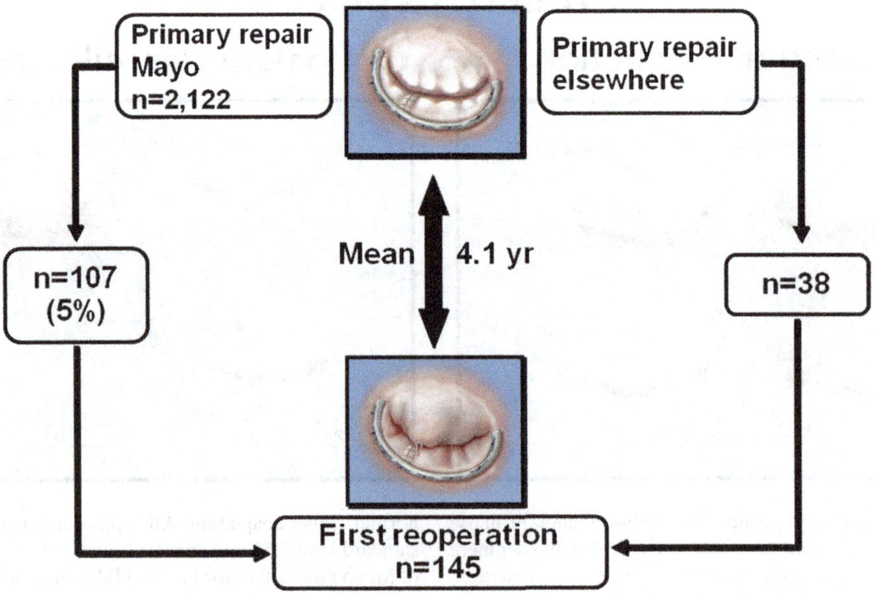

Fig. 11.3 Among 145 patients undergoing reoperation at Mayo clinic for recurrent MR following primary MV repair, 107 had prior repair at Mayo clinic and 38 had their first repair operation elsewhere. The mean interval between primary repair and reoperation was 4.1 years. By permission of Mayo Foundation for Medical Education and Research.

Mode of Failure

	Re-repair (%)	Replace (%)	*P*
New Pathology	42	65	0.005
Technical	56	31	0.002
Unclear	2	4	0.43

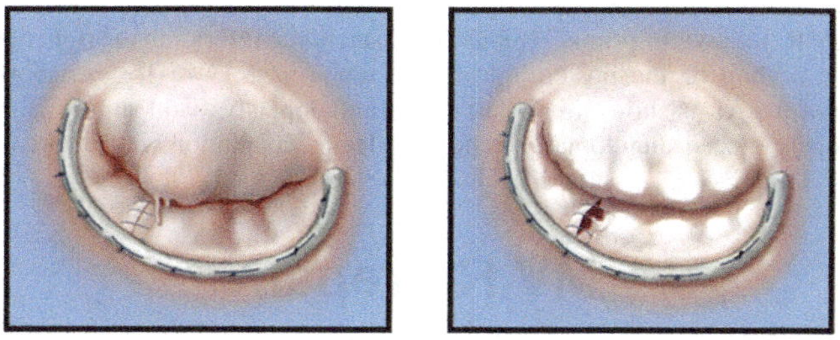

Fig. 11.4 The determination that new pathology caused repair failure more frequently led to mitral replacement whereas technical reasons for recurrent regurgitation more frequently led to re-repair in the Mayo series. By permission of Mayo Foundation for Medical Education and Research.

(56%) underwent replacement of the previously repaired valve. Concomitant procedures were performed in 38 patients including coronary artery bypass grafting (CABG) in 14 (10%), tricuspid valve repair in 12 (8%), aortic valve replacement in 8 (6%), Cox-Maze procedure in 4 (2.8%), atrial septal defect closure in 1 (0.7%), and patent foramen ovale closure in 1 (0.7%) patients.

Significant MR alone was the indication for reoperation in 109 patients (75%). Other indications were hemolytic anemia in 27 (19%), dynamic outflow tract obstruction caused by systolic anterior motion of the anterior mitral leaflet in 3 (2%), endocarditis in 3 (2%), and MV stenosis in 1 (1%) patients. Patients were more likely to have valve replacement at reoperation if the preoperative indication was MR alone and were more likely to have re-repair if hemolysis was the cause. Of the 27 patients with hemolytic anemia, the mean MR grade at reoperation was 3.4 and the mean interval from first operation to reoperation was 1.1 years. Patients having MV replacement were slightly more symptomatic and had greater left atrial dimensions prior to reoperation than patients having valve re-repair. All other aspects of the preoperative risk profiles were similar comparing those who had MV re-repair vs. prosthetic replacement [12].

In this experience, new valve pathology was the cause of recurrent MR in roughly half of patients (80, 55%), and technical failure of the primary repair led to recurrent MR in the other half (61, 42%). At operation, anterior leaflet abnormalities were identified in 65 (45%), posterior leaflet problems in 61 (42%), ring annuloplasty dehiscence in 42 (29%), and chordal rupture in 20 (14%) patients (Fig. 11.4). The etiology of MR at reoperation was unclear in four patients (3%). Patients having MV re-repair were more likely to have a specific anatomic cause for recurrent MR identified by the surgeon at reoperation, such as annuloplasty dehiscence or technical failure of the prior repair. Discovering new pathology was associated with a tendency to replace the MV. In some instances, a combination of new pathology and failure of primary repair were identified (Fig. 11.5a, b).

The finding that 44% patients had MV re-repair is consistent with the results of two recent series studying similar patient populations [13, 14]. During re-repair, an anterior leaflet procedure

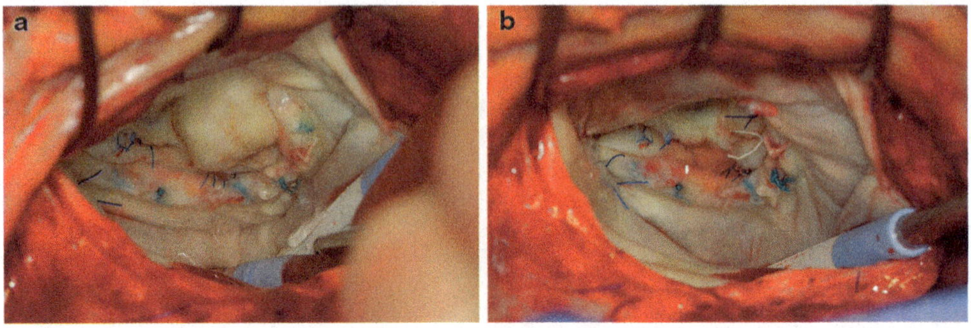

Fig. 11.5 Recurrent MR following primary repair of prolapse of the middle scallop of the posterior leaflet. (**a**) The medial scallop of the AL is shown to be flail and prolapsing. The previously placed annuloplasty band is anchored inferior to the right fibrous trigone. (**b**) Following repair with Gore-Tex neochordae and re-suturing of the annuloplasty band at the right fibrous trigone, normal leaflet coaptation was restored

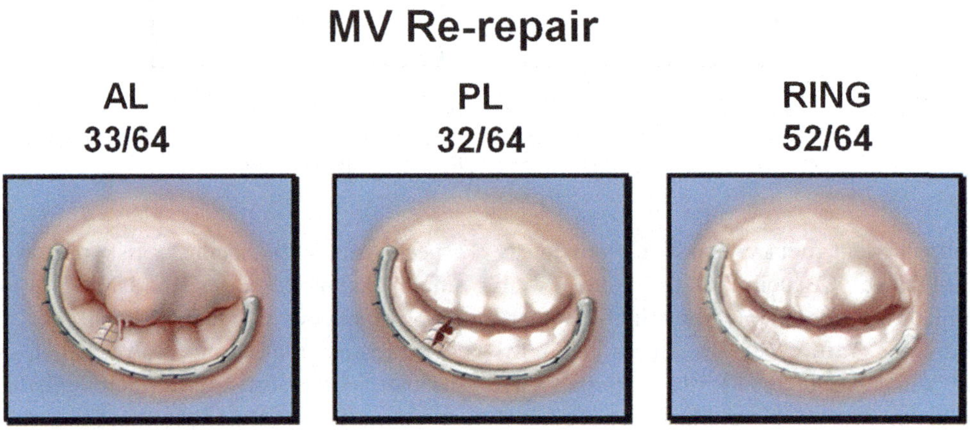

Fig. 11.6 Among 64 patients having MV re-repair, 33 had the AL addressed at reoperation, while 32 had the posterior leaflet (PL) corrected and 52 had an annuloplasty band (RING) placed, modified, or replaced. By permission of Mayo Foundation for Medical Education and Research.

was performed in 33 of the 64 patients, and the posterior leaflet was repaired in 32 patients; we revised the annuloplasty in 52 patients (Fig. 11.6).

Both the reason for reoperation and the surgical findings influence the decision for re-repair vs. replacement. In our experience, significant MR alone was associated with a tendency to perform valve replacement over re-repair (85 vs. 63%, $P=0.002$). Identification of technical reasons for failure of the primary MV more often led to re-repair (56%) vs. replacement (31%, $P=0.002$). More specifically, annuloplasty dehiscence was more prevalent in those having re-repair (47 vs. 15%, $P<0.001$). This observation emphasizes the importance of accurate echocardiographic assessment of MR [15].

Finding new valve pathology at reoperation may have influenced the decision to replace the MV, perhaps because of concern that disease progression in the remaining leaflet tissue would increase the likelihood of a third MV operation. Dumont et al. [13] reviewed 188 patients undergoing reoperation following MV repair and suggested that technical-related failures present earlier and are more amenable to re-repair. In their experience, patients with late failure of valve repair frequently had progression of valve disease and were more likely to undergo valve replacement.

Other authors have suggested that technical failure was the most common finding at reoperation [15, 16]; however, it is possible that the prevalence of rheumatic and ischemic MV disease in these studies may have influenced both the etiology of repair failure and the stated preference for valve replacement at reoperation. Zegdi et al. studied a population of 43 patients requiring reoperation after mitral repair using "Carpentier's techniques." They found that posterior leaflet tethering was a frequent cause of repair failure [14, 17] following primary repair of degenerative mitral disease. It is unclear whether the higher incidence of leaflet tethering in their series is related to their preference for quadrangular leaflet resection and sliding leaflet plasty.

Hemolysis is an important cause for reoperation after initial MV repair and was found in 19% of patients in our series who underwent reoperation. Lam et al. suggested that 90% of patients presenting with hemolysis following prior MV repair require MV reoperation [18]. In most instances, hemolysis is caused by a regurgitant jet of blood striking the annuloplasty ring, even though it may be small as measured by volume of regurgitation and effective regurgitant orifice (ERO). Evidence for a regurgitant jet is easily identified at reoperation by identifying the absence of endothelialization of the involved portion of the ring. If the leaflet abnormality cannot be corrected and the degree of valve leakage is not clinically important, hemolysis can be cured by simply excising the small portion of the ring that the regurgitant jet hits [18–21]. Although some surgeons [18] favor valve replacement, our experience indicates that re-repair for hemolysis is effective and is not a risk factor for a third mitral operation.

Outcomes of Reoperation for Recurrent Mitral Regurgitation

Overall operative mortality following valve replacement in our series was 3.4% and was higher following valve replacement (4.9%) compared with mitral re-repair (1.6%) [12]. Early after operation, Doppler echocardiography showed mild or less residual regurgitation in 97% of patients having valve re-repair and 98% of those having valve replacement. In a multivariate analysis, three independent factors were associated with improved survival, mitral re-repair (hazard ratio=0.44, $P=0.03$), younger age (hazard ratio=1.06, $P=0.001$), and an operative indication of MR alone (hazard ratio=0.31, $P=0.005$). It is important to emphasize that MV re-repair is an independent predictor of improved late survival compared with valve replacement, a finding similar to the outcomes of primary operations for MR. Other data support this finding. The series by Zegdi et al. [14] also demonstrated improved survival following MV re-repair, and Dumont's data suggests a similar trend [13].

Re-repair of the MV results in excellent functional improvement. At last contact, 100% of patients who had re-repair were in New York Heart Association (NYHA) class I/II vs. 91% of patients who underwent replacement. These functional outcomes correlated with reverse ventricular remodeling. Re-repair patients had significantly better LVEF ($P<0.001$) and smaller LV end-systolic dimension (LVESD) ($P=0.009$) during follow-up, as compared with those undergoing MV replacement. These same favorable features have been demonstrated following primary valve repair [12] and may explain the survival advantage observed during long-term follow-up [7, 22, 23]. These findings challenge the assumption that MV replacement is the "conservative" choice for correction of recurrent mitral regurgitation.

The major drawback to attempting re-repair is the risk of recurrent regurgitation prompting a third procedure. In our series, seven patients (six re-repair and one replacement) underwent a third MV operation, at a mean of 5.7 years after the second operation, and there was no perioperative mortality during valve replacement, which was performed in all seven patients. The actuarial survival free of subsequent reoperation after first MV reoperation was 93% at 5 years for all patients and 83% for patients having re-repair (linearized risk of reoperation was 3.4%/year). Surgical correction of the anterior leaflet during MV re-repair was performed in 33/64 (52%) of re-repair patients and was the only univariate risk factor associated with the need for a third mitral operation. Because the majority of the procedures in this report were carried out between 1980 and 2000, many patients had correction of anterior leaflet prolapse with methods that are now known to be less durable than chordal replacement [24, 25]. In the current era, the risks of reoperation following anterior leaflet repair approach those of repair of the posterior leaflet [4, 26, 27]. The improved durability of primary anterior leaflet repair will also likely influence the results of re-repair in the future. Indeed, a recent report by Dumont et al. [13] notes a freedom from second mitral reoperation of 93% at 10 years following valve repair, while Zegdi et al. [14] reported 95% freedom at 7 years following first reoperation.

Clinical Implications

Delaying surgery for recurrent severe MR following primary MV repair may harmful, and we would advise reoperation at the onset of symptoms or when there is clear evidence of progressive LV enlargement or systolic dysfunction. Approximately half of all patients are candidates for re-repair at reoperation, and factors that appear to favor repair include MV-related hemolysis, an anatomic abnormality of the prior repair, or technical failure of the prior repair evident at reoperation. Indeed, the proportion of patients who have anatomy amenable to re-repair is likely higher than is indicated by some published reports and is admittedly influenced by physician and patient expectations. Although some clinicians believe that MV replacement is the more "conservative" choice when reoperation is necessary following MV repair, our experience suggests otherwise. MV re-repair is advantageous in improving survival and facilitating more complete ventricular remodeling compared with valve replacement.

References

1. Cohn L et al. Long-term results of mitral valve reconstruction for regurgitation of the myxomatous mitral valve. J Thorac Cardiovasc Surg. 1994;107:143–50.
2. David TE. Outcomes of mitral valve repair for mitral regurgitation due to degenerative disease. Semin Thorac Cardiovasc Surg. 2007;19:116–20.
3. Galloway A et al. A comparison of mitral valve reconstruction with mitral valve replacement: intermediate-term results. Ann Thorac Surg. 1989;47:655–62.
4. Suri RM et al. Survival advantage and improved durability of mitral repair for leaflet prolapse subsets in the current era. Ann Thorac Surg. 2006;82:819–26.
5. Enriquez-Sarano M et al. Quantitative determinants of the outcome of asymptomatic mitral regurgitation. N Engl J Med. 2005;352:875–83.
6. Enriquez-Sarano M, Schaff HV, Frye RL. Early surgery for mitral regurgitation: the advantages of youth. Circulation. 1997;96:4121–3.
7. Enriquez-Sarano M et al. Echocardiographic prediction of left ventricular function after correction of mitral regurgitation: results and clinical implications. J Am Coll Cardiol. 1994;24:1536–43.
8. Bonow RO et al. ACC/AHA 2006 guidelines for the management of patients with valvular heart disease: A Report of the American College of Cardiology/American Heart Association Task Force on Practice Guidelines (Writing Committee to Revise the 1998 Guidelines for the Management of Patients with Valvular Heart Disease): Developed in Collaboration with the Society of Cardiovascular Anesthesiologists: Endorsed by the Society for Cardiovascular Angiography and Interventions and the Society of Thoracic Surgeons. Circulation. 2006;114:e84–231.
9. Bonow RO et al. Focused Update Incorporated into the ACC/AHA 2006 guidelines for the management of patients with valvular heart disease: A Report of the American College of Cardiology/American Heart Association Task Force on Practice Guidelines (Writing Committee to Revise the 1998 Guidelines for the Management of Patients with Valvular Heart Disease) Endorsed by the Society of Cardiovascular Anesthesiologists, Society for Cardiovascular Angiography and Interventions, and Society of Thoracic Surgeons. J Am Coll Cardiol. 2008;52:e1–142.
10. Ellis FH Jr, Frye RL, McGoon DC. Results of reconstructive operations for mitral insufficiency due to ruptured chordae tendineae Surgery. 1966 Jan;59(1):165–72.
11. Suri RM et al. Recovery of left ventricular function after surgical correction of mitral regurgitation caused by leaflet prolapse. J Thorac Cardiovasc Surg. 2009;137:1071–6.

12. Suri RM et al. Recurrent mitral regurgitation after repair: should the mitral valve be re-repaired? J Thorac Cardiovasc Surg. 2006;132:1390–7.
13. Dumont E et al. Reoperation after mitral valve repair for degenerative disease. Ann Thorac Surg. 2007; 84:444–50.
14. Zegdi R et al. Reoperation for failure of mitral valve repair in degenerative disease: a single-center experience. Ann Thorac Surg. 2008;86:1480–4.
15. Gillinov AM et al. Reoperation for failure of mitral valve repair. J Thorac Cardiovasc Surg. 1997;113:467–75.
16. Asmar B et al. Failures in reconstructive mitral valve surgery. J Med Liban. 1991;39:7–11.
17. Zegdi R, Achouh P, Fabiani J-N. Redo mitral valve repair. J Thorac Cardiovasc Surg. 2007;134:268.
18. Lam B-K et al. Hemolysis after mitral valve repair: mechanisms and treatment. Ann Thorac Surg. 2004;77:191–5.
19. Cerfolio RJ et al. Reoperation for hemolytic, anaemia complicating mitral valve repair. Eur J Cardiothorac Surg. 1997;11:479–84.
20. Lam B-K, Gillinov AM, Cosgrove I, Delos M. Failed mitral valve repair caused by polypropylene suture. Ann Thorac Surg. 2003;76:1716–7.
21. Schaff HV et al. Mechanisms of hemolysis after mitral valve repair: assessment by serial echocardiography. J Am Coll Cardiol. 1998;32:717–23.
22. Matsumura T et al. Echocardiographic prediction of left ventricular dysfunction after mitral valve repair for mitral regurgitation as an indicator to decide the optimal timing of repair. J Am Coll Cardiol. 2003;42:458–63.
23. Enriquez-Sarano M et al. Valve repair improves the outcome of surgery for mitral regurgitation: a multivariate analysis. Circulation. 1995;91:1022–8.
24. Mohty D et al. Very long-term survival and durability of mitral valve repair for mitral valve prolapse. Circulation. 2001;104(12 Suppl 1):I1–7.
25. Gillinov AM et al. Durability of mitral valve repair for degenerative disease. J Thorac Cardiovasc Surg. 1998;116:734–43.
26. De Bonis M et al. Similar long-term results of mitral valve repair for anterior compared with posterior leaflet prolapse. J Thorac Cardiovasc Surg. 2006;131:364–70.
27. Lawrie GM, Earle EA, Earle NR. Feasibility and intermediate term outcome of repair of prolapsing anterior mitral leaflets with artificial chordal replacement in 152 patients. Ann Thorac Surg. 2006;81:849–56.
28. Meyer SR et al. Reoperative mitral valve surgery by the port access minithoracotomy approach is safe and effective. Ann Thorac Surg. 2009;87:1426–30.
29. Loulmet DF et al. Less invasive intracardiac surgery performed without aortic clamping. Ann Thorac Surg. 2008;85:1551–5.

Reoperation for Prosthetic Mitral Valve Endocarditis

12

Kevin L. Greason and Hartzell V. Schaff

Introduction

Prosthetic valve endocarditis is a serious complication of mitral valve replacement with a reported incidence of 0.5% per patient-year [1]. Similar rates of infection are found with both biological and mechanical prostheses. Symptoms of infection are often variable with the diagnosis of prosthetic mitral valve endocarditis most often based upon blood culture data and echocardiographic evidence of vegetation or valve dysfunction. Despite advances in management of the condition, mortality associated with prosthetic mitral valve endocarditis remains high. As such, an aggressive surgical approach is required. This chapter will focus on the surgical management of the condition.

Pathology

Because of the significant differences sensitivity between the microbiology of prosthetic valve endocarditis observed within 1 year of operation and endocarditis observed a year or more after surgery, the cutoff between early and late prosthetic valve endocarditis has been arbitrarily classified at 1 year. Early prosthetic valve endocarditis is usually the result of perioperative contamination of the prosthesis. Staphylococci (including methicillin-resistant Staphylococci), fungi, and gram-negative bacilli are the main pathogens. Late prosthetic valve endocarditis more commonly includes Staphylococci, oral Streptococci, *Streptococcus bovis*, *Enterococcus*, and the HACEK group (*Heamophilus*, *Actinobacillus*, *Cardiobacterium*, *Eikenella*, and *Kingella*). Finally, culture results may be negative in ~11% of cases [2, 3].

Diagnosis

Because of the variable presentation, the diagnosis of prosthetic valve endocarditis is mainly based on positive blood cultures and findings noted at transesophageal echocardiography. Unfortunately, transesophageal echocardiography can be falsely negative in prosthetic valve endocarditis in up to 20% of patients with proven prosthetic mitral valve infection. Transesophageal echocardiography should be repeated in cases of high clinical suspicion. The Duke criteria were developed to aid in the diagnosis of infective endocarditis and are helpful for the diagnosis of native valve endocarditis with a sensitivity as high as 80%. Unfortunately, the criteria cannot be applied in clinical practice to prosthetic valve endocarditis because of their lower sensitivity in

K.L. Greason, MD (✉) • H.V. Schaff, MD
Division of Cardiovascular Surgery, Mayo Clinic, Rochester, MN, USA
e-mail: greason.kevin@mayo.edu

V.R. Machiraju et al. (eds.), *Redo Cardiac Surgery in Adults*,
DOI 10.1007/978-1-4614-1326-4_12, © Springer Science+Business Media, LLC 2012

this setting [2]. Infectious disease consultation is wise in all cases of suspected or confirmed prosthetic mitral valve endocarditis.

Indication for Operation

Most patients with prosthetic mitral valve endocarditis require operation to cure the infection. In the study of Sohail et al., only 40% of patients were treated with medical therapy alone and such treatment was associated with higher mortality [4]. The microbiology of early prosthetic valve endocarditis is dominated by *Staphylococcus*. Over 70% of these patients develop major complications, including paravalvular abscess or leak leading to congestive heart failure or septic embolism [4]. Other indications for operation include infection relapse and fungal infection [5]. The American College of Cardiology/American Heart Association (ACC/AHA) Practice Guidelines describing indications for operation in prosthetic valve endocarditis are listed in Table 12.1 [6]. There are a few subsets of patients for which medical therapy alone may be effective for the treatment of prosthetic valve endocarditis. Such patients usually have late biological valve endocarditis, infection by *Streptococcus* viridans, Enterococci, or HACEK bacteria, and the absence of invasive infection [3].

Table 12.1 Indications for operation in prosthetic valve endocarditis (ACC/AHA practice guidelines)

Class I
Operation is indicated for patients who present with heart failure (level of evidence: B)
Operation is indicated for patients who present with dehiscence evidenced by cine fluoroscopy or echocardiography (level of evidence: B)
Operation is indicated for patients who present with evidence of increasing obstruction or worsening regurgitation (level of evidence: C)
Operation is indicated for patients who present with complications (e.g., abscess formation; level of evidence: C)
Class IIa
Operation is reasonable for patients who present with evidence of persistent bacteremia or recurrent emboli despite appropriate antibiotic treatment (level of evidence: C)
Operation is reasonable for patients who present with relapsing infection

Modified from Ref. [6]

Timing of Operation

Early Prosthetic Valve Endocarditis

Bacteremia after mitral valve replacement is a serious finding and frequently is indicative of prosthetic valve endocarditis [7]. Antibiotics should be started at the earliest signs of infection. Patients without Staphylococcal bacteremia, without persistent bacteremia, and without heart failure are potentially curable with isolated medical management. Such patients should be considered to be at high risk for complicated prosthetic valve endocarditis and should have the diagnosis aggressively pursued with serial (probably weekly) transesophageal echocardiography. Reoperation should be undertaken at the earliest sign of failure of medical management to include development of perivalvular abscess or significant vegetation. In that setting, operation offers the best chance for successful treatment [7, 8].

Late Prosthetic Valve Endocarditis

Uncomplicated late prosthetic valve endocarditis may be managed medically. The typical patient for medical management would be one in whom the blood is easily sterilized (within 72 h) and who presents without Staphylococcal or fungal infection, has no evidence of significant heart failure, and no echocardiographic evidence of annular abscess or significant vegetation (>1 cm, or pedunculated). Such patients may be managed with antibiotics alone without an increase in the rates of reinfection, reoperation, or death [1]. Success is more likely in the setting of a biological prosthesis, as late endocarditis in mechanical prostheses is seldom cured by antibiotics alone and an aggressive surgical approach is justified [7].

Complicated late prosthetic valve endocarditis should be treated surgically soon after the diagnosis is established and appropriate antibiotics have been given. Ideally, one would delay operation until blood cultures are negative. Factors that complicate prosthetic valve endocarditis include large (>1 cm) or pedunculated vegetation, embolism, Staphylococcal or fungal pathogen, extravalvular extension, and congestive heart failure [1]. Patients in significant congestive heart failure should be operated on emergently.

Cerebrovascular Complications

Cerebrovascular complications occur in 22–40% of patients with left-sided heart valve endocarditis and are more common in patients with mitral valve involvement [9, 10]. The spectrum of clinical presentation includes silent cerebrovascular infarction, transient ischemic attack, and stroke. Given the high rate of occurrence, radiologic imaging (CT scan or MRI) is indicated in patients with prosthetic mitral valve endocarditis. Operation can be safely performed after silent cerebrovascular infarction and transient ischemic attack [10]. Patients with stoke have higher perioperative mortality and should have operation delayed for 2–3 weeks in an effort to prevent exacerbation of neurologic injury [9].

Operative Techniques

Surgical Approach

Operation for prosthetic mitral valve endocarditis may be challenging. Our standard approach to the mitral valve is via median sternotomy. Sternotomy allows complete access to all the cardiac chambers and great vessels. Cannulation for cardiopulmonary bypass, managing paravalvular abscess, managing aortic valve insufficiency, monitoring the left ventricle for distention, and evacuating air are all easier to do with the midline approach compared to lateral thoracotomy.

In the setting of reoperative median sternotomy, preoperative CT scan is a useful adjunct in planning sternal re-entry to identify areas of potential danger, such as coronary grafts, the aorta, or an enlarged right ventricle adherent to the back of the sternum. If there is concern about injury to one or more of these structures during sternotomy, we would institute extracorporeal circulation via cannulation of the femoral or axillary artery and femoral vein to allow decompression of the heart.

A useful technique for safe repeat sternotomy involves elevation of the sternum away from the mediastinal structures during bone division. Heavy needle drivers are used to lift up on both ends of a divided sternal wire, thus, elevating the sternum away from the heart. Additionally, the lungs are decompressed. The sternum is then divided with the microsagittal saw from the xiphoid up to the level of the respective wire. That wire is then removed and the needle drivers applied to the next most cephalad wire. The process is continued until all the wires are removed, usually leaving only a short segment of the manubrium left to divide.

After median sternotomy, the heart is dissected from the surrounding tissues. Maneuvers that help improve mitral valve exposure include traction on the right pericardial sutures, avoiding traction sutures on the left pericardium, and mobilizing the superior and inferior vena cavae. Freeing the apex of the heart from adhesions and opening the left pleural space allow the apex of the heart to fall posteriorly and, thus, improve exposure of the mitral valve.

Occasionally, a right anterolateral thoracotomy may be preferred for mitral valve surgery in a patient with multiple previous median sternotomies and anatomic considerations that make repeat median sternotomy risky. Typical patients include those with patent arterial coronary bypass grafts, especially if they cross the midline, and patients with other potential hazards, such as previous mediastinitis or a history of mediastinal radiation. However, exposure of the aorta for cannulation and cross-clamp placement via a right thoracotomy may be limited, and in some series, perioperative stroke was increased with this approach [11].

Institution of Cardiopulmonary Bypass

After median sternotomy is performed, cardiopulmonary bypass is instituted with cannulation of the aorta and the right atrium; bicaval cannulation may be helpful if adhesions are dense or a transseptal incision is contemplated. Typically, bicaval cannulation includes a right-angle superior vena cava cannula and a straight or right-angle inferior vena cava cannula. Adjuncts to improve myocardial cooling during cardioplegic arrest include opening the right atrium to drain all warm venous blood from the heart. Additionally, a suture tourniquet can be placed around the ostium of the coronary sinus and a retrograde cardioplegia cannula placed snug to the tourniquet. From this point on, intermittent doses of retrograde cardioplegia can be given without inhibiting the progress of the operation.

Atriotomy

In most patients, the mitral valve is exposed with an incision in the left atrium just posterior to the interatrial groove. Before making the atriotomy, the interatrial groove can be developed for several centimeters with sharp dissection. The incision begins on the anterior lateral left atrium near the junction of the right superior pulmonary vein and left atrium, posterior to Waterston's groove. It continues inferiorly between the right inferior pulmonary vein and the inferior vena cava. By developing the interatrial plane, the left atrial incision can be made approximately 2–4 cm from the right pulmonary veins, giving closer exposure of the mitral valve. More extensive exposure can be obtained by dividing the superior vena cava and rolling the heart to the patient's left side.

Other atrial incisions may be useful in circumstances where exposure is poor, as sometimes occurs in patients undergoing reoperation. For example, a simple transseptal incision provides excellent exposure of the mitral valve and is favored when a right atriotomy is necessary for the treatment of concomitant tricuspid valve disease. This approach is also useful in patients who have had multiple previous operations; after repeated left atriotomies, the tissue may be stiff and fibrotic making retraction and valve exposure difficult.

In rare situations, it may be impossible to adequately expose the mitral valve through a standard left atriotomy, and the surgeon may use additional incisions, such as the biatrial transseptal incision as described by Brawley or other modifications of the original Dubost technique [12]. Additionally, the extended vertical transatrial septal approach as described by Guiraudon opens both atria widely, giving excellent mitral valve exposure, even in the setting of a small left atrium [13].

As the surgeon approaches the mitral valve, it is important to understand the anatomic relationships that exist between the mitral valve and other structures that put those structures at risk during operation (Fig. 12.1). The anterior portion of the annulus is in direct continuity with the aortic valve, specifically portions of the left and noncoronary aortic valve cusps. The conduction bundle is susceptible to damage in the area of the right fibrous trigone. Vascular structures vulnerable to damage include the circumflex coronary artery, which courses parallel to the posterior annulus on the left, and the coronary sinus, which is superficial to the posterior annulus on the right. In a left dominant coronary artery system, the circumflex coronary artery is at risk for damage along the entire length of the posterior annulus [14].

Removal of the Prosthetic Valve and Debridement

The prosthetic mitral valve is explanted and the mitral annulus debrided of all foreign materials, including pledgets and sutures. Any tissue that appears inflamed or edematous may potentially contain bacteria or fungi and must be excised. Opening the aorta for inspection through the aortic valve can improve the exposure of the anterior mitral valve annulus. Radical debridement may result in removal of parts of the mitral annulus, fibrous trigones, and posterior ventricular wall. Aggressive debridement is indispensable to eradication of local sepsis [7]. We treat the debri-

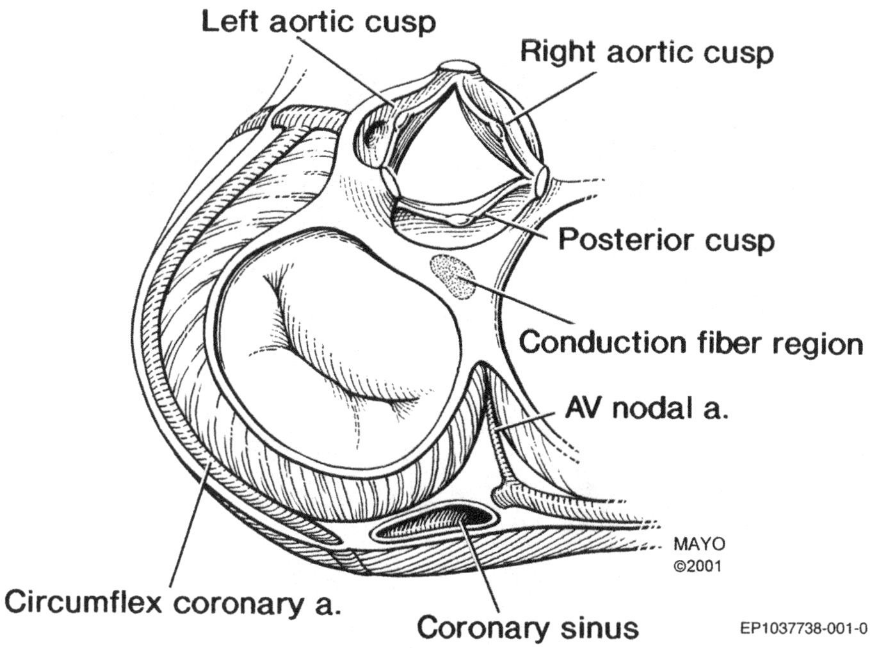

Fig. 12.1 Anatomical relationship of the mitral valve to other cardiac structures. By permission of Mayo Foundation for Medical Education Research. All Rights Reserved

ded annulus topically with a 10% phenol solution applied on a sterile Q-tip applicator. Phenol is a strong acid that acts both as an antiseptic and as a tissue fixative. The drug is left in contact with tissues for ~30 s, then copiously irrigated and suctioned with waste suction to remove any remaining phenol. Pledgeted 2-0 Ethibond sutures, with the pledgets on the ventricular side, are used to anchor the new prosthesis.

Reconstruction

Debridement of a posterior paravalvular abscess cavity may result in a defect that separates the left atrium, left ventricle, and mitral annulus. The defect in the annulus is reconstructed with a semicircular patch of bovine pericardium (Fig. 12.2a–c). The patch is approximately 2 cm larger than the defect in the mitral annulus. The circular margin of the patch is sutured to the endocardium of the left ventricle with a continuous 3-0 Prolene suture. The straight margin is used to secure the new prosthetic mitral valve. In cases of perforation of the atrioventricular groove, the straight margin of the patch is also sutured to the left atrium to seal the perforation completely [15].

More extensive destruction of the mitral annulus requires a circumferential reconstruction of the annulus (Fig. 12.3). A strip of pericardium 2 cm wide and 10–12 cm long (the length of the perimeter of the mitral annulus, which can be calculated by multiplying the diameter of the annulus by pi) is sutured to the endocardium of the left ventricle posteriorly and to the fibrous tissue underneath the aortic valve superiorly. The ascending aorta is opened to facilitate suturing underneath the aortic valve and to prevent damage to its noncoronary leaflet. A prosthetic mitral valve is sutured to the pericardial patch. To avoid a rocking movement of the prosthesis, no excessive patch material should be left between the two suture lines [15].

Extension of endocarditis into the intravalvular fibrosa/fibrous trigones may necessitate replacement of both mitral and aortic valves (Fig. 12.4a–d) [5]. In such circumstances, the fibrous trigones may be reconstructed with

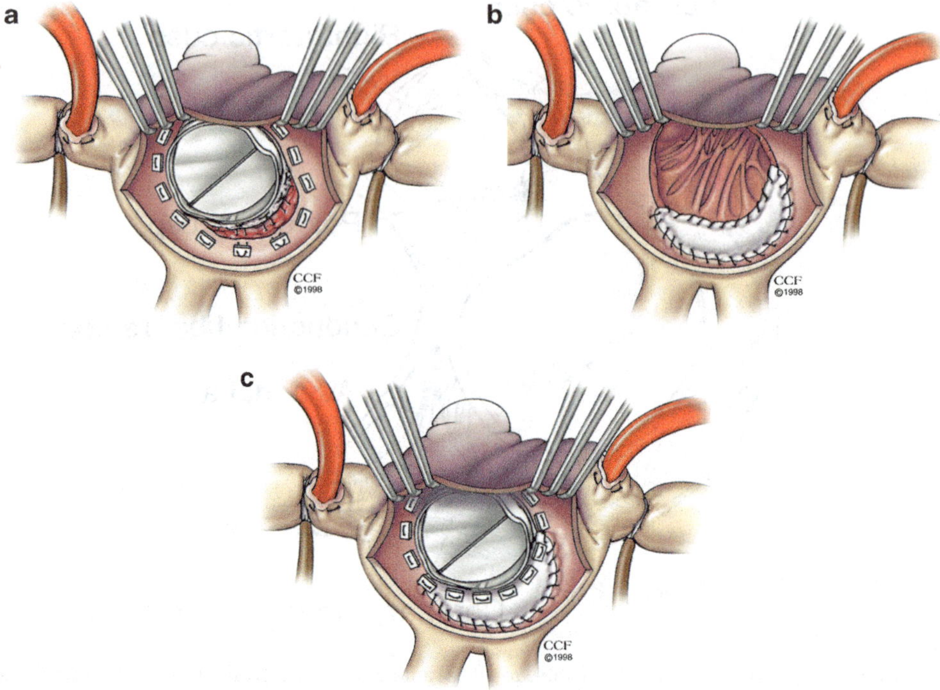

Fig. 12.2 (**a**–**c**) Reconstruction of the mitral annulus. Reprinted with permission, Cleveland Clinic Center for Medical Art & Photography ©1998–2011. All Rights Reserved

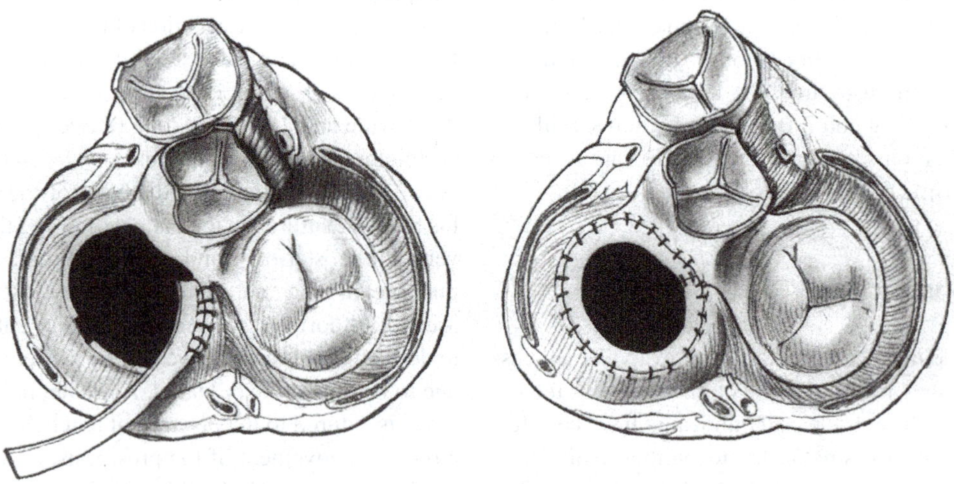

Fig. 12.3 Reconstruction of the entire mitral annulus. Reprinted from David et al. [10], Copyright (1995), with permission from Elsevier

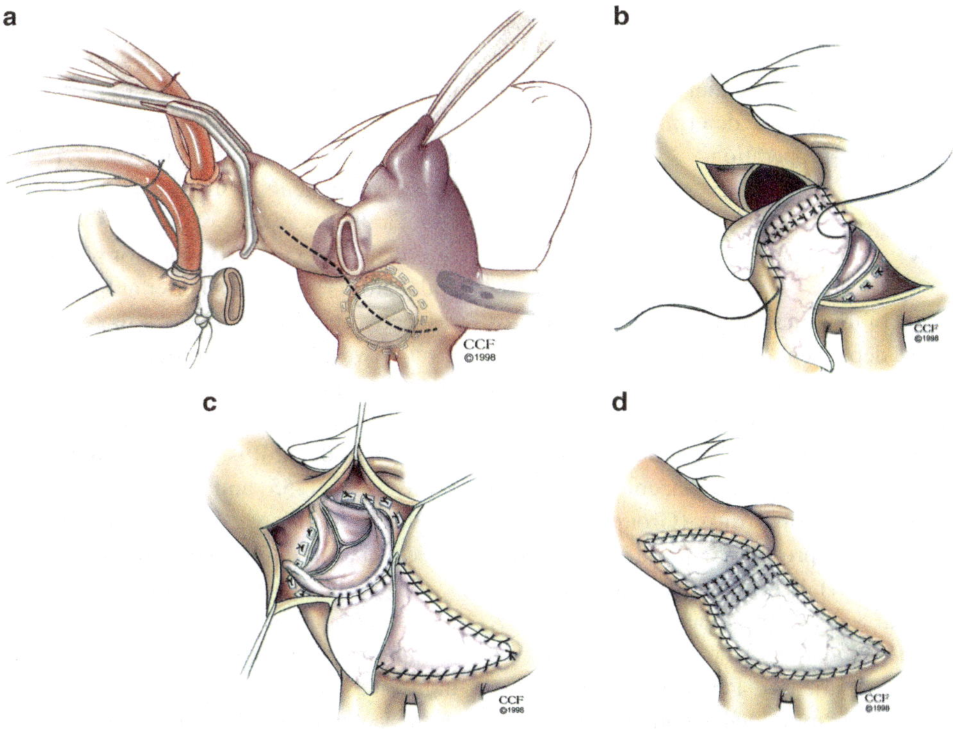

Fig. 12.4 (**a–d**) Reconstruction of the intravalvular fibrosa/fibrous trigones. Reprinted with permission, Cleveland Clinic Center for Medical Art & Photography ©1998–2011. All Rights Reserved

pericardium that is used to secure the new prostheses. Perfect exposure is mandatory whether it is provided by the extended transseptal approach or by dividing the superior vena cava and extending the left atriotomy from anterior to the right superior pulmonary vein toward the dome of the left atrium. This approach allows debridement of both valves and the fibrous trigones.

The prosthetic mitral valve is sutured to the annulus posteriorly, medially, and laterally, and the superior portion of the mitral valve annulus is reconstructed with a pericardial patch that replaces the fibrous trigones. The valve is sutured to the patch with horizontal mattress sutures. Once the mitral valve is secured in position, the aortic valve prosthesis is affixed to the aortic annulus. The pericardial patch is used to reconstruct the medial part of the aortic annulus. The aortic valve is sutured to patch. If the mitral prosthesis is too large, it can inhibit function of the aortic prosthesis. It is best not to oversize the mitral prosthesis [16].

Valve Choice

It is not known whether there are any important clinical advantages to using biological vs. mechanical valves for patients with prosthetic valve endocarditis. Moon and colleagues, from Stanford University, reported that prosthesis choice had no effect on perioperative mortality (biological 17% and mechanical 19%), 10-year survival (biological 51% and mechanical 50%), or 10-year freedom from reoperation (biological 56% and mechanical 74%, $p>0.64$). However, freedom from reoperation started to decline steeply 10 years after surgery for patients who received biological valves [17]. In the UK heart valve registry, of 322 infected prostheses explanted, there was no difference in 10-year survival by type of valve used for re-replacement (biological 44% and mechanical 33%) [18]. There is no clear evidence that type of prosthesis used for re-replacement determines survival or freedom from re-reoperation.

Results

The results of treatment of prosthetic valve endocarditis are dependent on many factors. The condition of the patient, timing of the operation, and the perioperative management all interact to affect outcome. Since 1972, we have performed prosthetic mitral valve replacement in 520 patients without endocarditis (Group A) and in 46 patients with prosthetic mitral valve endocarditis (Group B). In patients who received prosthetic mitral valve replacement for indications other than endocarditis, the mortality rate was 11% (58/520 patients). Perioperative mortality for the prosthetic mitral valve endocarditis group was higher (24%; 11/46 patients) and is consistent with other reported series [17, 18].

Long-term survival is reduced in patients treated with mitral valve replacement for prosthetic mitral valve endocarditis. Kaplan–Meier estimates for overall survival in our experience are shown in Fig. 12.5. Survival at 1, 5, and 10 years for patients with prosthetic mitral valve endocarditis was 66, 39, and 29%, respectively. Survival at 1, 5, and 10 years for patients without endocarditis was much better at 81, 66, and 43%, respectively. The difference between the two groups was highly significant ($p=0.006$). The UK heart valve registry reported similar poor late outcomes among patients requiring valve replacement for endocarditis with 1, 5, and 10 year survivals of 67, 55 and 38%, respectively [18]. Furthermore, type of valve implanted did not affect survival in our experience (Fig. 12.6).

Prosthetic valve endocarditis remains a serious complication of mitral valve replacement. Symptoms of infection are often variable, and a high index of suspicion is warranted in patients with bacteremia and a prosthetic mitral valve. Blood culture data and echocardiographic evidence of vegetation or valve dysfunction are the hallmarks of diagnosis. Most patients with an

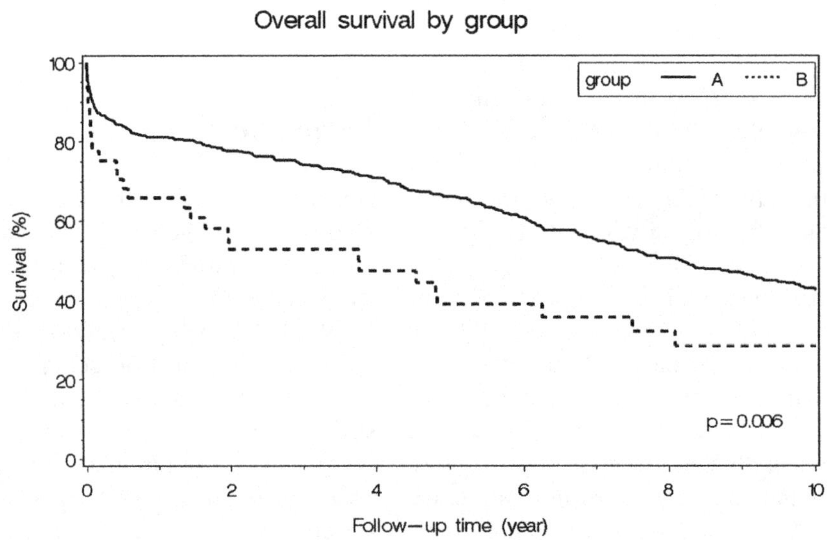

	0	2	4	6	8	10
A	520	339	287	215	164	127
B	46	20	17	12	9	8

Fig. 12.5 Kaplan–Meier estimates for overall survival. Group A: non-endocarditis-related prosthetic mitral valve replacement; Group B: endocarditis-related prosthetic mitral valve replacement

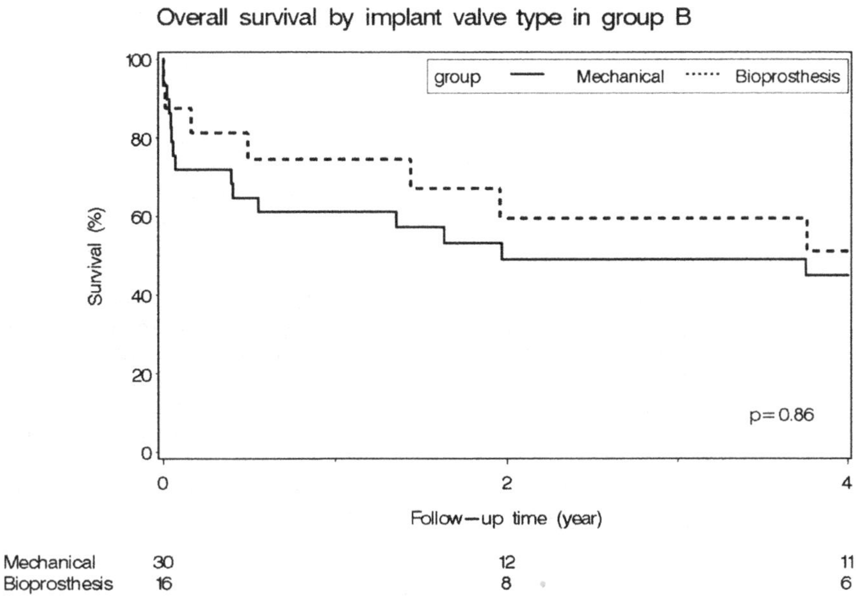

Fig. 12.6 Kaplan–Meier estimates for survival by implant valve type (mechanical vs. biological) of patients with endocarditis-related prosthetic mitral valve replacement

infected mitral prosthesis require operation. An aggressive surgical approach is required in this group of patients. Unfortunately, operation for prosthetic valve endocarditis carries a high associated mortality and reduced long-term survival.

References

1. Knott-Craig CJ, Trotter TH. Prosthetic valve endocarditis. In: Yang SC, Cameron DE, editors. Current therapy in thoracic and cardiovascular surgery. Philadelphia: Mosby Publishing; 2004. p. 640–4.
2. Habib G, Thuny F, Avierinos JF. Prosthetic valve endocarditis: current approach and therapeutic options. Prog Cardiovasc Dis. 2008;50:274–81.
3. Olaison L, Pettersson G. Current best practices and guidelines, indications for surgical intervention in infective endocarditis. Infect Dis Clin N Am. 2002;16:453–75.
4. Sohail MR, Martin KR, Wilson WR, Baddour LM, Harmsen WS, Steckelberg JM. Medical versus surgical management of *Staphylococcus aureus* prosthetic valve endocarditis. Am J Med. 2006;119:147–54.
5. Stamou SC, Petterson G, Gillinov AM. Surgical treatment of mitral valve endocarditis. In: Cohn LH, editor. Cardiac surgery in the adult. 3rd ed. New York: McGraw Hill Publishing; 2008. p. 1069–78.
6. American College of Cardiology/American Heart Association Task Force on Practice Guidelines; Society of Cardiovascular Anesthesiologists; Society for Cardiovascular Angiography and Interventions; Society of Thoracic Surgeons, Bonow RO, Carabello BA, Kanu C, de Leon AC Jr, Faxon DP, Freed MD, Gaasch WH, Lytle BW, Nishimura RA, O'Gara PT, O'Rourke RA, Otto CM, Shah PM, Shanewise JS, Smith SC Jr, Jacobs AK, Adams CD, Anderson JL, Antman EM, Faxon DP, Fuster V, Halperin JL, Hiratzka LF, Hunt SA, Lytle BW, Nishimura R, Page RL, Riegel B. ACC/AHA 2006 guidelines for the management of patients with valvular heart disease: a report of the American College of Cardiology/American Heart Association Task Force on Practice Guidelines (writing committee to revise the 1998 Guidelines for the Management of Patients With Valvular Heart Disease):developed in collaboration with the Society of Cardiovascular Anesthesiologists: endorsed by the Society for Cardiovascular Angiography and Interventions and the Society of Thoracic Surgeons. Circulation. 2006;114:e84–231.
7. David TE. Surgical management of prosthetic mitral valve endocarditis. In: Machiraju VR, editor. Redo cardiac surgery in adults. New York: CME Network Publishing; 1997. p. 90–2.
8. David TE. The surgical treatment of patients with prosthetic valve endocarditis. Semin Thorac Cardiovasc Surg. 1995;7:47–53.
9. Gillinov AM, Shah RV, Curtic WE, Stuart RS, Cameron DE, Baumgartner WA, et al. Valve replace-

ment in patients with endocarditis and acute neurologic deficit. Ann Thorac Surg. 1996;61:1125–30.
10. Thuny F, Avierinos JF, Tribouilloy C, Giorgi R, Casalty JP, Milandre L, et al. Impact of cerebrovascular complications on mortality and neurologic outcome during infective endocarditis: a prospective multicentre study. Eur Heart J. 2007;28:1155–61.
11. Svensson LG, Gillinov AM, Blackstone EH, Houghtaling PL, Kim KH, Pettersson GB, et al. Does right thoracotomy increase the risk of mitral valve reoperation. JTCVS. 2007;134:677–82.
12. Brawley RF. Improved exposure of the mitral valve in patients with a small left atrium. Ann Thorac Surg. 1980;29:179–81.
13. Guiraudon GM, Ofiesh JG, Kaushik R. Extended vertical transatrial septal approach to the mitral valve. Ann Thorac Surg. 1991;52:1058–60.
14. Burkhart HM, Zehr KJ. Mitral valve replacement. In: Yang SC, Cameron DE, editors. Current therapy in thoracic and cardiovascular surgery. Philadelphia: Mosby Publishing; 2004. p. 623–6.
15. David TE, Feindel CM, Armstrong S, Sun Z. Reconstruction of the mitral annulus. JTCVS. 1995;110:1323–32.
16. Maekawa A, Watanabe T, Usui A, Ohara Y, Takagi Y, Masumoto H, et al. Optimal size of prostheses for functioning of the aortic prosthetic valve in aortic and mitral valve replacement with annular enlargement through Manouguian's technique. Artif Organs. 2002;26:833–9.
17. Moon MR, Miller DC, Moore KA, Oyer PE, Mitchell RS, Robbins RC, et al. Treatment of endocarditis with valve replacement: the question of tissue versus mechanical prosthesis. Ann Thorac Surg. 2001;71:1164–71.
18. Edwards MB, Ratnatunga C, Dore CJ, Taylor KM. Thirty-day mortality and long-term survival following surgery for prosthetic endocarditis: a study from the UK heart valve registry. Eur J Cardiothorac Surg. 1998;14:156–64.

Surgical Management of Atrial Fibrillation in Redo Cardiac Operations

13

John M. Stulak and Hartzell V. Schaff

Reoperative Cardiac Surgery

With improving surgical care yielding better outcomes, patients who have undergone a cardiac operation are surviving longer, and surgeons will inevitably face an increasing number of reoperative procedures whether it is for surgical ablation of atrial fibrillation (AF) or other cardiac pathology. General approaches to reoperation and resternotomy are covered in other sections, but it is worth emphasizing that approximately 10% of all adult cardiac operations involve a redo sternotomy, which carries an 8% risk of significant hemorrhage [1]. Thus, it is important to weigh the potential risks and benefits of additional procedures, such as ablation of AF, in these patients who have higher than normal morbidity and mortality.

Indications

There are several distinct groups of patients who may require a redo cardiac operation and present with AF. Typically, AF is not the primary indication for operation in these patients, but is the result of underlying cardiac pathology. Because of structural alterations in the atria, sinus rhythm seldom returns after successful anatomic repair alone, and concomitant antiarrhythmic procedures yield the best chance of ablating AF. Concomitant ablation of AF during redo operations is especially important in patients who are highly symptomatic from tachyarrhythmias, especially younger patients with limiting symptoms and those who are intolerant to medications. Also, we are aggressive in performing surgical ablation of AF during reoperation in patients who have contraindications to anticoagulation with warfarin or those who have had thromboembolic stroke. Finally, there are selected patients with left ventricular dysfunction who may benefit from surgical treatment of AF in the setting of tachycardia-induced cardiomyopathy [2].

Conversely, we consider concomitant surgical ablation of AF less important in patients who have long-standing arrhythmias and those who will require anticoagulation with warfarin for other reasons, such as a mechanical prosthetic valve or a coagulation disorder. If concomitant ablation is undertaken during reoperation in such patients, we would, in general, prefer a lesser procedure, such as pulmonary vein isolation (PVI) with a radio frequency (RF) device or cryoprobe.

Another sizeable group of patients who require redo cardiac surgery and may benefit from surgical ablation of atrial arrhythmias during reoperative cardiac surgery are patients with congenital heart disease. Commonly, AF in these patients is associated with right atrial enlargement, and we have found that a right-sided maze procedure (incisions

J.M. Stulak, MD (✉) • H.V. Schaff, MD
Division of Cardiovascular Surgery, Mayo Clinic, Rochester, MN, USA
e-mail: stulak.john@mayo.edu

V.R. Machiraju et al. (eds.), *Redo Cardiac Surgery in Adults*,
DOI 10.1007/978-1-4614-1326-4_13, © Springer Science+Business Media, LLC 2012

limited to the right atrium and interatrial septum) at the time of intracardiac repair is effective in ablating AF.

Risk of thromboembolism increases with AF, and the loss of left atrial contraction impairs optimal hemodynamics. In addition, many patients undergoing reoperative procedures have reduced cardiac function and insufficient reserve to withstand the effects of continued AF, both from a hemodynamic and functional standpoint. For instance, the most common cause of repeat hospitalization in patients who have had repair of Ebstein anomaly was management of atrial tachyarrhythmias, thus, emphasizing the importance of performing a maze procedure at the time of tricuspid valve operation if AF or atrial flutter is present in these patients [3, 4]. This is especially important in reoperations in which the right atrium has undergone extensive structural and histologic changes due to significant tricuspid regurgitation after a prior repair has failed or during re-replacement of a degenerated bioprosthesis. These patients are at high risk of recurrent AF if intracardiac repair alone is undertaken. Similarly, arrhythmia surgery in patients undergoing Fontan conversion from an atriopulmonary to total cavopulmonary connection with an extracardiac conduit may be especially useful because AF causes significant functional disability, promotes thrombus formation, and the medications used for its treatment have significant adverse side effects [5]. Each subgroup of patients has its own special set of characteristics that must be considered when contemplating both resternotomy and what type of antiarrhythmic procedure is most appropriate to perform.

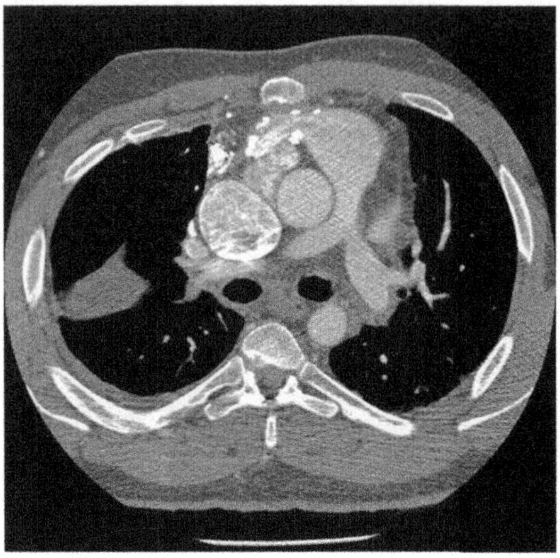

Fig. 13.1 Computerized tomography demonstrates a calcified atriopulmonary connection that is closely adherent to the posterior aspect of the sternum in a patient who underwent previous Fontan operation

Congenital Heart Disease

Many patients having palliation or correction of congenital defects during infancy or childhood will require later reoperation; it is estimated that there are approximately three million adults in the United States with congenital heart disease [6]. Repeat sternotomies in this patient population pose an increased risk of both potential cardiac injury and operative mortality. This risk increases as the number of redo sternotomies increases; 1.8% for patients with one previous operation and 8% in patients with four or more previous operations [6].

There are special technical considerations during reoperation in patients with congenital heart disease. For example, in patients with tetralogy of Fallot (TOF) or pulmonary atresia (PA) with ventricular septal defect (VSD) who had an extracardiac conduit used in the initial repair, the conduit lies to the left of the midline and the aorta is often enlarged and in the midline, frequently in close proximity to the posterior aspect of the sternum. In patients with transposition of the great arteries (TGA) who have undergone the Rastelli operation or repair of truncus arteriosus, the pulmonary conduit lies more in the midline and may be incorporated into the posterior side of the sternum. The atriopulmonary connection in patients who have undergone a Fontan operation may become calcified and adherent to the underside of the sternum (Fig. 13.1). Patients who have undergone the Ross procedure may have aneurysmal dilatation of their autograft, and this may be at risk during sternal reentry. Ebstein anomaly results in severely enlarged right-sided chambers, and the anterior position of the right ventricle places it at risk during reoperation (Fig. 13.2).

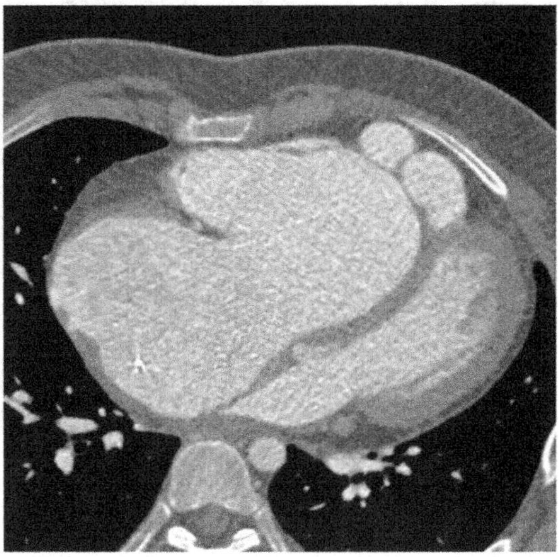

Fig. 13.2 Computerized tomography demonstrates a significantly enlarged right ventricle that is closely adherent to the posterior aspect of the sternum in a patient who underwent previous operation for Ebstein anomaly

A massively enlarged and thinned right atrium poses a risk during deeper mediastinal dissection. Some patients with congenital heart disease have residual, recurrent, or unrepaired septal defects, and this is important to consider during reoperation to avoid inadvertent air embolism. All these factors should be taken into account when deciding for or against an ablative procedure for AF and which method should be employed.

Valvular Heart Disease

Progression of native valve disease, failure of initial valve repair, and complications of valve prostheses including structural degeneration, paravalvular leakage, infection, and thrombosis are the most frequent and important causes of reoperation in patients with valvular disease. In many patients with these complications, dilatation and fibrosis of the left atrium are the substrate for the development and maintenance of AF. Indeed, the prevalence of AF in patients undergoing mitral valve reoperation may be as high as 52–62% and is greater than the prevalence of AF in patients undergoing primary mitral valve surgery [7, 8].

There is strong rationale for performing a concomitant maze operation during valve surgery in general, and these arguments may be more compelling in the reoperative setting because of a prolonged effect of valve pathology on the atria. First, valve repair or replacement alone cures AF in less than 50% of patients. An analysis of seven matched-controlled studies reported a 4–53% freedom from AF when only the valve pathology was corrected compared with 77–95% freedom from AF when a concomitant maze procedure was performed [9]. Furthermore, four randomized studies reported a 78–88% freedom from AF in the concomitant maze group compared with 29–40% freedom from AF in the control group with 1.5 years of follow-up [9]. Despite heterogeneity in definitions of AF and "success," studies clearly demonstrate that a concomitant maze procedure enhances control of AF compared with corrective valve surgery alone.

A second important reason to consider concomitant ablative procedures for patients with valvular heart disease and AF is risk of thromboembolic stroke. Improvement in rhythm status after the addition of a concomitant maze operation in the aforementioned studies was accompanied with a five to ninefold reduction in risk of embolic events or stroke [9]. Importantly, these beneficial effects of the maze procedure did not come at the expense of an increase in operative mortality or nonfatal morbidity, such as bleeding complications, infection, low cardiac output, reoperation, myocardial infarction, and renal failure. Furthermore, requirements for new permanent pacemaker implantation were similar in patients who had concomitant ablative procedures for AF compared with those who had valvular surgery alone. Thus, addition of a concomitant maze operation at the time of reoperative valvular surgery is associated with higher freedom from AF and stroke without a significant increase in morbidity or mortality. In addition, elimination of the arrhythmia in these patients offers the best chance for discontinuation of chronic warfarin anticoagulation if the valve is re-repaired or a bioprosthesis is used for re-replacement.

Another important reason to consider concomitant ablative procedures for patients with valvular heart disease and AF is to attempt to halt the progression of tricuspid valve regurgitation (TR). The course of TR after mitral valve surgery is difficult to predict [10, 11]; however, it is well documented that TR is associated with reduced late survival [12]. Furthermore, late reoperation for TR in this setting carries a high risk for mortality, and late functional improvement is poor [13].

Although correction of left-sided valvular pathology may decrease volume and pressure "back-up" through the pulmonary vasculature, TR may actually worsen during follow-up in some patients, especially those with rheumatic or ischemic heart disease, and persistent AF is an important predictor of late TR [14]. More recent data examining the role of AF in the progression of TR have demonstrated that the addition of a maze procedure at the time of correction of left-sided valvular pathology halted the progression of TR in 87–91% of patients compared with only 55–61% of patients after left-sided valve surgery alone ($p=0.001$) [15, 16]. Furthermore, significant late TR was present in only 15% of patients after the maze procedure compared to 40% after valve surgery alone ($p=0.001$). In both studies, the presence of late AF was the only factor that was associated with progression of TR late after correction of left-sided valvular pathology.

In contrast with the many reports of concomitant surgery for AF in patients undergoing primary operation for valvular disease, there are few studies that exclusively address outcome of concomitant procedures for AF in patients undergoing reoperation. Kobayashi and associates reported results of 42 patients who had a standard Cox-maze procedure at the time of mitral valve reoperation; there were no deaths in the series, and sinus rhythm was restored in 67% of patients [17].

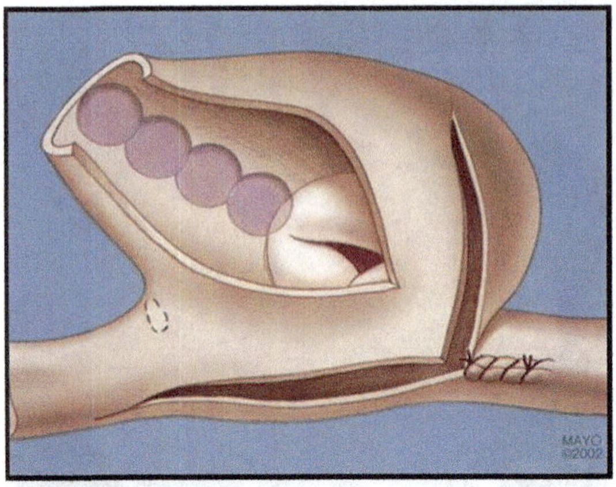

Fig. 13.3 On the medial aspect of the right atrium, we avoid an incision and apply a linear cryolesion from the cut edge of the appendage to the same area of the tricuspid valve as classically described. Depicted are sequential distinct cryolesions performed in the earlier years of our maze experience; as mentioned, in the current era, this is a continuous, linear cryolesion. By permission of Mayo Foundation for Medical Education and Research. All rights reserved

Surgical Techniques

Cut and Sew Biatrial Maze Procedure

After resternotomy and necessary mediastinal dissection, cardiopulmonary bypass is instituted with ascending aortic cannulation for arterial inflow and direct cannulation of the superior and inferior vena cavae for venous return. A tack vent is placed in the ascending aorta for cardioplegia administration and venting. Subsequent steps and choice of procedure are dictated by several factors including difficulty of the planned valve or congenital operation, quality of tissues, and anticipated difficulty in dissection.

If elimination of AF is of major importance, and if operative findings are favorable, we would proceed with a standard cut and sew biatrial maze procedure [18, 19]. The cavae are snared around the cannulas, and initial steps can be performed with the heart beating if the atrial septum is intact. Operation begins with amputation of the right atrial appendage, if it is present, and an incision is made from the base of the resected appendage inferolaterally toward the inferior vena cava. On the medial aspect of the right atrium, we avoid an incision and apply a linear cryolesion from the cut edge of the appendage to the same area of the tricuspid valve as classically described (Fig. 13.3). This avoids division of the frequently seen branch of the right coronary artery, which supplies the sinoatrial node. We have found that the risk of postoperative sinus node dysfunction can be

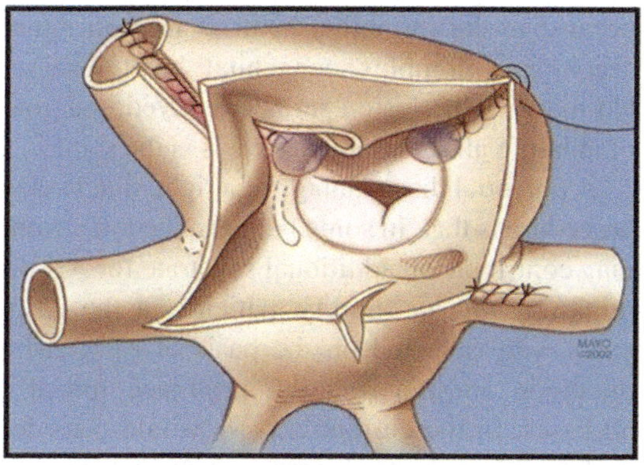

Fig. 13.4 The right-sided maze lesions are shown. A cryolesion is placed on the endocardial surface between the end of the epicardial incision and the tricuspid annulus. By permission of Mayo Foundation for Medical Education and Research. All rights reserved

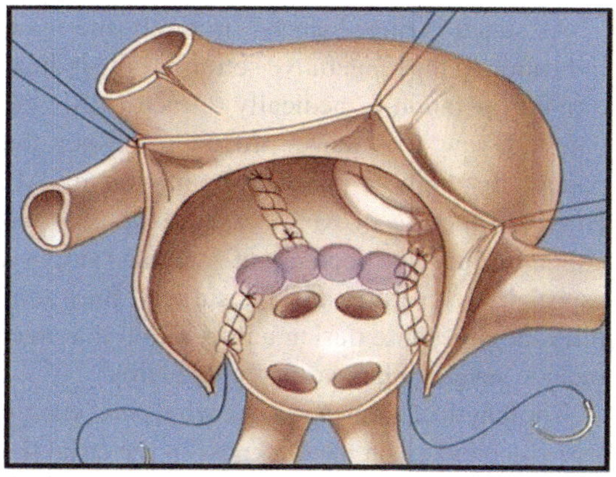

Fig. 13.5 The left-sided maze lesions are shown. A linear cryolesion can be utilized to complete isolation of the pulmonary veins if it appears that exposure of the left lateral portion of the left atrium will make suturing difficult. By permission of Mayo Foundation for Medical Education and Research. All rights reserved

reduced using a cryolesion instead of an incision in this location. The third incision is made from the superior vena cava to the inferior vena cava parallel to the plane of the atrial septum. A final incision is made perpendicular to the third incision and carried to the lateral tricuspid valve annulus. A cryolesion is placed on the endocardial surface between the end of the epicardial incision and the tricuspid annulus (Fig. 13.4).

After aortic cross-clamping, cardioplegia infusion, and opening of the left atrium, we incise the atrial septum staying just cephalad to the fossa ovalis and continuing toward the tendon of Todaro near the coronary sinus. For patients who have preoperative atrial flutter, the right atrial isthmus is cryoablated. The left atrial incision is carried laterally around the left pulmonary veins to intersect either below the orifice of the atrial appendage or in the orifice if the left atrial appendage is amputated. If the incision is carried below the appendage, we oversew the orifice; alternatively, if the appendage is amputated, we extend the encircling incision to the orifice and close the orifice with the same suture used for repairing the atrium (3-0 or 4-0 Prolene). An incision is made from the inferior encircling incision to the mitral valve annulus, and a cryolesion is placed on the coronary sinus and surrounding tissue.

A linear cryolesion can be utilized to complete isolation of the pulmonary veins if it appears that exposure of the left lateral portion of the left atrium will make suturing difficult (Fig. 13.5). A left reduction atrioplasty can be performed by resection of two segments, one inferior to the encircling incision and one superior to the encircling incision and then closing the encircling incision.

Alternate Energy Sources

Alternate energy sources are used by many surgeons to create atrial lesions, and indeed, some surgeons are attempting to cure AF by application of various energy sources to the epicardial atrial surface on the beating heart. The most frequently used method for ablation of atrial tissue is RF, which employs alternating current to transfer energy to atrial tissue. Another common method is cryoablation that freezes atrial tissue in contact with the cryotherapy probe. Although these alternate energy sources may simplify the procedure and potentially decrease the length of the operation, there are potential disadvantages including inconsistent depth of injury, leading to nontransmural lesions, and injury to surrounding mediastinal structures.

As stated earlier, lone AF is rarely the main indication in the reoperative setting. If the indication for operation is medically refractory AF, the cut and sew Cox-maze procedure offers the patient the highest chance of ablation of AF. However, the use of RF or cryoablation for AF ablation during concomitant cardiac surgery, especially reoperative cardiac surgery, may simplify the procedure during an operation that may include several other cardiac procedures.

The length of application of each type of energy varies depending on the thickness of the atrial tissue, presence of fibrosis, etc. Cryolesions are typically applied with the cryoprobe in contact with atrial tissue for approximately 1–2 min at −60°C. When bipolar RF is utilized, the device gives feedback when the lesion is transmural. This usually marks the end of creating the lesion; however, depending again on the quality and thickness of atrial tissue, a second application is sometimes used. The cryomaze or modified cryoablation procedure can be performed using a variety of Frigitronics cryoprobes (Frigitronics; CooperVision Inc, Lake Forest, CA), and more recently the CryoCath cryoprobe (Medtronic CryoCath, Pointe-Claire, Quebec). Bipolar RF ablation was performed using either the AtriCure device (AtriCure, Inc, Cincinnati, OH) or Medtronic device (Medtronic, Inc, Minneapolis, MN).

Cut and Sew Right-Sided Maze Procedure

Because many repairs for congenital heart disease are reoperations in patients with AF, the right-sided procedure has the advantage of minimizing dissection of adhesions, thus resulting in shorter cardiopulmonary bypass time when compared with the standard biatrial maze procedure [4, 20]. In addition, by avoiding suture lines in the left atrium, the total number of suture lines is limited and the risk of bleeding behind the heart is minimized while also preventing a possible postoperative noncontractile left atrium and the subsequent risk of systemic embolization. The right-sided maze procedure is often modified from the original description of the maze lesions because of the variability in atrial anomalies that accompany complex congenital heart disease. No matter what lesion set is employed, the goal of ablating all reentrant pathways is the same.

A potential disadvantage of a right-sided maze procedure is that, in some patients, the left atrium may contribute an additional substrate for AF. To minimize this possibility, patients in the early years were selected on the basis of right atrial dilatation, and a normal left atrial size in nearly all cases. In the current era, we would consider performing a biatrial maze procedure in any patient with evidence of atrial arrhythmias and any pathology leading to the development of a substrate for AF in the left atrium.

Alternate Lesion Sets

Increased understanding of the pathogenesis of AF coupled with the development of new ablation technologies have resulted in surgeons exploring simpler techniques and localized lesion sets. There are many alternate lesion sets described for ablation of AF using alternate energy sources, especially during surgery for mitral valve disease. Most include some combination of the following: left atrial appendectomy or exclusion, PVI, and some variation of linear connecting lesions [21]. The decision of which lesion set to employ is based upon patient factors, such as type of preoperative AF, concomitant procedures required, and goals of AF ablation. Furthermore, success of any particular lesion set depends on patient selection.

Although PVI is attractive because it is simple to perform and can be used “off pump,” isolated PVI is generally less effective compared with a more complete left atrial or biatrial lesion set, especially for patients with persistent or permanent AF [22] and patients requiring concomitant procedures [23]. Although a meta-analysis by Barnett and Ad [24] demonstrated greater efficacy with biatrial lesion sets when compared with left atrial lesion sets alone, certainly an isolated left atrial lesion set is better than no ablation at all. This stresses the importance of appreciating the anatomic substrate from which the AF is arising. A more complete left atrial lesion set generally includes a connecting lesion to the mitral valve annulus and excision of the left atrial appendage added to the PVI. Furthermore, regardless of surgical approach, the importance of particular left atrial lesions has been demonstrated in the literature. For example, patients with long-standing persistent AF have a higher frequency of recurrent AF if an isthmus lesion down to the mitral valve annulus is not performed [25], and isolation the entire posterior atrium around the pulmonary veins as a single unit ("box" lesion) increases freedom from AF and decreases antiarrhythmic medication use [26].

After weighing the risks and benefits, the ultimate choice of lesion set should be individualized toward the preoperative indications for AF ablation, anatomy encountered during the reoperation (dense adhesions, friable tissue, etc.), and need for concomitant operations. The success of any ablative procedure for AF in this or any other setting depends on individualized patient selection.

Prophylactic Maze Procedure

Although performing a maze procedure prophylactically has never been investigated or proven to be beneficial, it may play a role in patients with a markedly dilated right or left atrium. We believe that these patients are at high risk for subsequent development of atrial tachyarrhythmias. In addition, many of these patients have had multiple prior operations. Multiple prior incisions in the right atrium may also increase the late development of AF or "incisional" atrial tachycardias. In these patients, we would perform either the standard Cox-maze III procedure, or a modified cryoablation maze with lesions similar to those been previously described [18, 19].

Postoperative Management

There are variable protocols for the postoperative management of patients who have undergone a Cox-maze operation. For arrhythmia control, some centers utilize antiarrhythmic drugs, such as amiodarone, prophylactically in all patients and maintain this for 3 months. We prefer to use these medications selectively in patients who experience atrial or ventricular arrhythmias during hospitalization. We monitor potassium and magnesium levels and maintain these in the high normal range. Postoperative AF is treated promptly with amiodarone, and electrical cardioversion is used as needed. If AF occurs early after operation and is treated with amiodarone, we continue the drug for 3 months.

It is important to use diuretics liberally early after operation. Removal of the atrial appendages during the Cox-maze procedure eliminates an important source of atrial natriuretic peptide, and this along with elevations of aldosterone and antidiuretic hormone early postoperatively predisposes the patient to fluid retention [27].

We recommend systemic anticoagulation with warfarin (Coumadin) for 3 months postoperatively, but there is no consensus on the need for anticoagulation beyond this interval. Some clinicians prefer to continue warfarin believing that risk of thromboembolism is not reduced sufficiently to avoid systemic anticoagulation. Others argue that if AF is eliminated and ventricular function is normal, the risk of an intracardiac source of thromboemboli from a postoperative patient without a left atrial appendage is very low. Thus, the additional risk and inconvenience of using warfarin is not justified in this setting.

Patients who manifest junctional rhythm postoperatively may ultimately be discharged in this rhythm if hemodynamics are adequate. We do not routinely utilize medications or stimulants, such as theophylline, as is practice in other centers. A significant number of patients who have junctional bradycardia early after operation will regain a stable sinus rhythm; however, this may require weeks or months of convalescence. Persistent junctional rhythm may reflect sinus node dysfunction, and patients who have chronotropic incompetence because of this may require permanent transvenous pacing.

Mayo Clinic Experience

Patients

From January 1994 through May 2009, we performed surgery for AF in 245 patients who had at least one prior cardiac operation. All these procedures for ablation of AF were done in conjunction with other cardiac repairs. The median age was 45 years (range 1–75 years) and 134 (55%) were females. Preoperative AF was intermittent in 161 patients and persistent in 84 patients. Primary cardiac diagnoses are presented in Table 13.1; the three most common were Ebstein anomaly ($n=43$), TOF ($n=36$), and acquired valvular or ischemic heart disease ($n=35$). Prior procedures performed are listed in Table 13.2. Patients had a median of one prior procedure (maximum, 8) and one prior sternotomy (maximum, 6) before their redo operation with concomitant AF surgery. Overall, 144 patients had 1 prior procedure, 62 had 2, 25 had 3, and 14 had 4 or more prior operations. A permanent pacemaker was previously required in 30 patients, and 12 patients underwent a prior catheter-based ablation for treatment of AF

Table 13.1 Primary cardiac diagnoses

Cardiac diagnosis	No.
Ebstein anomaly	43
Tetralogy of Fallot	36
Acquired heart disease	35
Rheumatic heart disease	18
Tricuspid atresia	13
Partial atrioventricular septal defect	11
Congenital pulmonary stenosis	10
Pulmonary atresia/ventricular septal defect	9
Double-inlet left ventricle	8
Atrial septal defect	7
Pulmonary atresia/intact ventricular septum	6
Combined pulmonary stenosis, atrial septal defect	5
Double-outlet right ventricle	4
Partial anomalous pulmonary venous return	4
Combined transposition of great arteries, tricuspid atresia	4
Complete atrioventricular septal defect	3
Hypertrophic obstructive cardiomyopathy	3
Isolated transposition of great arteries	3
Congenitally corrected transposition of great arteries	3
Shone syndrome	2
Ventricular septal defect	2
Others	16

Results

The types of AF ablative procedures performed varied widely (Table 13.3) and depended heavily on the concomitant cardiac procedure being performed. The three most common were isolated right-sided cryomaze ($n=84$), isolated right-sided cut and sew maze ($n=39$), and biatrial maze ($n=52$; cut and sew in 26, cryoablation in 26). Isolated cryoablation of the right atrial isthmus was performed in 30 patients.

Concomitant procedures performed are presented in detail in Table 13.4; the three most common were tricuspid valve surgery ($n=114$; replacement in 73 and repair in 41), mitral valve surgery ($n=73$; replacement in 46 and repair in 27), and pulmonary valve surgery ($n=65$; replacement in 64 and repair in 1). The three most common nonvalvular procedures performed were Fontan conversion ($n=35$), right reduction atrioplasty ($n=34$), and atrial septal defect repair ($n=22$). There were 14 early deaths (5.7%), but none of these were directly related to performance of the ablative procedures for AF. Early nonfatal morbidity is presented in detail in Table 13.5; the three most common complications were acute renal insufficiency ($n=7$), respiratory failure requiring tracheostomy ($n=5$), and pleural effusion requiring thoracentesis ($n=4$). New permanent pacemaker was required in 39 patients (18%), but complete heart block was the indication in only nine patients.

Late Outcome

Median late follow-up was 6 months (mean 2.1 years, maximum 14.7 years). Late mortality occurred in 24 patients during the follow-up period, and late permanent pacemaker was required

Table 13.2 Prior procedures performed

Prior procedure	No.
Atrial septal defect repair	50
Mitral valve surgery	50
Repair	25
Commissurotomy	13
Replacement – bioprosthesis	8
Replacement – mechanical	4
Tricuspid valve surgery	40
Replacement	22
Repair	18
Blalock–Taussig shunt	36
Tetralogy of Fallot complete repair	35
Fontan operation	33
Pulmonary valvotomy	20
Right ventricle to pulmonary artery conduit	19
Ventricular septal defect repair	19
Aortic valve replacement	19
Coronary artery bypass grafting	12
Repair of partial atrioventricular septal defect	9
Septal myectomy/subaortic resection	9
Glenn anastomosis	8
Repair of pulmonary atresia/ventricular septal defect	7
Aortic coarctation repair	7
Pulmonary artery banding	6
Pott's shunt	5
Surgical division of accessory pathway	5
Waterston shunt	5
Pulmonary valvectomy	4
Fontan revision	4
Blalock–Hanlon septectomy	3
Repair of complete atrioventricular septal defect repair	3
Damus–Stansel–Kaye	3
Pulmonary valve replacement	3
Aortic root replacement	3
Closure patent foramen ovale	2
Right reduction atrioplasty	2
Unspecified shunt	2
Others	16

Table 13.3 Types of surgical AF ablation performed

Type of surgical AF ablation	No.
Isolated right-sided cryomaze	84
Isolated right-sided cut and sew maze	39
Isolated right atrial isthmus ablation	30
Biatrial cryomaze	26
Biatrial cut and sew maze	26
Concomitant right atrial isthmus ablation	11
Left-sided cryomaze	7
Isolated cryo pulmonary vein isolation	5
Isolated radio frequency pulmonary vein isolation	5
Biatrial maze – cut and sew, radiofrequency, and cryoablation	4
Biatrial radio frequency maze	3
Right-sided cryomaze + pulmonary vein isolation	3
Isolated cut and sew pulmonary vein isolation	2
Right-sided radio frequency maze	2
Focal cryoablation	2
Others	6

in nine patients. Rhythm at last follow-up in 229 late survivors who had follow-up was sinus in 117 (51%), pacemaker in 78 (34%), AF in 27 (12%), and junctional in 7 (3%) patients. Thus, overall freedom from AF at last follow-up was 88%.

Summary

Atrial fibrillation is common in patients undergoing cardiac reoperations, and concomitant procedures for ablation of AF can be performed with reasonable safety and success. As mentioned previously, the decision to combine AF ablation with reoperation for another cardiac problem depends on the severity of preoperative symptoms and, ultimately on the intraoperative findings including severity of adhesions and anticipated difficulty of

Table 13.4 Procedures performed during concomitant AF surgery

Procedure performed	No.
Tricuspid valve surgery	114
Replacement	73
Bioprosthesis	65
Mechanical	8
Repair	41
Mitral valve surgery	74
Replacement	46
Mechanical	35
Bioprosthesis	11
Repair	27
Commissurotomy	1
Pulmonary valve surgery	65
Replacement	64
Bioprosthesis	59
Mechanical	5
Repair	1
Fontan conversion	35
Right reduction atrioplasty	34
Atrial septal defect repair	22
Coronary artery bypass grafting	12
Closure patent foramen ovale	12
Pulmonary artery augmentation	8
Ventricular septal defect repair	7
Ascending aortic replacement	6
Aortic valve surgery	6
Repair	4
Replacement	2
Left reduction atrioplasty	4
Aortic root replacement	3
Baffle partial anomalous pulmonary venous return	3
Glenn anastomosis	3
Pulmonary artery aneurysm repair	2
Hemiarch replacement	2
Septal myectomy	2
Pericardiectomy	2
Others	6

Table 13.5 Early complications

Complication	No.
Acute renal failure	7
Respiratory failure requiring tracheostomy	5
Multisystem organ failure	4
Extracorporeal membrane oxygenation	4
Pleural effusion requiring thoracentesis	4
Reexploration for bleeding	4
Gastrointestinal bleeding	3
Wound infection	3
Clostridium difficile colitis	3
Pericardial tamponade	3
Pneumonia	3
Adult respiratory distress syndrome	3
Groin seroma/hematoma	3
Protein-losing enteropathy	2
Urinary tract infection	2
Others	15

the concomitant cardiac repair. Often, a planned procedure has to be modified because of intraoperative findings. For example, if the surgeon plans for a biatrial maze procedure, but exposure of the left side of the atrium is difficult, then completion of PVI using cryotherapy may be the safest option. Similarly, adhesions may prevent safe dissection of the left pulmonary veins, and an endocardial approach may be necessary rather than epicardial PVI. Despite these potential limitations, surgical management of AF during reoperation can control the arrhythmia in 80–85% of patients.

References

1. Ellman PI, Smith RL, Girotti ME, et al. Cardiac injury during resternotomy does not affect perioperative mortality. J Am Coll Surg. 2008;206:993–9.
2. Stulak JM, Dearani JA, Daly RC, Zehr KJ, Sundt TM, Schaff HV. LV dysfunction in atrial fibrillation: restoration of sinus rhythm by the Cox-maze procedure significantly improves systolic function and functional status. Ann Thorac Surg. 2006;82:494–500.
3. Mavroudis C, Deal BJ, Backer CL, et al. Arrhythmia surgery in the patients with and without congenital heart disease. Ann Thorac Surg. 2008;86:857–68.
4. Stulak JM, Dearani JA, Puga FJ, et al. Right-sided maze procedure for atrial tachyarrhythmias in congenital heart disease. Ann Thorac Surg. 2006; 81:1780–4.
5. Mavroudis C, Deal BJ, Backer CL, et al. 111 Fontan conversions with arrhythmia surgery: surgical lessons and outcomes. Ann Thorac Surg. 2007;84:1457–66.
6. Brown ML, Dearani JA, Burkhart HM. The adult with congenital heart disease: medical and surgical considerations for management. Curr Opin Pediatr. 2009;21:561–4. Electronic publication ahead of print.
7. Meyer SR, Szeto WY, Augoustides JG, et al. Reoperative mitral valve surgery the port access minithoracotomy approach is safe and effective. Ann Thorac Surg. 2009;87:1426–30.

8. Borger MA, Yau TM, Rao V, Scully HE, David TE. Reoperative mitral valve replacement: importance of preservation of the subvalvular apparatus. Ann Thorac Surg. 2002;74:1482–7.
9. Wong JWW, Mak KH. Impact of maze and concomitant mitral valve surgery on clinical outcomes. Ann Thorac Surg. 2006;82:1938–47.
10. Braunwald NS, Ross Jr J, Morrow AG. Conservative management of tricuspid regurgitation in patients undergoing mitral valve replacement. Circulation. 1967;35(Suppl):I63–9.
11. Matsuyama K, Matsumoto M, Sugita T, Nishizawa J, Tokuda Y, Matsuo T. Predictors of residual tricuspid regurgitation after mitral valve surgery. Ann Thorac Surg. 2003;75:1826–8.
12. Nath J, Foster E, Heidenreich PA. Impact of tricuspid regurgitation on long-term survival. J Am Coll Cardiol. 2004;43:405–9.
13. Hornick P, Harris PA, Taylor KM. Tricuspid valve replacement subsequent to previous open heart surgery. J Heart Valve Dis. 1996;5:20–5.
14. Koelling TM, Aaronson KD, Cody RJ, Bach DS, Armstrong WF. Prognostic significance of mitral regurgitation and tricuspid regurgitation in patients with left ventricular systolic dysfunction. Am Heart J. 2002;144:524–9.
15. Stulak JM, Schaff HV, Dearani JA, Orszulak TA, Daly RC, Sundt III TM. Restoration of sinus rhythm by the maze procedure halts progression of tricuspid regurgitation after mitral surgery. Ann Thorac Surg. 2008;86:40–5.
16. Kim HK, Kim YJ, Kim KI, et al. Impact of the maze operation combined with left-sided valve surgery on the change in tricuspid regurgitation over time. Circulation. 2005;112(Suppl):I14–9.
17. Kobayashi J, Kosakai Y, Isobe F, et al. Rationale of the Cox-maze procedure for atrial fibrillation during redo mitral valve operations. J Thorac Cardiovasc Surg. 1996;112:1216–22.
18. Cox JL, Jaquiss RDB, Scheussler RB, Boineau JP. Modification of the maze procedure for atrial flutter and atrial fibrillation. II. Surgical technique of the maze III procedure. J Thorac Cardiovasc Surg. 1995;110:485–95.
19. Stulak JM, Sundt 3rd TM, Dearani JA, Daly RC, Orszulak TA, Schaff HV. Ten-year experience with the Cox-maze procedure for atrial fibrillation: how do we define success? Ann Thorac Surg. 2007;83:1319–24.
20. Theodoro DA, Danielson GK, Porter CJ, et al. Right-sided maze procedure for right atrial arrhythmias in congenital heart disease. Ann Thorac Surg. 1998;65:149–54.
21. Gillinov AM. Ablation of atrial fibrillation with mitral valve surgery. Curr Opin Cardiol. 2005;20:107–14.
22. Edgerton JR, Edgerton ZJ, Weaver T, et al. Minimally invasive pulmonary vein isolation and partial autonomic denervation for surgical treatment of atrial fibrillation. Ann Thorac Surg. 2008;86:35–8.
23. Melby SJ, Zierer A, Bailey MS, et al. A new era in the surgical treatment of atrial fibrillation: the impact of ablation technology and lesion set on procedural efficacy. Ann Surg. 2006;244:583–92.
24. Barnett SD, Ad N. Surgical ablation as treatment for the elimination of atrial fibrillation: a meta-analysis. J Thorac Cardiovasc Surg. 2006;131:1029–35.
25. Gillinov AM, McCarthy PM, Blackstone EH, et al. Surgical ablation of atrial fibrillation with bipolar radiofrequency as the primary modality. J Thorac Cardiovasc Surg. 2005;129:1322–9.
26. Voeller RK, Bailey MS, Zierer A, et al. Isolating the entire posterior left atrium improves surgical outcomes after the Cox-maze procedure. J Thorac Cardiovasc Surg. 2008;135:870–7.
27. Albage A, van der Linden J, Bengtsson L, et al. Elevations in antidiuretic hormone and aldosterone as possible causes of fluid retention in the Maze procedure. Ann Thorac Surg. 2001;72:58–64.

Surgical Management of Tricuspid Valve Disorders

14

Venkat R. Machiraju

Introduction

In recent years, there has been more appreciation for intraoperative assessment of valvular heart disease by the routine use of transesophageal echocardiogram (TEE), and corrective measures have been adopted to repair moderately regurgitating mitral and tricuspid valves. As recently as 10 years ago, asymptomatic regurgitant mitral valves in ischemic heart disease were not repaired, let alone the tricuspid valves. The popular belief was that pulmonary hypertension decreases after surgical correction of mitral valve stenosis or regurgitation, and then tricuspid regurgitation (TR) automatically disappears. In the recent years, however, it has become clear that the regurgitant pathology not only does not get better but can also even get worse resulting in heart failure [1]. There are significant differences in the outcomes of patients treated for TR before they have developed symptoms and the outcomes of patients treated after they develop symptoms. An incidental TR noticed during routine TEE examination during cardiac surgery, when corrected, will carry a lower mortality and morbidity as compared with a patient admitted with peripheral edema, hepatomegaly, elevated bilirubin, and symptoms of congestive heart failure. In the latter group, mortality ranges from 15 to 30%. This is more true for reoperations to correct recurrent TR, mainly due to right ventricular enlargement. In addition, the hospital length of stay is significantly increased while correcting low cardiac output syndrome.

V.R. Machiraju, MD (✉)
Department of Cardiothoracic Surgery,
University of Pittsburgh Medical Center,
Pittsburgh, PA, USA
e-mail: machvr@upmc.edu

Pathology

Tricuspid valve pathology is divided into tricuspid valve stenosis and tricuspid valve regurgitation. This is best evaluated by transthoracic echocardiography performed preoperatively. Stenotic pathology is seen in patients who have associated rheumatic heart disease or a tumor or thrombus extending into the right atrium from inferior or superior vena cava. The majority of the patients with predominant regurgitation have left-sided valvular pathology, moderate pulmonary hypertension, and secondary tricuspid valve regurgitation. Primary tricuspid valve regurgitation in the western world is generally from endocarditis and rarely from congenital anomalies. The infection is typically due to either intravenous drug abuse or the presence of long-standing indwelling intravenous catheters.

Risk Factors

Pulmonary hypertension is associated with TR but not all patients with severe pulmonary artery systolic pressure (PASP) develop TR, including

V.R. Machiraju et al. (eds.), *Redo Cardiac Surgery in Adults*,
DOI 10.1007/978-1-4614-1326-4_14, © Springer Science+Business Media, LLC 2012

some patients with a PASP > 60 mmHg. Increased age, enlargement of the heart, atrial fibrillation, and the presence of indwelling pacing leads all contribute to the increased incidence of TR. Various risk factors for in-hospital operative mortality after surgical repair of TR have been identified including advanced age, male gender, the number of additional procedures performed, the length of cardiopulmonary bypass time, previous intracardiac repairs, the degree of hepatomegaly present, preoperative serum bilirubin level, mean pulmonary artery pressure >40 mmHg, New York Heart Association Classification > III, and emergent cardiac surgery. Symptoms of right-sided heart failure, including decreased appetite, the presence of ascites and peripheral edema, and decreased serum albumin, have all resulted in prolonged hospital stay even after successful surgical repair of TR. The presence of atrial fibrillation, secondary to enlargement of the right side of the heart, results in persistent low cardiac output syndrome. However, mortality is not increased by the duration of TR, concomitant aortic or mitral valve surgery, or radiographic evidence of congestive heart failure.

Tricuspid Regurgitation

Primary TR occurs in congenital conditions, like Ebstein's anomaly, and endocarditis but in adult redo cardiac surgical patients, most of the time TR is secondary to left-sided valvular pathology. Elevated systolic right ventricular pressure >55 mmHg, especially in patients with pulmonic stenosis, can cause TR. In such cases, the primary valvular problem should be corrected either by replacing or by repairing the pulmonary, mitral, or aortic valve before trying to correct the TR. Calafiore and associates [2] studied a group of patients that had ischemic mitral regurgitation and subsequent TR. In their study, the patients that had concomitant repair of the tricuspid valve did better than the group that did not have any repair. The patients that did not have tricuspid valve repair at the time of mitral valve surgery eventually developed symptomatic TR. Sometimes, there is no TR at the time of mitral valve replacement, but prosthetic valve changes the geometry of the fibrous trigone, which leads to the development of atrial fibrillation, and the patient slowly develops TR. Maintenance of the sinus rhythm after mitral valve surgery decreases the incidence of development of TR [3, 4]. Late onset TR after left-sided valve surgery is a sign of right-sided heart failure, and repairing such valves should be carefully judged as patient may go into further heart failure leading into higher surgical mortality. The normal tricuspid valve is oval shaped and generally measures 30–35 mm across the annulus. It is lowest at posteroseptal portion and highest at the anteroseptal portion. Any enlargement in this area changes the annulus to a circular configuration leading to tethering of the three leaflets and preventing the leaflets from coapting in the center. Tricuspid annular dilatation is the most important predictor of development of regurgitation. An annular dimension >30 mm or annulus size >70 mm will result in TR. An annuloplasty ring brings the valve to its original anatomical configuration. Although the De Vega annuloplasty was used several years ago, we have switched to an established ring annuloplasty to reduce the valve annular dimension to <30 mm. With a significantly dilated tricuspid valve, a cloverleaf repair technique along with an annuloplasty ring can decrease the regurgitant jet without replacing the valve. The American College of Cardiology/American Heart Association (ACC/AHA) 2006 Guidelines for Management of Patients with Valvular Heart Disease make the several recommendations for surgical management of TR. Specifically, the guidelines state that tricuspid valve repair is beneficial with mitral valve disease requiring mitral valve repair or replacement (class I recommendation, level of evidence: B); tricuspid valve repair is reasonable for primary TR when the patient is symptomatic (class IIa recommendation, level of evidence: C); tricuspid valve replacement is reasonable for severe TR when valve leaflets are not amenable for repair (class IIa recommendation, level of evidence: C); and correction of moderate TR may be considered during mitral valve surgery when pulmonary artery hypertension is present (class IIb recommendation, level of evidence C).

Symptomatic Tricuspid Valve Regurgitation

Management of Patients with Decompensated TR

Symptoms and signs of heart failure are evident in patients with decompensated TR with increased venous pressure, enlarged jugular veins, and enlarged veins over the chest wall. The presentation of TR can vary depending on preload, afterload, and right ventricular systolic function. Patients may be on anticoagulation therapy prior to surgery because of atrial fibrillation. Also, there may be hepatic congestion and an abnormal prothrombin time or low platelet count. Especially in a redo cardiac surgical setting, these patients are notorious for bleeding after surgery, even though the prothrombin time has been reversed back to its normal level. Most of the time, the perioperative bleeding is seen from the chest wall, the bone marrow from the sternum, and the raw mediastinal surface. Multiple transfusions of blood and blood products and the use of multiple inotropic agents to maintain adequate cardiac output are typically required. Multiple re-explorations for bleeding control have resulted in increased perioperative morbidity. The subsequent development of renal failure and further development of multisystem failure have contributed to higher mortality. In patients with severe TR and congestive heart failure, some surgeons prefer replacing the tricuspid valve rather than repairing it with an annuloplasty ring for fear of recurrence of regurgitation, even though the regurgitation appears to have been corrected with the ring annuloplasty surgical procedure [5]. I have seen worsening peripheral edema of both lower extremities extending all the way up to the umbilicus in spite of satisfactory repair of the tricuspid valve. These patients required higher doses of diuretic therapy to resolve their pedal edema.

Management of Tricuspid Valve Endocarditis

Tricuspid valve endocarditis is seen most frequently in intravenous drug users and in patients who have long-term indwelling catheters. Patients receiving hemodialysis are more prone to such infections. The most commonly involved organisms are *Staphylococcus aureus* and gram-negative rods, such as *Pseudomonas aeruginosa*. Fungal infections from *Candida albicans* also cause tricuspid valve endocarditis in immune suppressed patients. Whenever there is significant damage to the structure of the valve tissue, valve replacement has typically been performed. However, with improved surgical techniques and various successful cases reported following valve repairs, there is more impetus to repair partially or totally destroyed valves. Excision of vegetation on the valve leaflets and repair of the hole with a piece of pericardium or an opposing leaflet transfer has been successful. Even partial replacement of the tricuspid valve with a mitral homograft has been reported. The presence of ongoing sepsis and the possibility of prosthetic valve endocarditis, in addition to the initial native valve endocarditis, have encouraged more surgeons to pursue repair techniques in lieu of replacement.

When replacement of the tricuspid valve has been necessary, both mechanical and tissue valves have been used. There has been controversy about the benefit of one type of replacement valve over the other, but in the current era, tissue valves have been used more frequently to avoid high-dose anticoagulation protocols [6]. Valve replacement has a higher incidence of complete heart block, compared with valve repair, as the annuloplasty ring generally excludes the septal area while sutures need to be placed circumferentially to secure the prosthetic valve. If a patient already has an endocardial ventricular lead, it can be left outside the prosthetic ring instead of replacing it with an epicardial lead. Patients requiring a permanent pacemaker after tricuspid valve replacement fare better with an epicardial pacemaker lead.

Conclusions

Though the surgical techniques for fixing tricuspid valve pathology are relatively simple compared with mitral and aortic valve surgical procedures, the morbidity and mortality are much higher for correcting tricuspid valve pathology. This is mainly because right-sided heart failure may develop for various reasons. Incidental echocardiographic findings of TR during cardiac surgical procedures warrant attention, and repair of such valves will lead to better outcomes. Untreated TR will continue to worsen and eventually will lead to right-sided heart failure, even after correcting mitral valve pathology.

References

1. McGrath LB, Gonzalez-Lavin L, Bailey BM, Grunkemeier GL, Fernandez J, Laub GW. Tricuspid valve operations in 530 patients. Twenty-five-year assessment of early and late phase events. J Thorac Cardiovasc Surg. 1990;99(1):124–33.
2. Calafiore AM, Gallina S, Iaco AL, et al. Mitral valve surgery for functional mitral regurgitation: should moderate-or-more tricuspid regurgitation be treated? A propensity score analysis. Ann Thorac Surg. 2009;87(3):698–703.
3. Bianchi G, Solinas M, Bevilacqua S, Glauber M. Which patient undergoing mitral valve surgery should also have the tricuspid repair? Interact Cardiovasc Thorac Surg. 2009;9(6):1009–20.
4. Stulak JM, Suri RM, Dearani JA, Sundt 3rd TM, Schaff HV. When should prophylactic maze procedure be considered in patients undergoing mitral valve surgery? Ann Thorac Surg. 2010;89(5):1395–401.
5. Rogers JH, Bolling SF. The tricuspid valve: current perspective and evolving management of tricuspid regurgitation. Circulation. 2009;119(20):2718–25.
6. Shiran A, Sagie A. Tricuspid regurgitation in mitral valve disease incidence, prognostic implications, mechanism, and management. J Am Coll Cardiol. 2009;53(5):401–8.

Reoperation for Aortic Valve Disease

15

Lars G. Svensson

Introduction

Reoperation for aortic valve dysfunction or aortic disease can represent a challenge. In this section, experts address how they approach different types of aortic reoperations, depending on the underlying pathology.

Reoperation on the Aortic Valve After Coronary Bypass, Aortic Valve Repair, and Percutaneous Options

The most common reason for reoperation on the aortic valve is valve failure in patients who either had previous coronary artery bypass grafting (CABG), or a previous aortic valve replacement or repair [1–7]. Essentially, the techniques for reoperation fall into two broad groups: either the patient is placed on cardiopulmonary bypass before opening the chest or the patient undergoes a dissection out of the heart, and, when appropriate, the internal mammary artery (IMA) is clamped.

L.G. Svensson, MD (✉)
Department of Thoracic and Cardiovascular Surgery, Cleveland Clinic Foundation, Cleveland, OH, USA
e-mail: svenssl@ccf.org

Cardiopulmonary Bypass Before Sternotomy

The approach of placing the patient on cardiopulmonary bypass is best used in those patients who have either pseudoaneurysms pressing against the back of the sternum, multiple previous cardiac operations, difficulty in isolating the IMA, or the presence of ascending aneurysms, particularly if an arch repair is also contemplated. The caveats of the cardiopulmonary bypass technique are the longer pump time, the possibility of increased bleeding, and the inability be used easily with cooling when there is an incompetent aortic valve.

Certainly, on the positive side, the approach is straightforward. The right axillary/subclavian artery is dissected out, the right femoral vein exposed, and the sternal wires removed [1]. The patient is fully heparinized and, then, the cannula (side graft) is attached to the axillary artery. Next, the femoral vein cannula is inserted and fed, using echocardiographic guidance, into the right atrium. In our opinion, placing the tip of the cannula at the junction of the superior vena cava and right atrium works best. While the patient is being cooled to the desired temperature, the sternum is opened with an oscillating saw, being careful not to plunge with the blade. The adhesions around the aorta, right ventricle, and right atrium are then dissected to expose both the aorta for clamping and, if needed, the right atrium for a retrograde cardioplegia cannula. The IMA can be dissected out and clamped, or the patient can be cooled to

V.R. Machiraju et al. (eds.), *Redo Cardiac Surgery in Adults*,
DOI 10.1007/978-1-4614-1326-4_15, © Springer Science+Business Media, LLC 2012

22°C, being careful to check that ventricular distention does not occur. Of note, cooling to deeper temperatures is often used for circulatory arrest procedures but one needs to be aware of the likelihood that as much as 10% of the ejection fraction will be lost with this approach.

In more complex situations, where the patient's aorta cannot be clamped and retrograde cardioplegia cannot be given for severe aortic regurgitation, the strategy needs modification. In this subset of patients, lidocaine, atropine, and ammiodarone are given before opening the chest, and the patient is cooled more slowly. We have also observed that these patients usually present with large aneurysms. Once the heart fibrillates, pump pressures are reduced, the chest is rapidly opened, and the aneurysm sac is opened. Perfusion catheters are then inserted into the innominate artery and left carotid artery, and perfusion via the axillary cannula graft and left carotid artery is started. In these patients, we advise the anesthetist to place a transjugular retrograde cardioplegia cannula. This step is important to avoid wasting valuable time, and the heart is protected while the arch is being repaired.

In most patients, the aorta can be clamped and antegrade cardioplegia given followed by retrograde cardioplegia, as needed. The aorta is then exposed, and optimal cardioplegia is further given if the patient has severe regurgitation.

Next, the valve or root procedure is performed. In subsequent chapters, more complex issues are reviewed. Sundt discusses surgery for previous homograft insertions, and Pettersson discusses aortic valve endocarditis.

If a patient has not had a previous valve replacement, valve replacement is no more difficult than in a primary case. When the valve has been replaced previously, care needs to be taken that the annulus is not destroyed and a hole is not made, particularly posteriorly, when removing the old valve. The left ventricular outflow tract also needs to be carefully inspected for any hypertrophy or scar tissue. Great attention needs to be taken in removing all potentially embolic materials, particularly in the setting of endocarditis. Most biologic valves fail from calcification, degeneration, or endocarditis. Mechanical valves usually fail due to tissue in-growth or endocarditis. A useful figure shows durability of the biological valves by age (Fig. 15.1). A discussion of valve selection in these patients is beyond the purpose of this chapter but a reference is included [2].

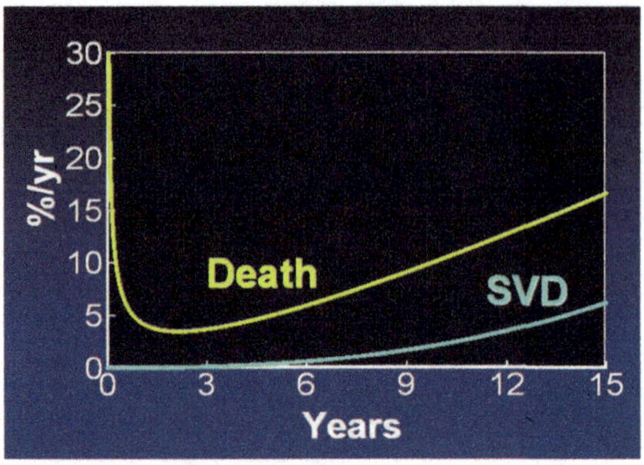

Fig. 15.1 Computing risks of death and structural valve disease. *SVD* structural valve deterioration

Patients who have had previous aortic valve repairs, mostly for bicuspid valves, or valve-sparing procedures, such as remodeling, generally will need a new replacement valve. However, the durability of repairs has been excellent, and most repairs after reimplantation were for endocarditis in our series of 234 modified David reimplantations (up to May 2009). For bicuspid valves, the failures are usually because of progression of aortic valve stenosis with calcification of the bicuspid valve tissue over time, or less so for regurgitation (Figs. 15.2 and 15.3) [3, 4].

Cardiopulmonary Bypass After Sternotomy

Placing the patient on cardiopulmonary bypass after sternotomy is the standard approach for most patients who have had previous cardiac surgery unless other factors pertain, as discussed previously. Clearly, we advise that special care needs to be taken on reentry. The aorta and right atrium are dissected out, making sure that the vein grafts are not disturbed. The lateral left ventricle is dissected out on pump after standard cardiopulmonary bypass and, if needed, after

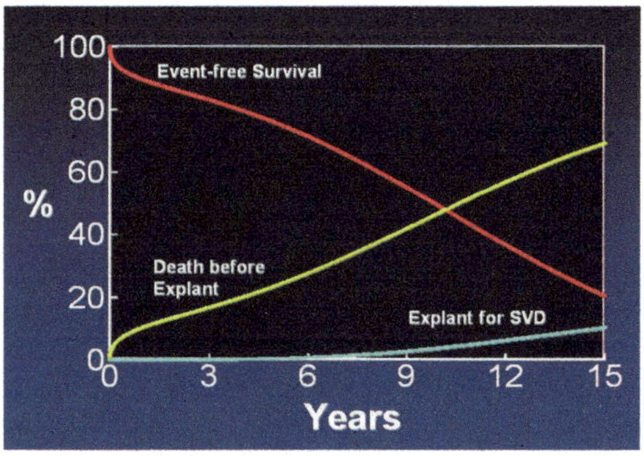

Fig. 15.2 Computing events. *SVD* structural valve deterioration

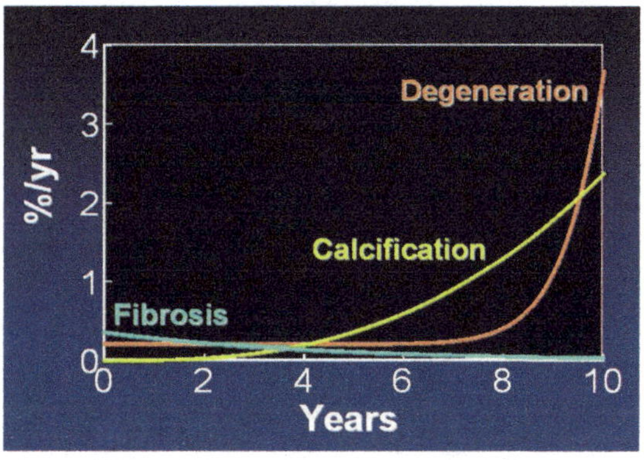

Fig. 15.3 Modes of structural valve deterioration

cardioplegia administration. Unless the IMA cannot be isolated, significant cooling is not needed for myocardial protection.

Results

We previously demonstrated that a cannula graft on the right subclavian/axillary artery reduced the risk of stroke by 40%. We also found that with cannulation of the femoral artery, the risk of stroke was higher [5]. Age and reoperation have an influence on risk of death as shown in Table 15.1. The results show that for those patients undergoing reoperation over the age of 80 years, the risk of death increases to >5%. Hence, these are the patients who are potentially good candidates for percutaneous valve insertion. Table 15.2 shows the influence of reoperation with aortic valve insertion and peripheral vascular disease on the risk of stroke and death. The importance of this is that in the United States, the transapical approach is only used in patients with poor peripheral access and as the table shows, then patients are at greater risk of death or stroke.

Percutaneous Valve Insertion After Previous Cardiac Operations

Following animal experiments, the technique of placing a tissue valve inside a wire stent was patented by Dr. H.R. Andersen of Denmark. This was bought by the PVT Company and later, after Cribier further developed the technology, was sold to Edwards Life Sciences Company (Irvine, CA) [6, 7]. Currently, there are two systems that are used extensively and have been inserted in over 8,000 patients. To date, the Edwards system with the Sapien valve is undergoing FDA-approved assessment in the United States, and the Core valve, now owned by Medtronics (Minneapolis, MN), is likely to follow in about 8 months time.

Thus, there are two groups of patients who are potential candidates for percutaneous valve insertion: first, those as indicated earlier, who are at high risk for conventional surgery and, second, those who are inoperable by conventional measures. Thus, by implication, a large proportion of the potential candidate patients are elderly and have had prior CABG. The entry criteria for the Edwards PARTNERS trial (Placement of Aortic Transcatheter Valve trial) are as follows: valve area ≤0.8 cm^2, Society of Thoracic Surgeons (STS) score >10 and surgeon-expected risk of death >15%, not a bicuspid valve, expected survival greater than 1 year, native aortic annulus size (as estimated by left ventricular outflow tract) of 1.7–2.4 cm, transvalvular velocity >4 m/s, and creatinine <2.5 mg/dL. In the PARTNER trial, there are two arms, namely Group A, comprising patients with high-risk surgical risk, and Group B,

Table 15.1 Death rates for aortic valve procedures, including complex aortic procedures, at Cleveland Clinic: 2001 to December 2007 (Modified from Ref. [5])

Group	*N*	Death rate (%)
Primary AVR < 70 years	720	0.28[a]
Primary AVR > 70 years	426	1.6[a]
Primary AVR > 80 years	139	1.4[a]
Primary AVR > 90 years	3	0[a]
Reoperative AVR < 70 years	217	2.3[a]
Reoperative AVR > 70 years	238	2.9[a]
Reoperative AVR > 80 years	89	5.6
Reoperative AVR > 90 years	3	0
Valve-sparing technique	418	1.4[b]
Repair of ascending aorta	2,812	4.2[c]
Repair of ascending aorta and aortic arch	985	4.6[c]
Use of "elephant trunk" technique	275	7.3[c]

AVR aortic valve replacement
[a] Including those with endocarditis but excluding those with coronary artery disease
[b] Including those with aortic dissection
[c] Including those with dissection and endocarditis involving the aorta

Table 15.2 Outcome for aortic valve replacement with or without other procedures of coronary bypass

Primary aortic valve replacement			
N=4214	PVD=2,039	No PVD=2,175	
Stroke	PVD=2.5%	No PVD=1.6%	*P*=0.02
Death	PVD=2.5%	No PVD=1.6%	*P*=0.006
Reoperative aortic valve replacement			
N=1967	PVD=1,219	No PVD=748	
Stroke	PVD=3%	No PVD=2.9%	*P*=0.5
Death	PVD=6.5%	No PVD=3.8%	*P*=0.007
Outcome for all 6,181 patients			
Stroke	PVD=2.7%	No PVD=1.9%	*P*=0.03
Death	PVD=4.2%	No PVD=2.2%	*P*<0.0001

comprising inoperable patients. Subjects were then randomized to either open surgery or a device procedure, namely transfemoral aortic valve insertion (TF-AVI) or transapical valve insertion (TA-AVI) (Figs. 15.4–15.8). The allocation of TF-AVI vs. TA-AVI was based on whether a patient had femoral access. By default, TF-AVI was the method of insertion if access was available and, if not, TA-AVI was the alternative. For patients in Group B, TA-AVI was not an alternative.

In the PARNTER trial, most patients are in their 80s with comorbidity and undergoing

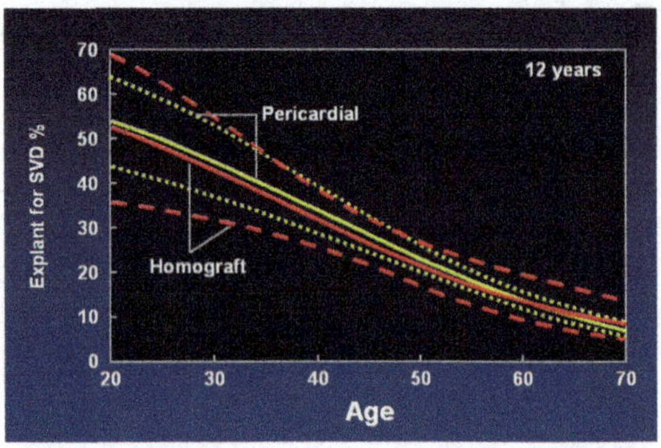

Fig. 15.4 Curve of relationship to risk of reoperation according to age

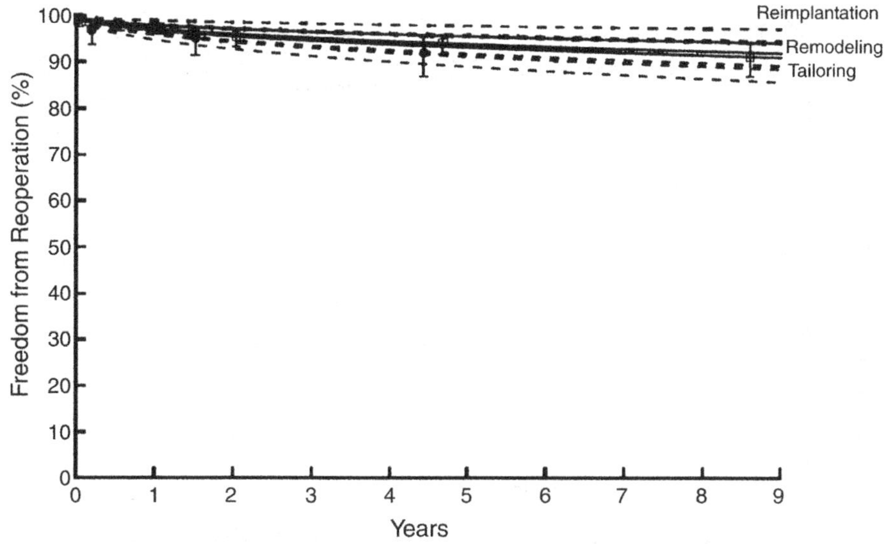

Fig. 15.5 Risk of reoperation according to repair

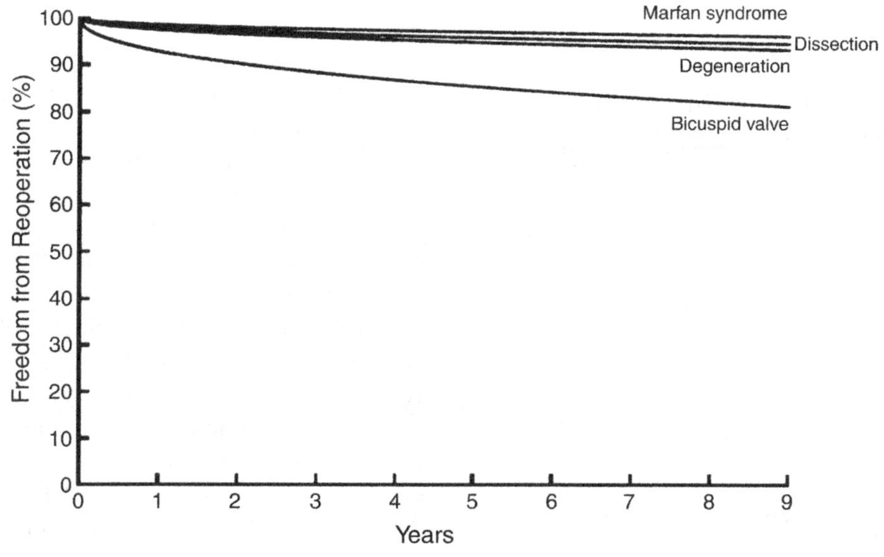

Fig. 15.6 Risk of reoperation

reoperation. Even patients in their early 90s and having a reoperation without comorbidity (e.g., pulmonary, vascular, or renal disease) were not eligible based on STS calculations. Of interest, of the approximately 1,000 patients who we evaluated for the study by our group, less than 20% have been enrolled. Approximately 20% have undergone conventional surgery, and it has been gratifying to see how well the elderly patients have done, particularly with the minimally invasive "J" incision. Approximately 20% of the patients have balloon valvulotomies as a physiological "test," and their long-term survival has been strongly influenced by their response to valvuloplasty, and whether they have had an open, mini AVR, TF-AVI, or TA-AVI.

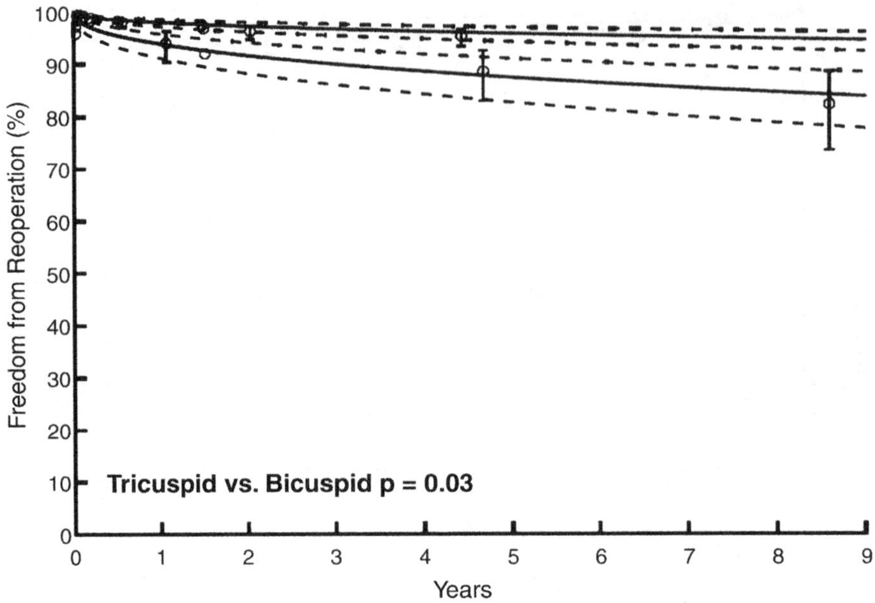

Fig. 15.7 Risk of procedure reoperation by leaflet number: tricuspid vs. bicuspid

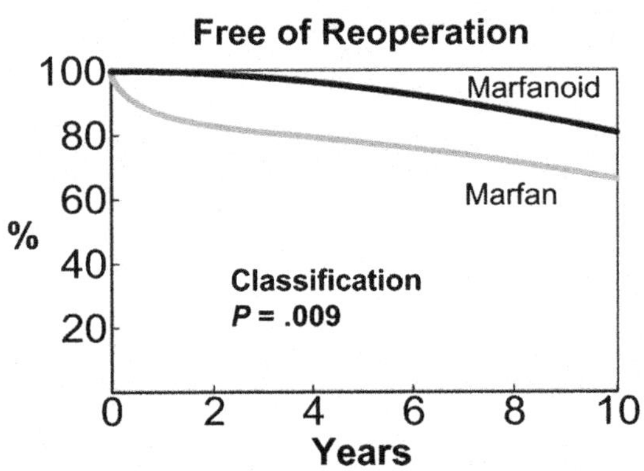

Fig. 15.8 According to pathology risk of reoperation for Marfan and marfanoid patients

We reported our early experience with the transapical approach in 40 patients as part of the U.S. feasibility study [6]. Since then, after the initial learning curve and also because the patients were at greater risk in the feasibility study (e.g., STS > 15%), our results have improved and our own experience compares favorably with the best reported transapical results (<10% 30 day/in-hospital mortality).

In the TF-AVI feasibility study in 55 patients in the United States, the mortality rate was 7% and stroke rate was 9% [6]. In our own experience, the results have been better. Currently, the Group B arm of the PARTNER trial is completed and patients are now being enrolled without randomization in the Group A arm in the continued access part of the study as an extended registry. The Group A arm with randomization was completed on August 28, 2009, and the data will be presented to the FDA for evaluation after 1-year follow-up. In addition, valve-in-valve approaches are being used. At this time, we have done six valve-in-valve procedures with TF-AVI or TA-AVI using the Sapien valve for failure.

TA-AVI and TF-AVI have clearly succeeded beyond our expectation and should prove to be a useful additional option for certain high-risk patients who are not good candidates for undergoing conventional reoperation.

References

1. Svensson LG, Blackstone EH, Rajeswaran J, Sabik 3rd JF, Lytle BW, Gonzalez-Stawinski G, et al. Does the arterial cannulation site for circulatory arrest influence stroke risk? Ann Thorac Surg. 2004;78:1274–84.
2. Svensson LG, Blackstone EH, Cosgrove 3rd DM. Surgical options in young adults with aortic valve disease. Curr Probl Cardiol. 2003;28:417–80.
3. Svensson LG. Ortic valve stenosis and regurgitation: an overview of management. J Cardiovasc Surg (Torino). 2008;49:297–303.
4. Svensson LG, Deglurkar I, Ung J, Pettersson G, Gillinov AM, D'Agostino RS, et al. Aortic valve repair and root preservation by remodeling, reimplantation, and tailoring: technical aspects and early outcome. J Card Surg. 2007;22:473–9.
5. Svensson LG. Evolution and results of aortic valve surgery, and a 'disruptive' technology. Cleve Clin J Med. 2008;75:802–4.
6. Svensson LG, Dewey T, Kapadia S, Roselli EE, Stewart A, Williams M, et al. United States feasibility study of transcatheter insertion of a stented aortic valve by the left ventricular apex. Ann Thorac Surg. 2008;86:46–54.
7. Kapadia SR, Goel SS, Svensson L, Roselli E, Savage RM, Wallace L, et al. Characterization and outcome of patients with severe symptomatic aortic stenosis referred for percutaneous aortic valve replacement. J Thorac Cardiovasc Surg. 2009;137:1430–5.

16 Reoperation Following Homograft Aortic Valve Replacement

Thoralf M. Sundt III

Human allografts, most often referred to as "homografts" in the cardiac surgical literature, were introduced in the orthotopic position as a prosthetic option almost simultaneously by Mr. Donald N. Ross and Sir Bryan Barratt-Boyes. Mr. Ross reported, in the September 8, 1962 issue of The Lancet, a single case of an orthotopic aortic valve replacement using a freeze-dried homograft implanted in a manner that would now be termed the subcoronary position [1]. Mr. Ross graciously acknowledged the input of Mr. A. Gunning and Mr. G. Duran of Oxford for their suggestions concerning the preparation and dissection of the valve in preparation for replacement. This clinical work followed on preliminary experimental work as well as human implantation of homograft valves in the descending thoracic aorta. Subsequently, Sir Barratt-Boyes reported, in the March 19, 1964 issue of *Thorax,* his experience with orthotopic homograft aortic valve replacement between August 1962 and November 1963 in 21 patients with aortic incompetence, 17 patients with calcific aortic stenosis, and six with multivalvular disease [2]. Interestingly, in that report, Barratt-Boyes notes that his first case was in August 1962 "before receiving the report of a similar procedure performed by Ross (1962) at about the same time." It is, perhaps, not surprising that both occurred so close together as multiple discovery is the rule, not the exception, in all scientific endeavors. In 1976, Yacoub first reported the free-standing root technique for aortic homografts, a technique that has gained popularity over the more complex subcoronary approach employed by both Ross and Barratt-Boyes as a more reproducible technique with superior freedom from postimplantation aortic regurgitation [3]. Numerous studies comparing long-term outcome of the two techniques have been published and are beyond the scope of our discussion here; however, it would be a fair generalization to say that the subcoronary technique has been all but supplanted by the root technique in most practices [4]. Sadly, and relevant to our discussion here, the root technique also leads to a more complex reoperation.

In today's practice, homografts are principally used in the setting of active infection [5]. In this circumstance, the greater technical complexity of homograft implantation relative to stented xenograft valves or mechanical valves is offset by their greater flexibility and conformability to complex root pathology, and the apparent resistance of homografts to infection. While homografts are not immune to recurrent or persistent infection, there are numerous studies supporting a lower risk of these complications when homograft valves are used.

Apart from infection, some stalwart advocates of homograft valve replacement argue for their use in younger, more active patients based on the benefits of freedom from anticoagulation, superior hemodynamics, and the potential for superior

T.M. Sundt III, MD (✉)
Massachusetts General Hospital,
Boston, MA, USA
e-mail: tsundt@partners.org

V.R. Machiraju et al. (eds.), *Redo Cardiac Surgery in Adults*,
DOI 10.1007/978-1-4614-1326-4_16, © Springer Science+Business Media, LLC 2012

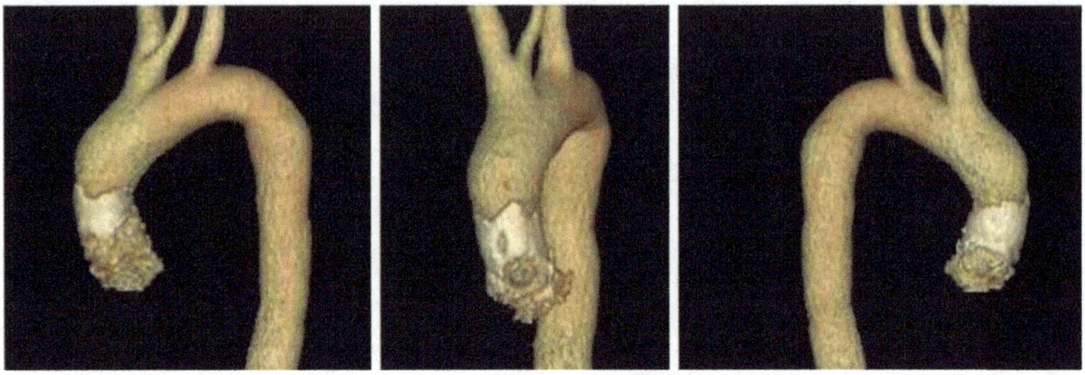

Fig. 16.1 "Stove-pipe" calcification of a homograft used for root replacement

durability over xenograft valves. On a theoretical basis, superior durability has been argued on the basis of viability of the stromal cells. The cryopreservation process is undertaken in such manner as to optimize cellular viability, including a carefully controlled slow rate of freezing and inclusion of dimethylsulfoxide (DMSO) in the cryopreservation solution. Dr. Mark O'Brien was a strong advocate of the cryopreserved allograft, reporting initial results suggesting durability far superior to xenografts. Unfortunately, subsequent follow-up studies revealed late degeneration [6]. Subsequent efforts to improve late durability have most recently included a reversal of approach entailing a careful decellularization process intended to reduce the allogeneic response to the transplanted valve, while preserving the extracellular structure such that it may serve as a matrix within which circulating stem cells may take root [7]. There are data to support reduced antibody production after implantation of such valves, but thus far, little evidence to support superior durability. Professor Sir Magdi Yacoub has argued in favor of fresh "homovital" valves harvested from transplant recipients and implanted, preferably within hours to days, after storage in an antibiotic solution [8]. In most instances, however, all these homografts have proven no more durable than current-generation tissue prostheses.

The mode of degeneration of homografts, regardless of treatment, appears to be typically extensive calcification of the aortic wall with torn leaflets and resulting aortic regurgitation. Stenosis, when it occurs, is less often secondary to calcification of the leaflets themselves than obstruction of the lumen by exuberant calcification of the aortic wall and surgical annulus. Both these factors, mural calcification and valvular incompetence, enter into the strategic considerations surrounding reoperation. Particular consideration must be given to myocardial management during reopening and dissection as the aortic regurgitation, which is often torrential, will wreak havoc if the heart fibrillates before aortic cross-clamping can be performed. Furthermore, the calcium may present challenges, both in terms of cross-clamping the aorta and in the technical aspects of excising the homograft. Cross-clamping the aorta is particularly of importance when the homograft has been used for replacement of the entire ascending aorta and proximal arch, as it is sometimes performed in the setting of infection. It is always most prudent to consider the reoperation when performing the initial procedure. Stovepipe calcification (Fig. 16.1) of the entire ascending aorta will present significant challenges at the time of reoperation.

Preoperative Evaluation

As is the case for any reoperation, details of the prior surgery should be sought. The patient may not be fully aware as to whether or not a subcoronary or root replacement was performed. While either can be dealt with at the time of surgery, it is often helpful to the surgeon, particularly one with less experience reoperating on homografts, to have a clear idea of what to expect. A subcoronary homograft itself is often covered with a shiny white pseudointima, which may make it, in fact, quite challenging to tell where the homograft ends and native aorta begins. What is billed as a subcoronary valve may look all the world like a root replacement at first glance. If the patient had a root replacement, it is helpful to know whether it was a true free-standing root replacement or some modification thereof, such as the mini-root procedure. Again, this is of importance as one addresses mobilization of the coronary arteries. Details regarding the coronary reconstruction are similarly helpful. Finally, forewarning of the use of Teflon felt may better prepare the surgeon for debridement of the surgical annulus. Prior use of surgical adhesives may be particularly problematic as they have been associated with significant tissue destruction in some cases. Most surgical adhesives, including agents intended for cross-linking of the glue itself, can, over time, leak out of the glue into the surrounding tissues and be quite toxic. We have seen instances of complete aortoventricular disruption that we have attributed to the use of such agents during complex prior operations. Unfortunately, details regarding the use of these agents are often missing from the operative note.

Preoperative imaging is particularly helpful in the setting of prior homograft replacement. This is particularly true when homografts have been used to treat prosthetic endocarditis as this means the sternotomy for replacement of the homograft will be a tertiary sternotomy at a minimum. It is clear from multiple series that the number of prior sternotomies is a significant risk factor for injury during sternal reentry. As noted earlier, inadvertent injury, while always problematic, is particularly so here where the functional pathology most often includes significant aortic regurgitation. Therefore, as always, careful preoperative planning is important.

Preoperative echocardiography is routine. Indeed, in most instances, a preoperative echocardiogram demonstrating significant aortic regurgitation was the stimulus for evaluation for surgical reoperation. It is important to look at the echocardiogram for the degree of aortic regurgitation as well as left ventricular function, right ventricular function, and evidence of pulmonary hypertension. As always, one should be attentive to concomitant pathology of other valves.

Coronary arteriography is routine in most instances, as much to define the coronary ostial anatomy as to define the distal atherosclerotic disease. Coronary buttons may be small leading to ostial stenosis. Alternatively, buttons may have been left large leading to button aneurysms. Views of the course of any prior bypass grafts, with particular attention to immobility of any segment against the chest wall, should be requested at the time of coronary arteriography. Angiographers more often focus on the distal anastomoses without attention to the course of the grafts. Direct posterior–anterior (PA) and lateral views should be requested.

Preoperative computed tomography (CT) scanning is also particularly helpful in the setting of prior homograft replacement. As always, for any reoperation, one should be attentive to the location of the aorta, vis-à-vis the sternum itself (Fig. 16.2). One should also be attentive to the

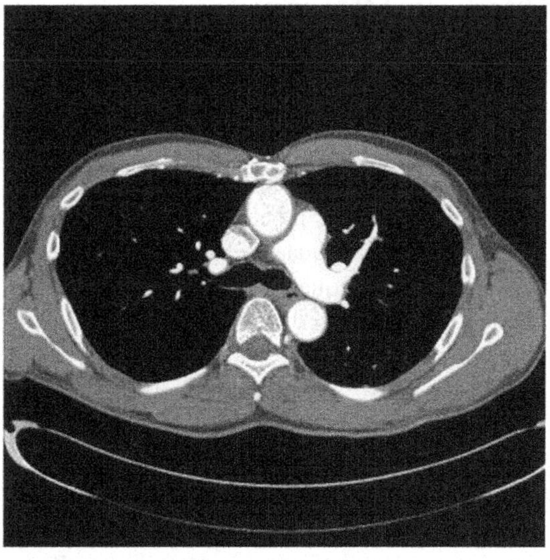

Fig. 16.2 The homograft in this case is adherent to the posterior table of the sternum and is at great risk of injury at resternotomy. Peripheral (axillary) artery cannulation is advisable in this circumstance

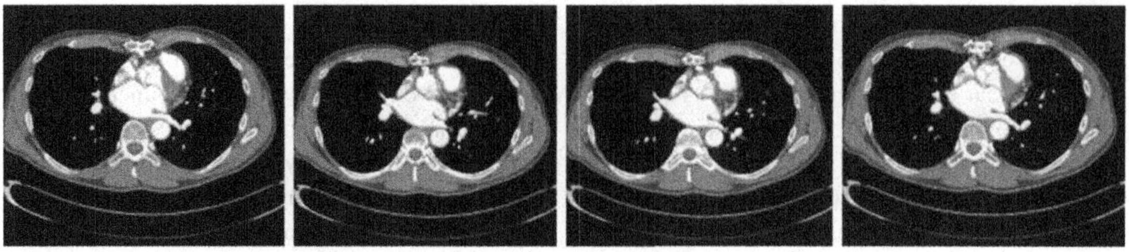

Fig. 16.3 The course of the right coronary artery is immediately behind the sternum in the midline

course of the right coronary artery, which may lie directly below the sternum in harm's way, as well as, of course, the course of any previous bypass grafts (Fig. 16.3). Finally, CT scanning, particularly noncontrast studies, is helpful in identifying calcification of the aortic wall and potential sites for aortic cross-clamping. If the prior homograft extends to the base of the innominate artery or, even worse, has been used for hemiarch replacement, consideration must be given to alternative peripheral cannulation sites for arterial inflow and potentially to alternative strategies for control of the aorta including balloon occlusion of the aorta itself using a Foley catheter or coda balloon.

Operative Strategy

Broadly, the operative strategy is dictated principally by the extent and approach in the original operation [9]. If the prior operation was a subcoronary aortic valve replacement, repeat valve replacement alone is most likely the appropriate operation. With adequate debridement of the old homograft, an adequate annulus should remain. While this may seem daunting, the calcium is, as Professor Yacoub used to say, "noninvasive" and therefore, careful debridement of all calcium should reveal an intact and often remarkably normallooking annulus. In this case, the art is to actually achieve complete debridement of the old homograft itself. The homograft may be covered with a pseudointima, which makes this challenging at first, but if one can get into the appropriate plane between the homograft and the native aortic wall, the dissection often proceeds quite easily. The first maneuver I make is to try and find that plane with a dural elevator. An alternative is to seat a new valve within the homograft itself; however, this may lead to an implantation of a smaller prosthesis than might be desired. Furthermore, the calcified homograft itself will not heal to the sewing ring of the new valve, likely with an increased risk of late perivalvular leak. Often, just a little bit of patience in debriding the old homograft can be quite gratifying in terms of the very normal looking annulus left behind.

If the prior operation was a root replacement, the reoperation is more challenging. Not only is the root itself typically adherent to the pulmonary artery, but also coronary buttons may be challenging to mobilize. For this reason, one may wish to consider, in the setting of prior root replacement, implantation of a new valve within the old homograft if the homograft itself is not significantly calcified. This has been previously reported and one can, on occasion, get away with this. If, however, the entire homograft is calcified, one is often committed to its entire removal.

The actual conduct of the operation can be considered in three phases: first, control of the aorta, such that it may be cross-clamped; second, debridement of all calcified materials; finally, reconstruction. In general, as the calcification is noninvasive, a focus on debriding all calcified material will leave behind sufficient native tissue to permit reconstruction (Fig. 16.4). The calcification of the wall may appear quite imposing initially (Fig. 16.5); however, with patience and a focus on just removing the calcified material, a satisfactory annulus will become apparent if one

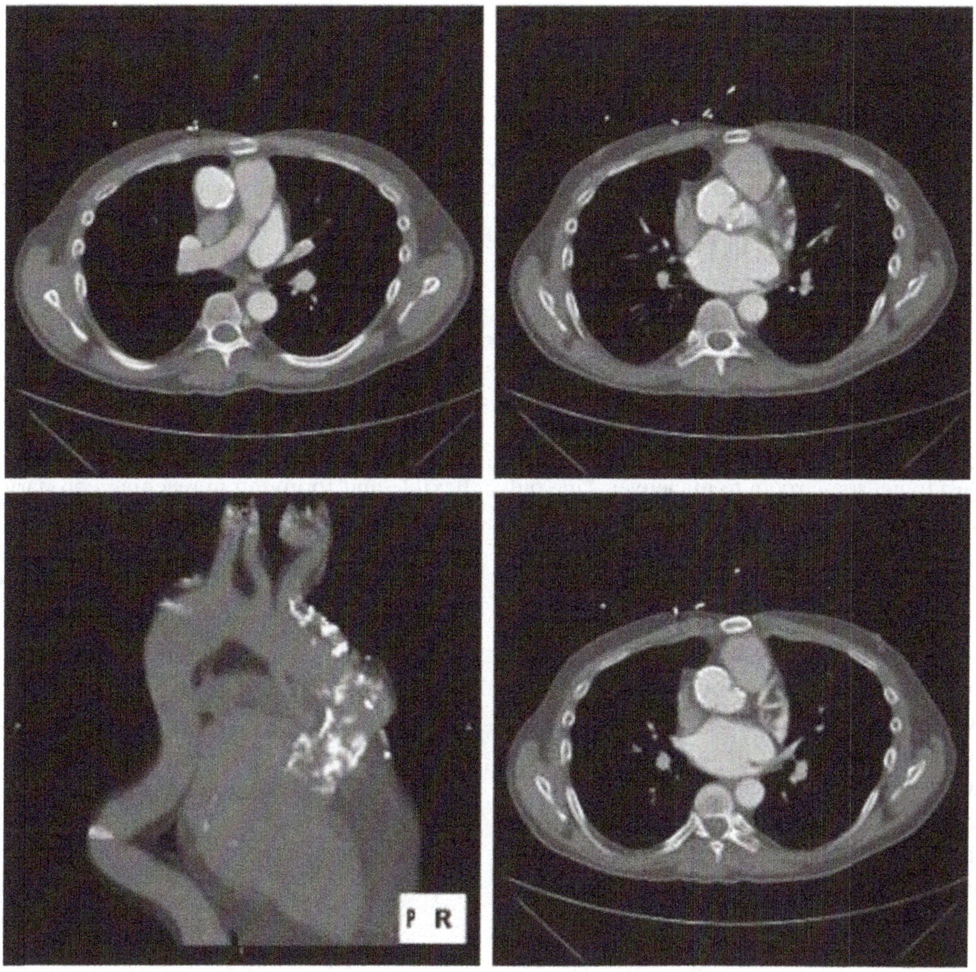

Fig. 16.4 Preoperative CT scan demonstrating scattered calcification of a previously implanted homograft root

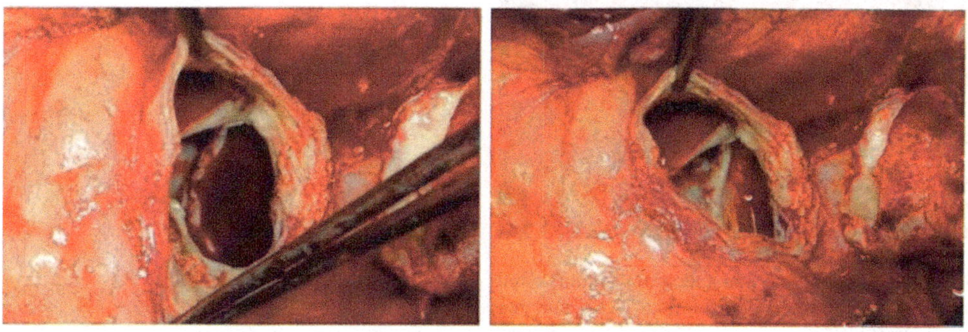

Fig. 16.5 The wall of the homograft may be quite stiff, making visualization of the annulus and coronary ostia difficult. Patiently debriding the calcified material will reveal underlying normal anatomy

existed at the time of homograft implantation (Fig. 16.6). Of course, if the homograft was implanted for prosthetic endocarditis and there was annular destruction at that time, one will need to leave behind sufficient fibrous material to which to sew. Also of note, if the homograft wall around the coronary buttons is itself not calcified, some of that material can be left behind to facilitate reconstruction. There is no need to remove all the homograft if it is not itself calcified. However, the secondary suture line should extend into the native button tissue.

I should note that if one enters the pulmonary artery – and on occasion I have done so intentionally just to get some room to maneuver – the pulmonary artery should be repaired with a patch rather than repaired primarily. Bleeding from behind the homograft revision is troublesome, to say the least, and placing an ample patch is often time well spent. Occasionally, at the time of debridement of the calcium, one will find a significant amount of Teflon felt at the level of the annulus. In this circumstance, it can be quite challenging to know how much felt to remove and how much to leave behind. In general, I try to remove as much felt as feels safe and as much as is required to implant a new prosthetic valve of adequate size.

My preferred reconstructive option in the setting of a failed homograft is a mechanical valve conduit if the patient is younger than 65 years of age, as coronary buttons just get smaller each time one reoperates for a root replacement and their mobilization is increasingly difficult. Repeated root replacements are increasingly complex and, in my view, the most definitive procedure possible is certainly the preferred one. One can facilitate mobilization of the coronary buttons by passing the coronary probe to witness their course, and, as noted earlier, occasionally simply entering the right pulmonary artery to gain access to the transverse and sinus. An alternative is to use a conduit with a "Sinus of Valsalva" component, which may be a bit more flexible and forgiving in reaching coronary ostia that have not been mobilized. One can also reconstruct the coronary arteries without mobilizing them by utilizing a Cabrol graft (Fig. 16.7). This is particularly useful for the left coronary button. In the setting of root replacement, I am

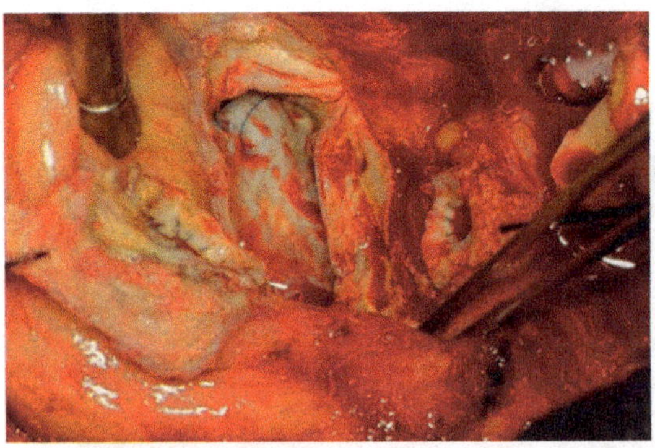

Fig. 16.6 A remarkably normal appearing annulus often lies under the calcified homograft material. Also note that if the homograft wall is not calcified around the coronary buttons, some of that material can be left behind to buttress the new suture line. From my point of view, one must, however, pass the new sutures through the native button and not rely on the homograft material

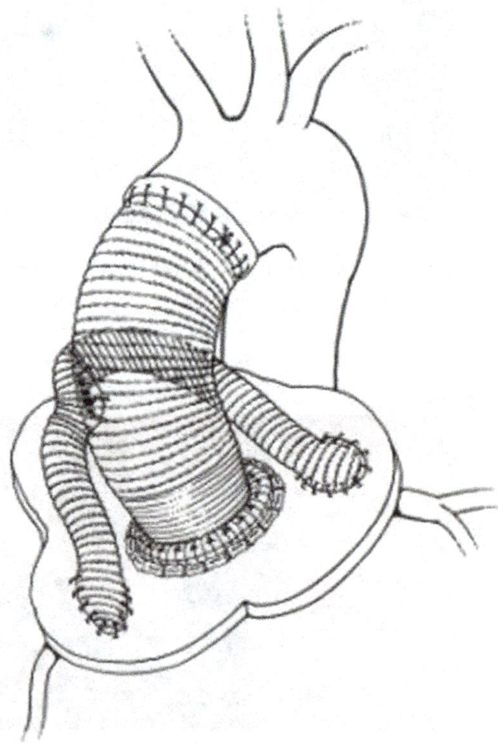

Fig. 16.7 Reconstruction of the coronary arteries using a Cabrol graft. By permission of Mayo Foundation for Medical Education and Research.

reluctant to use surgical adhesives for the reasons noted earlier. My experience is that with the use of surgical adhesives, the scarring becomes increasingly dense and I worry about the integrity of the tissues left behind as the tissue can become necrotic. One certainly does not want to be back for repair of an aortoventricular disruption or pseudoaneurysm following redo root replacement.

Postoperative Management

The postoperative management of patients following root replacement is routine in most regards. I routinely obtain predischarge imaging that includes a CT scan of the root. It is particularly helpful at late follow-up to have this imaging of the immediate postoperative anatomy. From my point of view, Echocardiography prior to discharge, as well as on an annual basis, is also of value.

Reoperation Following the Ross Procedure

Finally, a few words regarding reoperation following the Ross operation may be of value to the reader. Reoperation following the Ross operation may be extraordinarily complex as the autograft and pulmonary homograft are frequently densely adherent to one another; it may not be possible to separate the two. However, on the positive side, the pulmonary autograft seldom calcifies. If the pulmonary autograft becomes aneurysmal, a reoperation is more straightforward as one can conduct the operation essentially within the autograft with a coronary reconstruction, et cetera, as noted earlier. The pulmonary homograft more frequently becomes calcified and can be problematic. Its excision may be difficult and implantation of a stented prosthesis with ample patch closure of the pulmonary homograft may be preferable. Details concerning reoperation following failed right ventricular outflow reconstruction are dealt with elsewhere.

References

1. Ross DN. Homograft replacement of the aortic valve. Lancet. 1962;2(7254):487.
2. Barratt-Boyes BG. Homograft aortic valve replacement in aortic incompetence and stenosis. Thorax. 1964;19:131–50.
3. Yacoub M, Gula G, McKay R, Pomerance A. Proceedings: surgical treatment of aneurysms of ascending aorta. Br Heart J. 1976;38:874.
4. Dearani JA, Orszulak TA, Daly RC, et al. Comparison of techniques for implantation of aortic valve allografts. Ann Thorac Surg. 1996;62:1069–75.
5. Dearani JA, Orszulak TA, Schaff HV, et al. Results of allograft aortic valve replacement for complex endocarditis. J Thorac Cardiovasc Surg. 1997;113:285–91.
6. O'Brien MF, Stafford EG, Gardner MA, et al. Allograft aortic valve replacement: long-term follow-up. Ann Thorac Surg. 1995;60(2 Suppl):S65–70.
7. Hogan PG, O'Brien MF. Improving the allograft valve: does the immune response matter? J Thorac Cardiovasc Surg. 2003;126:1251–3.
8. Yacoub MH, Knight E, Towers M, Somerville W. Aortic valve replacement using fresh unstented homografts. Br Heart J. 1973;35:555–6.
9. Sundt III TM, Rasmi N, Wong K, et al. Reoperative aortic valve operation after homograft root replacement: surgical options and results. Ann Thorac Surg. 1995;60(2 Suppl):S95–9; discussion S100.

Prosthetic Aortic Valve and Root Endocarditis

17

Gosta B. Pettersson, Rajesh Ramankutty, Brian Griffin, and Thomas Fraser

Introduction

Prosthetic aortic valve endocarditis is a progressive and serious disease. Today, with good diagnostic methods, antibiotic regimens, and improved surgical techniques and experience, most patients are expected to survive and be cured. Cure requires prompt and aggressive diagnosis, optimal antibiotic treatment, and, most often, well-timed and executed surgery. These operations are difficult and require experience, as illustrated by the wide variations in outcomes in different series. Operations for prosthetic valve endocarditis (PVE) require understanding of the pathology and familiarity with all the tools necessary to reconstruct the heart.

G.B. Pettersson, MD (✉) • R. Ramankutty, MD
Department of Thoracic and Cardiovascular Surgery, Surgical Director of Lung Transplant Unit, Cleveland Clinic, Cleveland, OH, USA
e-mail: petterg@ccf.org

B. Griffin, MD
Department of Cardiovascular Medicine, Cleveland Clinic, Cleveland, OH, USA

T. Fraser, MD
Division of Cardiac Infections, Department of Infections Diseases, Cleveland Clinic, Cleveland, OH, USA

Pathophysiology and Pathology

Prosthetic Aortic Valve Endocarditis

Prosthetic aortic valve endocarditis (Fig. 17.1) can appear at any time after implantation of a prosthetic valve. The literature distinguishes between early and late occurrence, with some disagreement about the defining interval – 3, 6, or 12 months after implantation. From an etiologic (source-of-infection) standpoint, early PVE may be the result of perioperative contamination of the prosthesis in the surgical field; bacteremia in the postoperative course, such as from line sepsis; direct contamination, such as from wound infection or mediastinitis; or, if the original operation was also for endocarditis, failure to eradicate the infection because of incomplete debridement or insufficient antibiotic treatment. Bioprostheses and mechanical prostheses are equally prone to infection. Allografts seem to be more resistant, and the same may be true for pulmonary autografts.

Bloodstream bacteria adhere to thrombotic material formed on defects in the endothelial and endocardial lining where vegetations develop. Endocarditis on a bioprosthesis or allograft can be limited to cusps; most often, however, the infection involves the sewing ring. Involvement of the sewing ring starts locally but eventually becomes circumferential. Enzymatic disintegration of the tissue holding the sutures results in dehiscence of the prosthesis. Progression of dehiscence invasion is decided by the specificity

V.R. Machiraju et al. (eds.), *Redo Cardiac Surgery in Adults*,
DOI 10.1007/978-1-4614-1326-4_17,

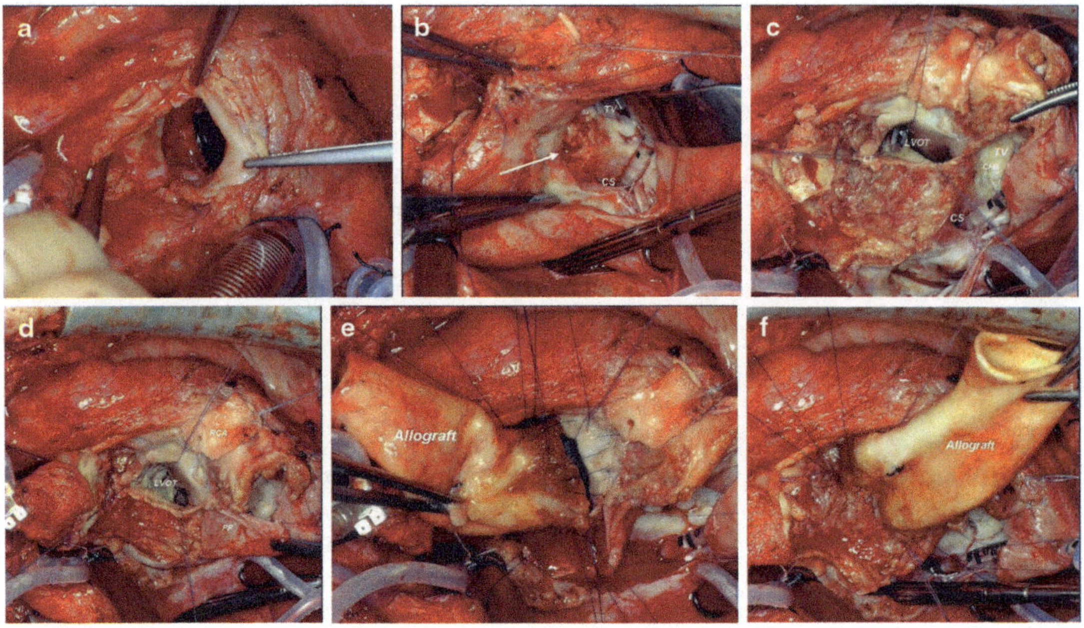

Fig. 17.1 Step-by-step (**a–f**), images from a case of advanced prosthetic valve endocarditis presenting with complete heart block (*TV* tricuspid valve; *CS* coronary sinus; *AVNode* atrioventricular node; *RCA* right coronary artery; *LVOT* left ventricular outflow tract; *LT* lateral trigone; *CFB* central fibrose body; *LCA* left coronary artery; *PP* pericardial patch). (**a**) The appearance of the prosthesis with vegetations after aortotomy. (**b**) Right atrium view of fistula (*arrow*) from the aortic root with destruction of the AV node. (**c**) The aortic root following radical debridement demonstrating circumferential infection is different stages suggesting a counter clockwise spread and progression of the infection. The left ventricular outflow tract is well preserved and ready for reconstruction. (**d**) The defect in the right atrium wall is closed using a piece of autologous pericardium. (**e**) The allograft is sutured with running monofilament suture to the LVOT. (**f**) The allograft tied down leaving the debrided areas draining to the pericardium

and potency of the enzymes produced by the microorganism. *Staphylococcus aureus,* with the most aggressive enzymes, causes dehiscence of a valve prosthesis in days. Less vascularized tissue, like fat and connective tissue, is more susceptible to bacterial destruction than well-vascularized tissue, like muscle. Invasion and destruction develop through four stages: cellulitis, tissue necrosis, abscess formation, and formation of pseudoaneurysms or fistulas. It is unusual to find large collections of pus during surgery, suggesting that the process is more that of "mining," with the bacteria working at the end of a "tunnel" as the tissue behind disintegrates and is constantly irrigated away by the blood flow. The consequences of extra-aortic invasion depend on where the invasion starts and in which direction it progresses: Invasion toward the right into the right atrium and Koch's triangle causes heart block by destruction of the atrioventricular (AV) node (Fig. 17.1b, c); invasion posteriorly/inferiorly may result in a fistula to the left atrium or destruction of the intervalvular fibrosa and the base of the anterior mitral valve leaflet; invasion to the left results in a subpulmonary abscess or pseudoaneurysm; invasion anteriorly under the right coronary artery is more often shallow, but occasionally larger abscesses and cavities are formed in this area as well. Although rare, perforation to the right ventricle is most often seen close to the membranous septum, and rupture to the pericardium may also occur in this area.

Ascending Aorta and Arch Graft Infection

A patient with an infected ascending aorta graft presents with sepsis and fluid collection around the graft. The source can be perioperative contamination, external infection from sternal infection, or blood-borne infection. Fluid around an ascending aorta graft in the absence of sepsis can occasionally be a sterile purulent reaction to glue or felt.

Microbiology

The likelihood of a particular organism causing infective endocarditis is the result of an interaction between that organism's predilection to adhere to defects in the valvular endothelium or endocardium (e.g., presence of a prosthetic valve) and the patient's immune status. Clinical circumstances determine the risk of exposure to infection and bacteremia. In the majority of cases, the cause of PVE is one of a core group of organisms: *S. aureus,* coagulase-negative staphylococci, viridans group streptococci, and *Enterococcus* species. These organisms account for nearly 65% of infections. The interval between the preceding valve surgery and onset of the infection influences the likelihood of recovering a particular organism. Although the definition of "early PVE" can vary, staphylococci are consistently the leading cause. The importance of *S. aureus* in the etiology of infective endocarditis must be appreciated, as we see more patients with clinical characteristics, such as diabetes mellitus, end-stage renal failure on hemodialysis, presence of an indwelling vascular catheter, and intravenous drug abuse, which place them at risk for *S. aureus* infection. *S. aureus* is also the leading cause of surgical site infections. A patient with a prosthetic valve who becomes bacteremic with this organism has a 50% risk of developing PVE.

Another group of organisms that merit specific mention are fungal pathogens. The most common fungi to cause PVE are *Candida* species. This genus of yeast is an increasingly recognized cause of hospital-acquired bloodstream infection, and defined risk factors for candidemia are well established. One series found the prevalence of fungal PVE after development of nosocomial candidemia to be 25%.

Diagnosis

Diagnosis is by clinical picture, blood cultures, and echocardiography (Table 17.1). Blood cultures should be secured before antibiotic treatment is started.

Table 17.1 Definition of infective endocarditis according to the proposed modified Duke criteria

Definite infective endocarditis
Pathologic criteria
Microorganisms demonstrated by culture or histologic examination of a vegetation, a vegetation that has embolized; or
An intracardiac abscess specimen; or
Pathological lesions; vegetation, or intracardiac abscess confirmed by histologic examination showing active endocarditis
Clinical criteria
Two major criteria[a]; or
One major criterion and three minor criteria; or
Five minor criteria
Possible infective endocarditis
One major criterion and one minor criterion; or
Three minor criteria
Rejected (not infective endocarditis)
Firm alternative diagnosis explaining evidence of infective endocarditis; or
Resolution of infective endocarditis syndrome with antibiotic therapy for less than 4 days; or
No pathologic evidence of infective endocarditis at surgery or autopsy, with antibiotic therapy for less than 4 days; or
Does not meet criteria for possible infective endocarditis, as noted earlier

[a] Major and minor criteria are defined in Li et al. [1]. Major criteria include positive blood culture, evidence for endocardial involvement, and positive echocardiogram. Minor criteria include predisposing heart condition, fever, vascular phenomena, immunologic phenomena, and microbiological evidence not meeting the standards for major criteria (Modified from Li et al. [1])

Echocardiography

Doppler echocardiography (Figs. 17.2–17.4) is the imaging technique of choice in establishing a diagnosis of prosthetic or allograft endocarditis. Transthoracic echocardiography (TTE) is effective in detecting PVE in its later stages, but transesophageal echocardiography (TEE) is better for early detection. TEE should be performed whenever a diagnosis of PVE is entertained, and especially when aortic abscess is suspected. Endocarditis is unlikely in the absence of abnormalities on TEE. Because TTE is usually superior in estimating valve gradients, it remains an important part of the diagnostic work-up.

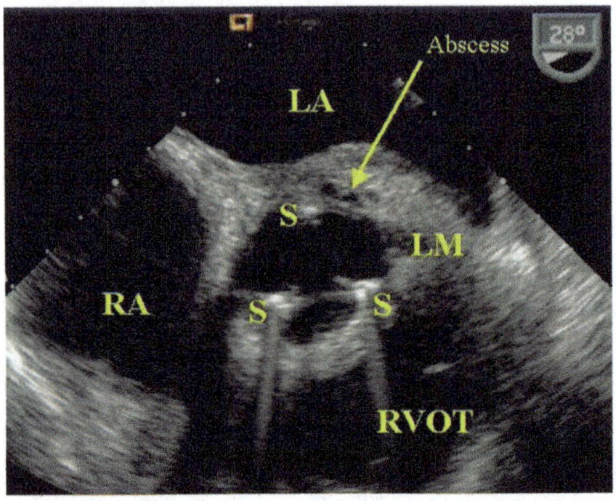

Fig. 17.2 TEE short-axis image of aortic abscess and perivalvular thickening seen around a bioprosthesis whose struts are indicated by S. *RA* right atrium; *RVOT* right ventricular outflow tract; *LM* left main; *LA* left atrium

The appropriate views in the detection of aortic endocarditis by TEE include a mid-esophageal short-axis view of the aortic valve at 30–60° with the multiplane probe. In this view, the cusps and sewing ring are usually well visualized, and abnormal regurgitation around the sewing ring is detected. Vegetations manifest as mobile echodensities attached to the valve cusps or adjacent structures with a motion independent of the valve and are one of the cardinal signs of endocarditis. In more advanced endocarditis, an abscess cavity may be seen as an echolucent area in an area of thickening around the prosthesis (Fig. 17.2). This is most often posterior to the prosthesis, but may eventually become circumferential and communicate with the left ventricular (LV) outflow tract. Before abscess formation, only thickening may be evident. When an abscess communicates with the LV outflow tract, to-and-fro flow may be seen by color Doppler into the cavity. Occasionally, an abscess may also communicate back into the aorta above the valve, allowing flow to enter the left ventricle through this fistulous communication, which is usually apparent by color Doppler. Fistulous communication to other chambers, including the left atrium, may also be seen in this view, often by means of the anterior mitral valve leaflet and more rarely the right atrium.

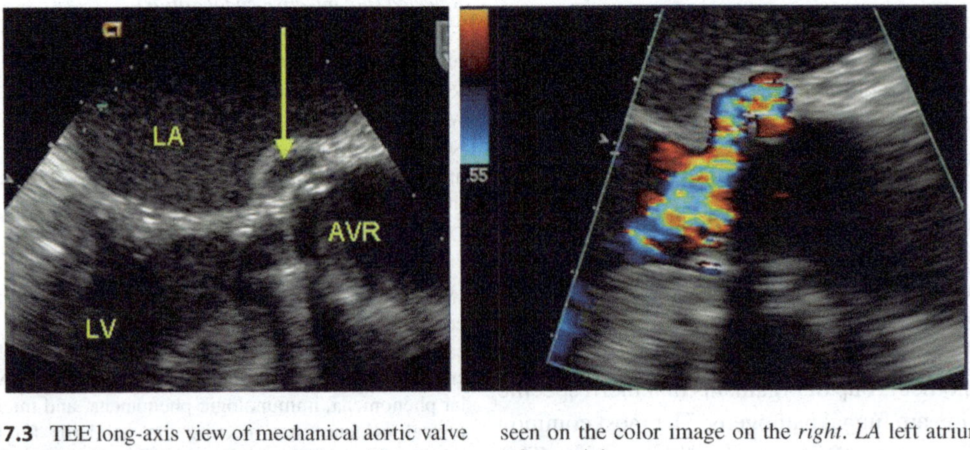

Fig. 17.3 TEE long-axis view of mechanical aortic valve prosthesis (AVR) with abscess cavity indicated by *arrow*. Flow through the abscess cavity into the left ventricle is seen on the color image on the *right*. *LA* left atrium; *LV* left ventricle

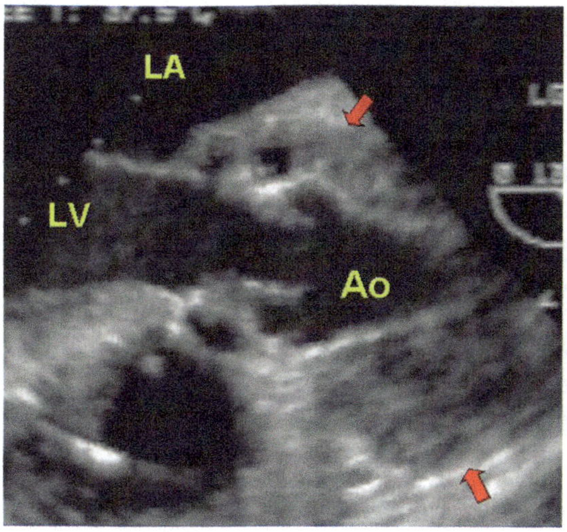

Fig. 17.4 Abscess at homograft in long-axis TEE view of aorta and left ventricular outflow tract. The abscess cavity is indicated by the *red arrows*. *LV* left ventricle; *Ao* aortic homograft; *LA* left atrium

The long-axis view of the aortic valve and aorta, seen at 110–150° with the multiplane probe, is particularly helpful in detecting vegetation on the valve cusps and in diagnosing the site and extent of abnormal regurgitation around the valve. Abscess formation and extent of the abscess are usually apparent. In the setting of a composite graft or allograft infection, dehiscence of the valve results in pseudoaneurysm formation (Figs. 17.3–17.5). In more advanced cases of endocarditis, dehiscence may be seen as a rocking motion of the valve itself, associated with severe regurgitation. Fistula formation may also be apparent in this view (Fig. 17.5). Once infection or abscess has been adequately documented at the aortic valve or graft, involvement of other cardiac structures, such as the mitral or tricuspid valve, and of any intracardiac catheters or pacing wires should be investigated.

Although echocardiography, especially TEE, is highly sensitive and specific for the diagnosis of PVE, false negatives and false positives nevertheless occur. False negatives may occur early in the course of endocarditis, before vegetations have become large enough to be visualized by echocardiography. Shadowing and reverberation, though usually more of an issue with TTE, may also render full evaluation of the aortic prosthesis by TEE difficult, especially when a mitral prosthesis is also present. False negatives can be avoided by a comprehensive evaluation of the valve from multiple views and by repeating TEE later if the diagnosis seems reasonable. False-positive diagnosis occurs because sutures or fibrin strands may look like vegetation. Aortic abscess may be simulated by the Cabrol method of implanting coronary arteries in a graft by small conduits. To the unwary, these coronary extension grafts may suggest abscess in short-axis views. Postoperative hematoma may simulate the thickening of an early abscess. False positives may be prevented by comparing the current echocardiography study with the immediate postoperative TEE study when this is available.

Coronary Angiography

Coronary angiography is performed for normal indications, although this procedure may be associated with an increased risk of embolic events when large foci of vegetation are present on the prosthesis. A coronary angiogram is particularly important if the patient has undergone previous coronary artery bypass grafting.

Brain Imaging

Stroke is a common and serious complication of endocarditis and, irrespective of obvious clinical neurologic symptoms, patients with PVE should have an examination of the brain by computed tomography (CT) scan or magnetic resonance imaging (MRI) within 24–48 h of surgery for detection of cerebral infarctions and mycotic aneurysms. Neither CT nor MRI is sensitive enough to diagnose smaller mycotic aneurysms, and if these are suspected, cerebral angiography is required.

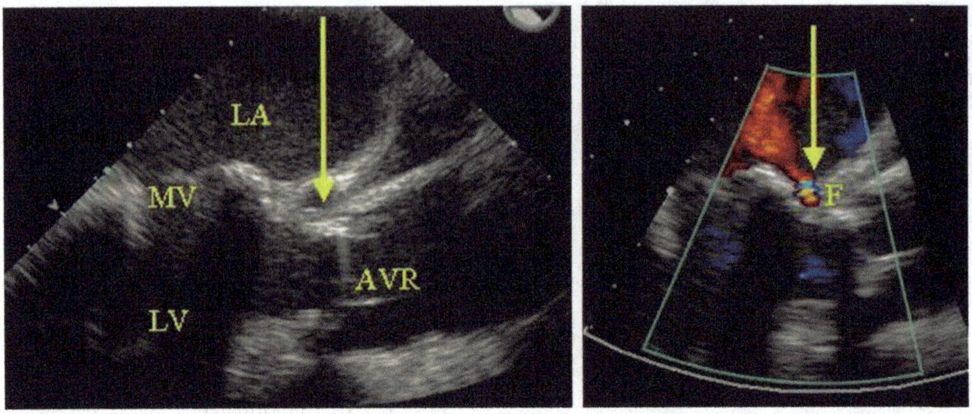

Fig. 17.5 TEE long-axis of aorta and LVOT with abscess cavity (*arrow*) around bioprosthesis (AVR). A fistula (F) is seen on the color Doppler display on the *right*. *LA* left atrium; *LV* left ventricle; *MV* mitral valve

CT and MRI of the Chest

Operations for PVEs are reoperations, and appropriate imaging is important not only for diagnosis but also for planning the surgery and safe sternal reentry. Anatomic relationships, calcifications, fluid collections, and pseudoaneurysms and other cavities may be diagnosed.

Additional Diagnostic Tests are Performed as Clinically Indicated

Body screening for metastatic infection is performed based on clinical suspicion and symptoms.

Indications for Surgery

Most patients with PVE will require surgery, because cure with antibiotics alone is unlikely and progression, further destruction, and invasion are likely even when the patient is on adequate antibiotic treatment. When caused by *S. aureus,* PVE is always a surgical disease. Endocarditis on a bioprosthesis or an allograft can be limited to cusps and, when this is true, curable by antibiotics alone. Surgery is not indicated if complications (severe embolic cerebral damage) or comorbid conditions make the prospect of recovery remote (Table 17.2).

Timing of Surgery and Preoperative Considerations

Once there is an indication to operate, there are few reasons to delay the operation. Knowing the organism and its sensitivity pattern makes certain that the patient is treated with adequate antibiotics at the time of surgery, but treatment with adequate antibiotics might not prevent progression of invasive disease to allow safe delay of surgery. Delaying surgery also allows more time for embolic events. The presence of a hemorrhagic cerebral infarction on the CT or MRI of the brain increases the risk of intracerebral bleeding during and after the operation and worsening of existing neurologic deficits and is a reason to postpone surgery 1–2 weeks if hemodynamically tolerated.

Table 17.2 AHA/ACC Recommendations for Surgery for Prosthetic Valve Endocarditis (Modified from American College of Cardiology/American Heart Association Task Force on Practice Guideline [2])

Class I
Consultation with a cardiac surgeon is indicated for patients with infective endocarditis of a prosthetic valve (Level of Evidence: C)
Surgery is indicated for patients with infective endocarditis of a prosthetic valve who present with heart failure (Level of Evidence: B)
Surgery is indicated for patients with infective endocarditis of a prosthetic valve who present with dehiscence evidenced by cine fluoroscopy or echocardiography (Level of Evidence: B)
Surgery is indicated for patients with infective endocarditis of a prosthetic valve who present with evidence of increasing obstruction or worsening regurgitation (Level of Evidence: C)
Surgery is indicated for patients with infective endocarditis of a prosthetic valve who present with complications (e.g., abscess formation; Level of Evidence: C)
Class IIa
Surgery is reasonable for patients with infective endocarditis of a prosthetic valve who present with evidence of persistent bacteremia or recurrent emboli despite appropriate antibiotic treatment (Level of Evidence: C)
Surgery is reasonable for patients with infective endocarditis of a prosthetic valve who present with relapsing infection (Level of Evidence: C)
Class III
Routine surgery is not indicated for patients with uncomplicated infective endocarditis of a prosthetic valve caused by first infection with a sensitive organism (Level of Evidence: C)

Operative Technique

Preparing for the operation, the surgeon should obtain the best possible understanding of the pathology and anatomic relationships and their technical implications with regard to reentry of the chest, cannulation, myocardial protection, and need for reconstruction of the heart. This requires careful review of all available imaging, echocardiograms, CT scans, and MRIs of the chest and the cardiac catheterization.

Sternal Reentry and Myocardial Protection

When dealing with an ascending aorta graft surrounded by fluid, sternal reentry that opens the fluid collection may result in catastrophic bleeding; caution is justified. An aortic pseudoaneurysm in contact with the sternum requires deep hypothermia and circulatory arrest or control of the aorta and cardioplegic cardiac arrest using percutaneous techniques normally used for minimal access and robotic cardiac surgery (Fig. 17.6). When extrathoracic arterial cannulation is indicated, axillary artery cannulation is preferred over femoral artery cannulation unless the patient is young enough not to have important atherosclerosis. Dual arterial cannulation may occasionally be considered. The difficulty of the mediastinal dissection depends on the interval from the previous operation and the severity of the periaortic inflammation, and this fact must be taken into consideration when deciding on operative strategy to avoid prolonged duration of circulatory arrest. The key to a clean dissection is to identify and stay in the correct plane. Bicaval cannulation and open placement of the retrograde cardioplegia cannula in the coronary sinus is routine and gives automatic access to the right atrium, tricuspid valve, and right ventricle for inspection. Cold blood cardioplegia is repeated every 15–20 min.

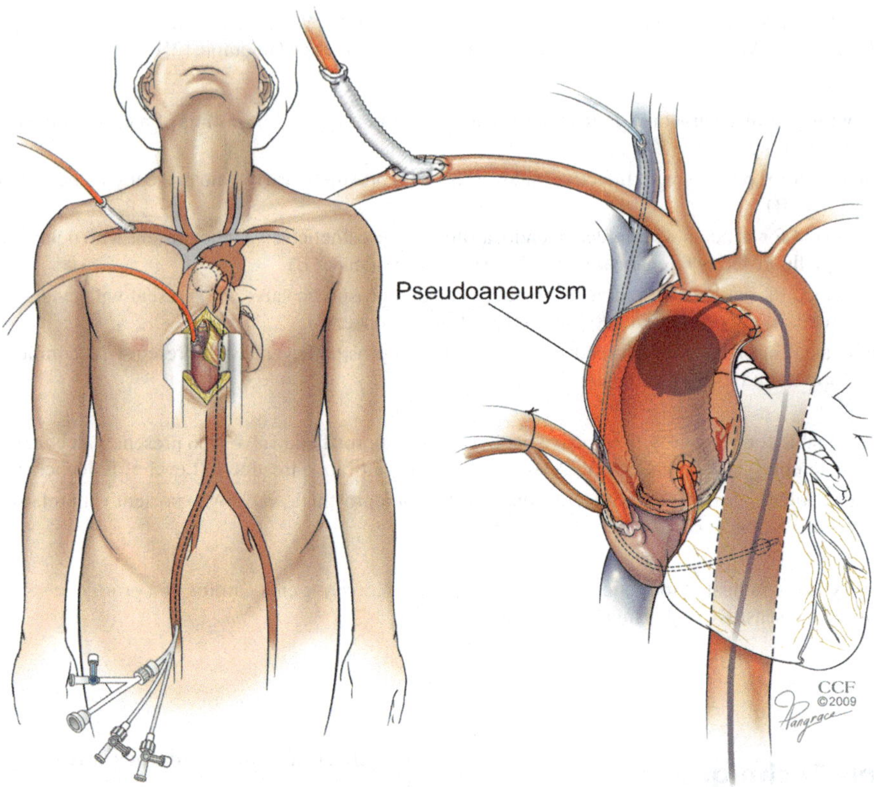

Fig. 17.6 Schematic illustration of the strategy for extrathoracic arterial cannulation, balloon aortic cross clamp, and delivery of antegrade and retrograde cardioplegia to avoid catastrophic bleeding when opening a periaortic pseudoaneurysm. Reprinted with permission, Cleveland Clinic Center for Medical Art and Photography ©2009–2011. All Rights Reserved

Radical Debridement

Radical debridement of all infected necrotic tissues and foreign materials is the first step toward curing the infection. The LV outflow tract is usually well preserved even after extensive invasion and destruction (Fig. 17.1c). Occasionally, a patient with an infected ascending aorta graft might not initially have involvement of the aortic valve prosthesis (the same can be true for the mitral valve in cases of previous double valve replacement); however, at a later time, they may present with an infected aortic prosthesis. Whenever there is heart block, invasion into right atrium and the triangle of Koch with destruction of the AV node is the most likely cause; to recognize this, the right atrium must be opened and the atrial septum and area around the membranous septum inspected (Fig. 17.1b). Whether local antibiotics or antiseptics, beyond generous irrigation, are of value to sterilize the field is disputable, but nevertheless used by many surgeons.

Replacement Choice for the Aortic Valve and Root

When there is minimal destruction of the aortic annulus and root, any replacement valve can be used. This is seldom true for PVE, and whenever the sewing ring is involved, the infection can be considered invasive. Whenever there is invasion and destruction, allograft root replacement is our preferred choice for reconstruction for technical reasons, low operative risk, and low risk of persistent and recurrent infection. The LV outflow tract is usually preserved well enough to allow direct implantation of an allograft without use of additional material for reconstruction. The coronary buttons are cut out (U-shaped for orientation) and mobilized. An allograft with an internal annulus diameter of 1–3 mm less than the patient's annulus diameter is ideal (cryopreserved allografts are not always accurately sized). The allograft is implanted in anatomic orientation using running monofilament sutures for all anastomoses, avoiding any other foreign material (Fig. 17.1e, f). If additional material is needed for the reconstruction, autologous pericardium is our preferred material. Invasion into the right atrium leaves a defect after debridement, which is easy to close with an autologous pericardial patch (Fig. 17.1d). The use of bovine pericardium for reconstruction in between the LV outflow tract and an allograft has resulted in dehiscence and development of pseudoaneurysm. Dead tissue to dead tissue does not heal.

Other centers have used other valved conduits to reconstruct the LV outflow tract with excellent results, possibly paying the price of a higher rate of heart block. The Ross operation has also been used in cases of active endocarditis, with good results. PVE in patients on dialysis has a very high risk of recurrence, but also a high probability of early calcification of an allograft or other bioprosthesis; thus, use of a mechanical valve should be given consideration.

Double Valve Endocarditis with Destruction of the Intervalvular Fibrosa

Although reconstruction of hearts with double valve endocarditis and destruction of the intervalvular fibrosa may be a formidable challenge, the principles are the same as other reconstructions: radical debridement of both valves and the intervalvular fibrosa followed by reconstruction, rebuilding from the bottom up. Access to the left atrium is guided by severity of the pathology and the prospects for preservation of the intervalvular fibrosa, but most of the time, a direct dome access works well. The mitral valve prosthesis is implanted first, placing sutures posteriorly from trigone to trigone and tying down the valve. An intervalvular fibrosa is reconstructed using available living tissue, autologous pericardium, or an aortic wall flap, or by direct anatomic implantation of the aortic allograft by suturing it directly to the mitral valve prosthesis.

Surgical Specimens

Specimens are divided between pathology and microbiology. Although it should be unusual for a patient to go to the operating room without therapeutic antibiotics initiated, careful processing of suspect tissue by culture and histopathology are complementary and should be done in all cases. Molecular diagnostic testing offers the potential to make a microbiologic diagnosis in cases deemed culture negative, whether due to the fastidious nature of the organism or prior antibiotic therapy.

Postoperative Management, Antibiotic Treatment, and Follow-Up

Decisions regarding antimicrobial therapy are substantially easier when the offending pathogen and its antimicrobial susceptibility sensitivity have been determined. Blood cultures at the time of initial presentation are particularly important to secure the microbiologic diagnosis.

The recommended antibiotic management of patients with PVE treated surgically is not substantially different from that of patients treated with antibiotics only. Although targeted therapy is preferred, a broad-enough regimen to provide coverage for all likely pathogens is necessary in "culture-negative" cases. For active cases, our practice is to provide intravenous antimicrobial therapy for 6 weeks postoperatively, timed from the day of operation. It is less well established that combination antimicrobial therapy is necessary in patients treated surgically if cultures from the operating room are negative. The potential benefits of additional agents must be weighed against the established risks of antibiotics such as gentamicin (nephrotoxicity) and rifampin (drug interactions).

Late relapse of fungal PVE, despite aggressive surgical debridement and intensive medical management, has been observed, and for these patients, we recommend lifelong suppressive therapy with an antifungal of the azole class, such as fluconazole.

Outcomes

Cleveland Clinic's overall mortality for PVE remains significant at 15%. In our practice, the use of allografts for LV outflow tract and aortic root reconstruction has made a difference with regard to both hospital mortality and medium-term survival. When an allograft was used for reconstruction, mortality was 3.9% for prosthetic aortic valve endocarditis and 3.7% for infected ascending and arch prosthetic grafts. Although other groups have presented good results with other alternatives for reconstruction, we remain convinced that short- and intermediate-term outcomes after the use of allografts is unparalleled.

Recommended Readings

1. Li JS, Sexton DJ, Mick N, et al. Proposed modifications to the Duke criteria for the diagnosis of infective endocarditis. Clin Infect Dis. 2000;30:633–8.
2. American College of Cardiology/American Heart Association Task Force on Practice Guideline; Society of Cardiovascular Anesthesiologists; Society for Cardiovascular Angiography and Interventions; Society of Thoracic Surgeons, Bonow RO, Carabello BA, Kanu C, de Leon AC Jr, Faxon DP, Freed MD, Gaasch WH, Lytle BW, Nishimura RA, O'Gara PT, O'Rourke RA, Otto CM, Shah PM, Shanewise JS, Smith SC Jr, Jacobs AK, Adams CD, Anderson JL, Antman EM, Faxon DP, Fuster V, Halperin JL, Hiratzka LF, Hunt SA, Lytle BW, Nishimura R, Page RL, Riegel B. ACC/AHA 2006 guidelines for the management of patients with valvular heart disease: a report of the American College of Cardiology/American Heart Association Task Force on Practice Guidelines (writing committee to revise the 1998 Guidelines for the Management of Patients With Valvular Heart Disease): developed in collaboration with the Society of Cardiovascular Anesthesiologists: endorsed by the Society for Cardiovascular Angiography and Interventions and the Society of Thoracic Surgeons. Circulation. 2006;114:e84–231. Erratum in: Circulation. 2007;115:e409.
3. Lytle BW, Sabik JF, Blackstone EH, Svensson LG, Pettersson GB, Cosgrove III DM. Reoperative cryopreserved root and ascending aorta replacement for acute aortic prosthetic valve endocarditis. Ann Thorac Surg. 2002;74:S1754–7; discussion S1792-9.
4. Sabik JF, Lytle BW, Blackstone EH, Marullo AG, Pettersson GB, Cosgrove 3rd DM. Aortic root replacement with cryopreserved allograft for prosthetic valve endocarditis. Ann Thorac Surg. 2002;74:650–9; discussion 659.
5. Gillinov AM, Diaz R, Blackstone EH, Pettersson GB, Sabik JF, Lytle BW, et al. Double valve endocarditis. Ann Thorac Surg. 2001;71:1874–9.
6. Pettersson G, Tingleff J, Joyce F. Treatment of aortic valve endocarditis with the Ross operation. Eur J Cardiothorac Surg. 1998;13:678–84.
7. Olaison L, Pettersson G. Current best practices and guidelines: indications for surgical intervention in infective endocarditis. Infect Dis Clin N Am 2002;16:453–75 and Cardiol Clin 2003;21:235–51.
8. Wang A, Athan E, Pappas PA, Fowler Jr VG, Olaison L, Paré C, et al. Contemporary clinical profile and outcome of prosthetic valve endocarditis. JAMA. 2007;297:1354–61.
9. Fowler VG Jr, Miro JM, Hoen B, Cabell CH, Abrutyn E, Rubinstein E, Corey GR, Spelman D, Bradley SF, Barsic B, Pappas PA, Anstrom KJ, Wray D, Fortes CQ, Anguera I, Athan E, Jones P, van der Meer JT, Elliott TS, Levine DP, Bayer AS; ICE Investigators. *Staphylococcus aureus* endocarditis: a consequence of medical progress. JAMA 2005;293:3012–21. Erratum in: JAMA 2005;294:900.
10. Baddour LM, Wilson WR, Bayer AS, Fowler VG Jr, Bolger AF, Levison ME, Ferrieri P, Gerber MA, Tani LY, Gewitz MH, Tong DC, Steckelberg JM, Baltimore RS, Shulman ST, Burns JC, Falace DA, Newburger JW, Pallasch TJ, Takahashi M, Taubert KA; Committee on Rheumatic Fever, Endocarditis, and Kawasaki Disease; Council on Cardiovascular Disease in the Young; Councils on Clinical Cardiology, Stroke, and Cardiovascular Surgery and Anesthesia; American Heart Association; Infectious Diseases Society of America. Infective endocarditis: diagnosis, antimicrobial therapy, and management of complications. Circulation 2005;111:e394–433. Erratum in: Circulation. 2005;112:2373.

18 Reoperation on the Aortic Arch

Lars G. Svensson

Introduction

In previous chapters, Doctors Pettersson and Sundt described reoperation techniques in patients exhibiting complex pathologies, such as root and ascending involvement. In this chapter, various approaches will be discussed for repairing the aortic arch [1–5]. Based on our experience, when possible, we use axillary/subclavian cannulation with a side graft for patients undergoing reoperation on the aortic arch [1]. This includes femoral vein cannulation with the cannula being fed upward into the right atrium while using transesophageal echocardiography for positioning. We recommend this because of the lower risk of stroke with deep hypothermia and circulatory arrest, and this procedure also offers the ability to both perfuse the innominate artery and run antegrade brain perfusion (Figs. 18.1–18.5). Next, the patient is placed on-pump, and cooling is begun immediately as the chest is being opened. As discussed in a previous chapter, if the patient has severe aortic valve regurgitation, further plans have to be instigated to deal with this problem.

L.G. Svensson, MD (✉)
Department of Thoracic and Cardiovascular Surgery, Cleveland Clinic Foundation, Cleveland, OH, USA
e-mail: svenssl@ccf.org

Hemiarch

In most patients, if a hemiarch is being replaced, the ascending aorta can be clamped during cooling and then, the valve or coronary artery disease dealt with at the time of cooling. Once the patient is cold enough, the circulation is arrested, after the administration of sodium pentothal [2] (Fig. 18.6). If deemed necessary, retrograde brain perfusion through the superior vena cava is then commenced and the aortic arch opened. Typically, with hemiarch reconstructions, the aorta is transected and a graft sewn into the under-surface of the aortic arch. Once the graft is sewn into position, it is tested under pressure and a proximal root procedure performed as needed. Retrograde brain perfusion helps with evacuating any potentially embolic material or air from the aortic arch as does using the axillary side graft for perfusing the arch. In most patients, this hemiarch repair can be achieved with a brief period of circulatory arrest.

Extended Aortic Arch Replacement Including the Proximal Descending Aorta with a Long Tongue

Often patients requiring extended aortic arch replacement will have had previous aortic root and ascending aortic surgery, for example, for bicuspid valves where aneurysms have extended into the aortic arch. As a rule, these patients can

V.R. Machiraju et al. (eds.), *Redo Cardiac Surgery in Adults*,
DOI 10.1007/978-1-4614-1326-4_18, © Springer Science+Business Media, LLC 2012

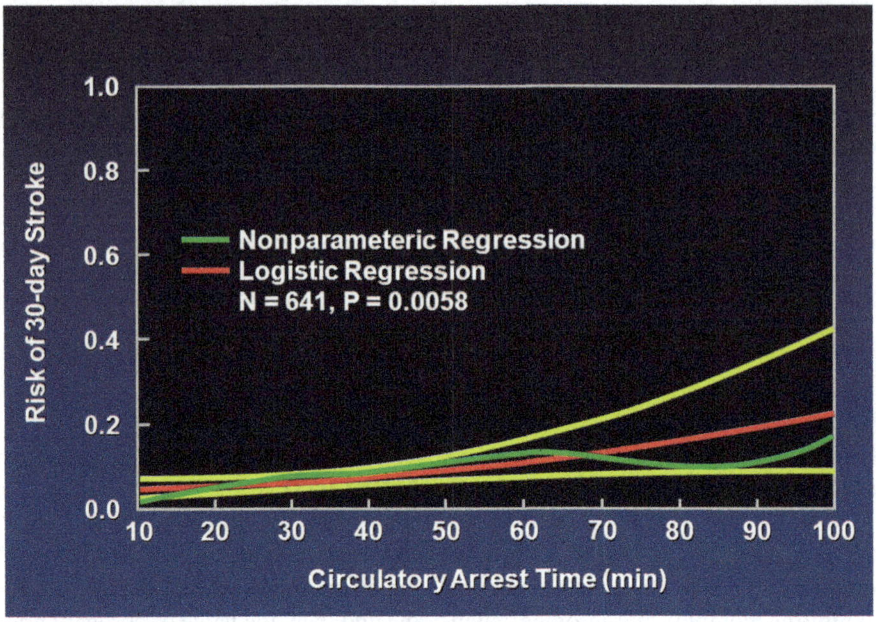

Fig. 18.1 Deep hypothermia circulatory arrest and risk of stroke (from Svensson et al. J Thorac Cardiovasc Surg. 1993;106(1):19–31)

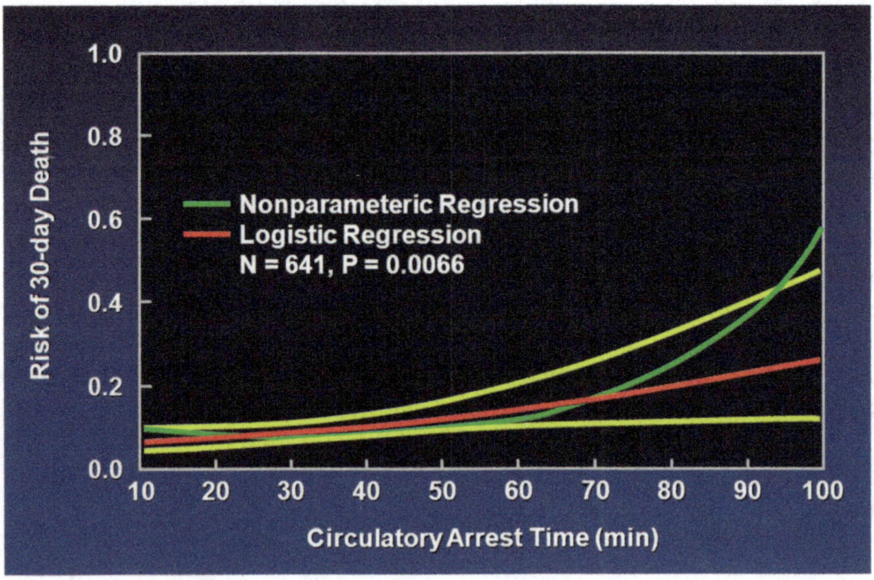

Fig. 18.2 Deep hypothermia circulatory arrest and risk of death (from Svensson et al. J Thorac Cardiovasc Surg. 1993;106(1):19–31)

often be treated by extending a long tongue of graft down into the descending aorta with the tongue being centered around the greater vessels and reaching up to the proximal innominate artery. This is a relatively quick and easy operation with minimal risk to the patient of either death or stroke. Of note, care should be taken not to damage the phrenic nerve.

Replacement of the Aortic Arch and Insertion of an Elephant Trunk into the Descending Aorta

The majority of patients who undergo reoperation for the aortic arch have previously undergone surgery for aortic dissection, typically as an acute procedure. These patients later present with either a descending or an aortic arch aneurysm that needs to be treated. For these patients, cannulation is similar with a side graft sewn onto the axillary subclavian artery and the femoral vein cannulated. Next, the patient is placed on cardiopulmonary bypass while the chest is opened on-pump. If severe aortic valve regurgitation is present, the procedure is done without cooling or with minimal cooling; whereas if there is no severe aortic valve regurgitation, the patient can be cooled. Once the patient's body temperature has been adequately lowered, the circulation is arrested, the aortic arch opened, and the previously prepared elephant trunk sewn into position beyond the left subclavian artery or, if the distal arch is particularly large, between the left carotid and subclavian arteries [4].

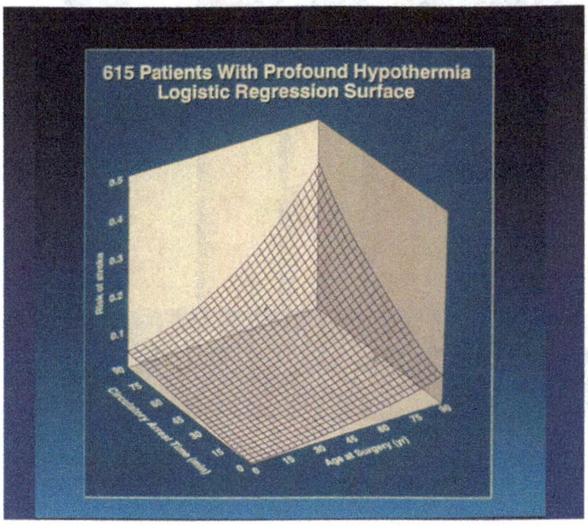

Fig. 18.3 Circulatory arrest and risk of death by age (from Svensson et al. J Thorac Cardiovasc Surg. 1993; 106(1):19–31)

With chronic dissection, care has to be taken that part of the septum is cut back so that the elephant trunk perfuses both the true and false lumens. The greater vessels are then attached to the side of the graft. The graft is clamped and perfusion to the brain is reestablished. The proximal anastomosis is then performed as needed. An alternative is to place a stent in the descending aorta and then sew an interposition graft

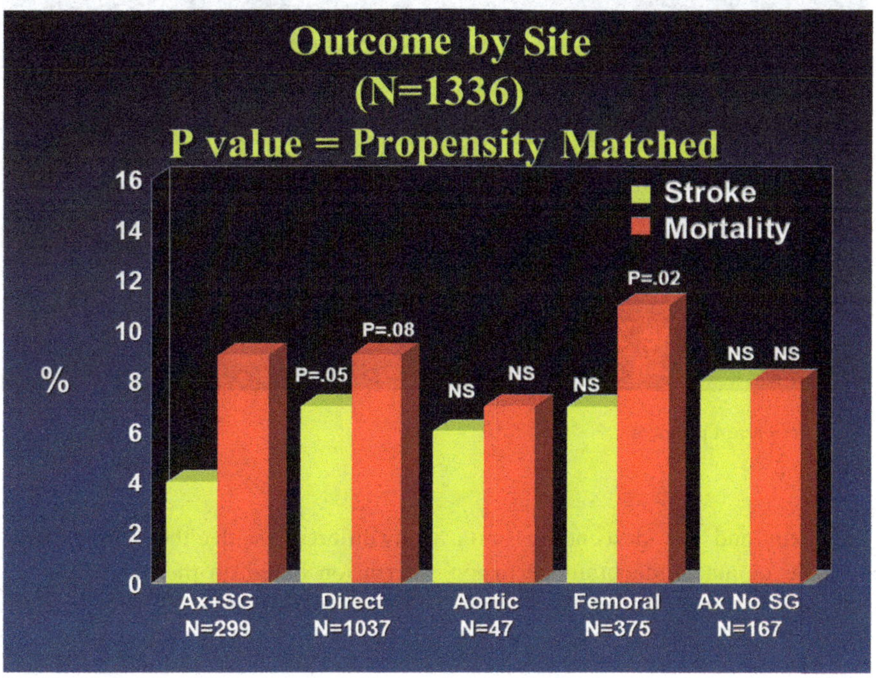

Fig. 18.4 Risk of stroke by cannulation site

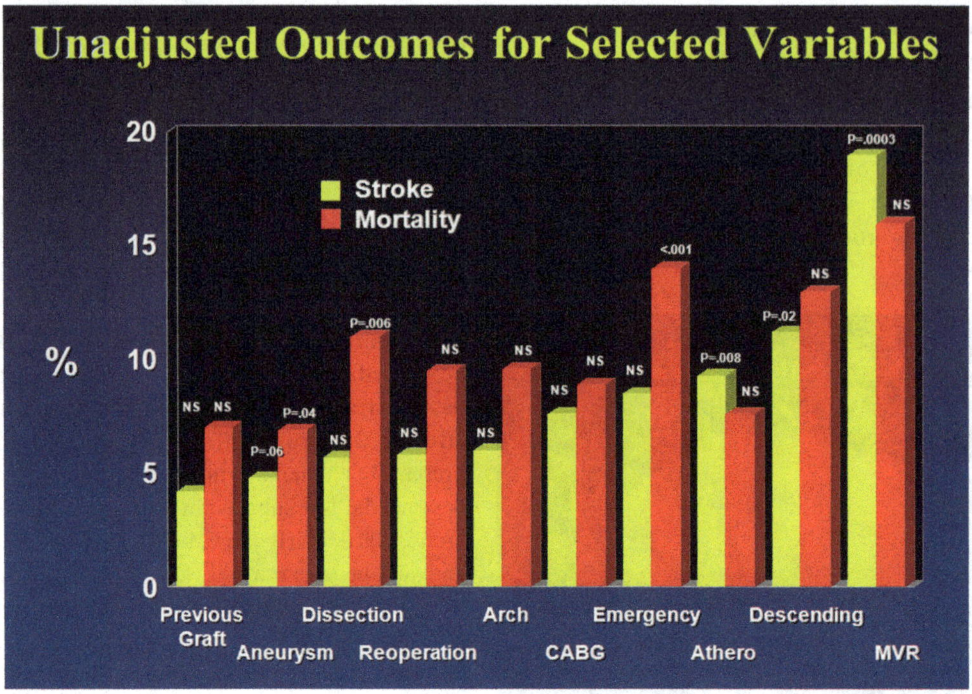

Fig. 18.5 Risk of stroke by procedure with circulatory arrest

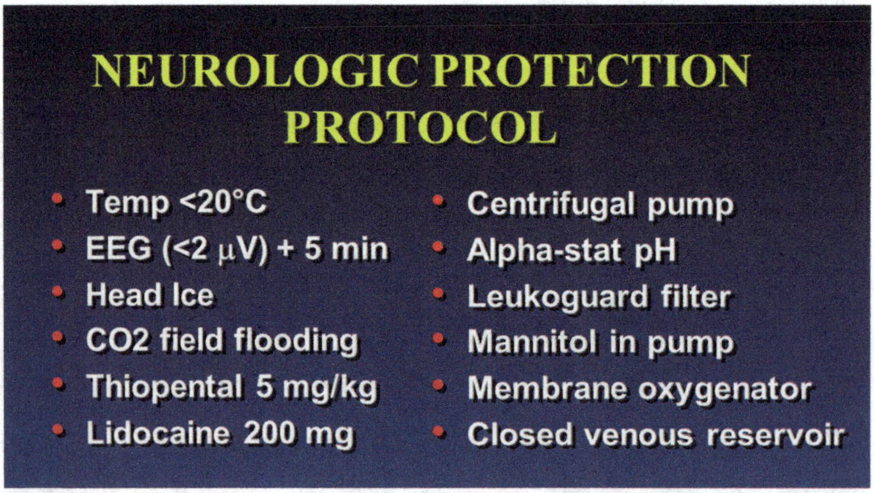

Fig. 18.6 Circulatory arrest protocol

between the stent and the descending aorta. Either retrograde or antegrade brain perfusion can be run at the same time as deep hypothermic circulatory arrest, although our data did not show any difference with either retrograde or antegrade perfusion based on the incidence of stroke [5]. A forthcoming study of neurocognitive deficits may elucidate the benefits of either approach.

Aortic Arch Replacement with Individual Bypasses to the Greater Vessels and the Elephant Trunk Procedure

When performing aortic arch replacement with individual bypasses to the greater vessels and an elephant trunk procedure, once again, cannulation is similar to other arch reoperations, with a side graft sewn onto the axillary subclavian artery and the femoral vein cannulated. The patient is then cooled. Circulation is arrested, and the innominate and carotid arteries transected. The first part of the operation is sewing a graft to the transected innominate artery and then clamping the graft and reperfusing the right side of the brain. The left carotid artery is similarly transected, another tube graft is sewn to it, and then the graft is clamped proximal to the bifurcation for the innominate and carotid arteries, enabling reperfusion of both vessels. To do this operation, there are custom-made grafts that can be used to reattach the greater vessels, including one with three limbs made out of a gel-impregnated graft material. A decision needs to be made about the left subclavian artery. In most cases, the left subclavian artery is also bypassed but if there is difficulty gaining access then, it can be oversewn and, if needed, a later carotid subclavian bypass performed. Alternatively, an ascending aorta to axillary bypass via the left second interspace can be attempted. Once the greater vessels have been reperfused, the elephant trunk is placed in the descending aorta and sewn into position and then withdrawn and sewn to the graft going to the greater vessels. The proximal anastomosis is then performed as needed. Of note, this operation is often the procedure of choice for patients with Marfan syndrome, patients with a bicuspid aortic valve, or patients with an aortic dissection in whom there is some risk, over time, that the aortic valve patch may enlarge if not replaced. This is also the preferred operation for Takayasu disease because it results in the individual vessels being bypassed and if a later stenosis occurs distal to the anastomosis, then the problem can be addressed without reopening the chest.

Debranching of the Aortic Arch Without Replacement of the Aortic Arch and Proximal Descending Aorta via Open Methods

Debranching of the aortic arch is achieved by various methods involving the use of stents, either at the same time as debranching or later. The first option is to place a side graft on the ascending aorta with branch grafts that are then sewn to the innominate and carotid arteries with or without the subclavian artery, hence avoiding the need to replace the ascending aorta. The aortic arch can then be stented into a normal-sized ascending aorta. If required, a wrap can be sewn around the ascending aorta to further aid anchoring and prevent later expansion. The second method is replacing a short bit of the ascending aorta with a debranching graft coming off the ascending aorta graft and then subsequent stenting of the aortic arch. Once again, the stenting can be performed at the same operation or at a subsequent operation using either antegrade or retrograde perfusion. The third option is to replace the ascending aorta and aortic arch with a tube graft of varying extents and then, under circulatory arrest, place a stent graft into the descending aorta, which is used to do a graft-to-graft anastomosis. The fourth option is to arrest the circulation, place a stent graft into the descending aorta, and sew it into position beyond the left subclavian artery. Of course, multiple other options can be devised to accommodate individual patients. For example, debranching operations are usually performed for complex repairs, for those patients who do not tolerate heparinization, or patients on cardiopulmonary bypass in whom an off-pump procedure can be done. The latter example includes those patients with traumatic injuries and multiple complex injuries or patients with cirrhosis.

In many of these patients, the second-stage operation includes either doing an open repair or stenting the descending aorta or the descending and thoracoabdominal aorta. In most patients with chronic dissection, an open second-stage procedure is performed, particularly if the patient has Marfan syndrome. If the patient does not have chronic aortic dissection but a degenerative aneurysm, then typically, the patient will undergo stenting of the descending aorta or thoracoabdominal aorta.

In summary, the important issues to keep in mind, as far as brain protection is concerned, include use of the subclavian artery, which reduces the risk of stroke by 40%, and cooling the patient at this stage, which affords the best brain protection with or without antegrade brain perfusion or retrograde brain perfusion [1] (Figs. 18.4 and 18.5). A few years ago, with careful attention to detail, we reviewed our series of elephant trunk procedures, and in these patients, we reported a 30-day survival of 98% [4]. Thus, the approach of various debranching operations will continue to develop and maybe, with time, less invasive operations for the aortic arch will be achieved, particularly for patients who require reoperations. The most critical issues will be finding a proximal anchoring place and preserving blood supply to the greater vessels without causing a stroke. Clearly, percutaneous aortic valves have become very useful in treating those patients with aortic valve disease who require reoperations and, undoubtedly, the technology of endovascular procedures will also evolve.

References

1. Svensson LG, Blackstone EH, Rajeswaran J, Sabik 3rd JF, Lytle BW, Gonzalez-Stawinski G, et al. Does the arterial cannulation site for circulatory arrest influence stroke risk? Ann Thorac Surg. 2004;78:1274–84.
2. Svensson LG, Nadolny EM, Kimmel WA. Multimodal protocol influence on stroke and neurocognitive deficit prevention after ascending/arch aortic operations. Ann Thorac Surg. 2002;74:2040–6.
3. Hirose H, Svensson LG, Lytle BW, Blackstone EH, Rajeswaran J, Cosgrove DM. Aortic dissection after previous cardiovascular surgery. Ann Thorac Surg. 2004;78:2099–105.
4. Svensson LG, Kim KH, Blackstone EH, Alster JM, McCarthy PM, Greenberg RK, et al. Elephant trunk procedure: newer indications and uses. Ann Thorac Surg. 2004;78:109–16.
5. Svensson LG, Nadolny EM, Penney DL, Jacobson J, Kimmel WA, Entrup MH, et al. Prospective randomized neurocognitive and S-100 study of hypothermic circulatory arrest, retrograde brain perfusion, and antegrade brain perfusion for aortic arch operations. Ann Thorac Surg. 2001;71:1905–12.
6. Svensson LG et al. Deep hypothermia with circulatory arrest. Determinants of stroke and early mortality in 656 patients. J Thorac Cardiovasc Surg. 1993;106(1):19–31.

19 Descending and Thoracoabdominal Aortic Reoperations

Edward Soltesz

Introduction

Patients with thoracic aortic aneurysms are at significant risk of developing aneurysmal disease in other areas of their aortas [1]. Reoperations on the descending and thoracoabdominal aorta have become more common as both the safety of the initial aneurysm repair has increased and subsequent radiologic surveillance with computed tomography (CT) scanning has improved. Patients with previous repairs are requiring further replacement of untreated aortic segments, underscoring the chronic nature of aortic disease. Reoperations requiring a repeat left thoracotomy or thoracoabdominal incision carry risks similar to primary operations on the same segments of aorta with the added morbidity of significant lung injury and bleeding. This has often led surgeons to delay or decline surgery even when an operation is clearly indicated. Elective surgical repair in patients with aortic disease is the only effective treatment to eradicate the potential risk of rupture. Here, we will review our approach to reoperative repair of descending and thoracoabdominal aneurysms and highlight the literature associated with this surgical practice. We also will highlight endovascular and hybrid techniques for managing certain high-risk patients.

E. Soltesz, MD, MPH (✉)
Department of Thoracic and Cardiovascular Surgery, Cleveland Clinic, Cleveland, OH, USA
e-mail: SOLTESE@ccf.org

Classification of Descending and Thoracoabdominal Aortic Aneurysms

The extent of aortic disease is paramount to predicting outcome and discussing surgical strategy for descending and thoracoabdominal aortic aneurysms. In general, a distinction should be made between descending and thoracoabdominal aortic disease resulting from progressive aneurysmal growth alone and aneurysmal degeneration in the setting of a chronic aortic dissection. The exact extent of the dissection should be noted in addition to the extent of aneurysmal dilatation.

Thoracoabdominal aneurysms have been classified by Crawford and colleagues [2] into four extents (Fig. 19.1). Two key anatomic landmarks in this organizational scheme are the sixth rib and the diaphragm, both of which can be accurately identified on any CT scan. Type I thoracoabdominal aneurysms involve the descending aorta proximal to the level of the sixth rib to above the renal arteries; type II thoracoabdominal aneurysms extend from the aorta proximal to the sixth rib to beyond the renal arteries; type III thoracoabdominal aneurysms involve the region below the sixth rib to any level in the abdominal aorta, and type IV thoracoabdominal aneurysms involve the visceral segment of the abdominal aorta without involvement of the descending thoracic aorta. The extent of previous aortic involvement should be noted, but the present region of aortic involvement should determine the classification.

V.R. Machiraju et al. (eds.), *Redo Cardiac Surgery in Adults*,
DOI 10.1007/978-1-4614-1326-4_19, © Springer Science+Business Media, LLC 2012

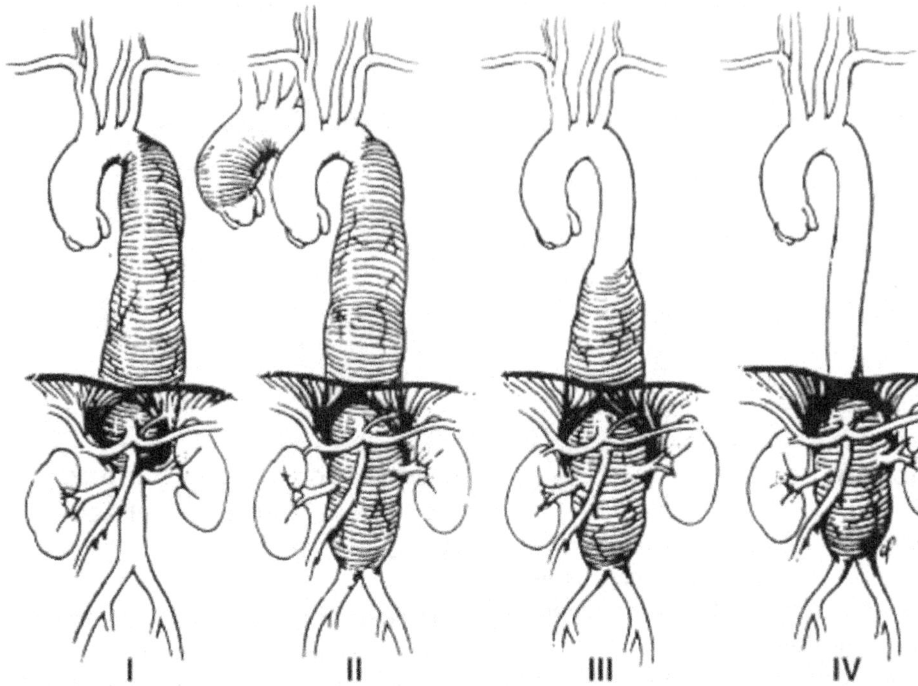

Fig. 19.1 Crawford classification of thoracoabdominal aortic aneurysms. Type I aneurysms extend from the proximal descending thoracic aorta to the renal arteries. Type II aneurysms extend from the proximal descending thoracic aorta above T6 to below the renal arteries. Type III aneurysms extend from below the level of T6 in the descending thoracic aorta into the abdomen in varying extents. Type IV aneurysms involve predominantly the abdominal aorta

Etiology

The majority of descending and thoracoabdominal aneurysms are degenerative and result from thinning of the media layer with associated loss of collagen and elastin. Pathologically, there is loss of smooth muscle cells, infiltration of inflammatory macrophages, and a variable extent of concomitant atherosclerosis. As these fusiform aneurysms enlarge, they develop increasing amounts of atheromatous material, which can lead to distal embolization. Familial clustering of aneurysms is apparent since 20% of patients with thoracic aortic aneurysms have one or more first-degree relatives with a thoracoabdominal aneurysm. Marfan's syndrome, an inherited connective tissue disorder, is the most well-known genetic disorder that causes aneurysms. Occurring at a frequency of 1:5,000, the syndrome is characterized by skeletal, ocular and cardiovascular abnormalities. Patients with Marfan's develop aortic aneurysms because of a deficiency of fibrillin, a large extracellular glycoprotein that is a major constituent of the aortic medial layer. Other genetic syndromes that predispose patients to aortic aneurysms include Turner's syndrome, Ehlers–Danlos syndrome, and polycystic kidney disease.

Patients with previous thoracic aortic aneurysms have a proclivity for developing further aortic pathology in nonrepaired segments. Crawford and Cohen [3] reported that multiple aneurysms developed in 60% of patients who originally presented with aortic aneurysms involving the ascending, transverse arch, or descending aortic segments, while multiple aneurysms developed in only 12% of patients who had previous abdominal aneurysms. Carrell and colleagues [4] noted that 28% of 130 thoracic aortic reoperations performed in their series of 120 patients were due to new or recurrent aortic aneurysms. Finally, Svensson et al. [5] showed that 181 patients (12%) of Crawford's 1,509 thoracoabdominal aortic aneurysm patients had undergone a previous proximal aortic operation. Thus, extension of aortic disease to nonoperated aortic segments is a significant cause for reoperation.

Another area of recurrent aneurysmal dilation is the area of native aorta that remains surrounding an aortic patch. Typically, reimplantation of intercostal and lumbar arteries below the T7–T8 level at the initial aortic operation is accomplished with the Crawford inclusion technique, wherein a side-to-side anastomosis between the graft and the aorta surrounding the intercostal vessels is made, or with a Carrel patch, where an end-to-side anastomosis is performed between prosthetic graft and full-thickness aortic patch. The risk of visceral artery patch aneurysm after thoracoabdominal aortic aneurysm repair with these techniques is 4–8%. Recently, Kulik et al. [6] have reported an incidence of intercostal patch aneurysms of 7% of a series of 155 descending and thoracoabdominal aortic aneurysm repairs. Marfan's syndrome and other connective tissue diseases predispose to the formation of both intercostal and visceral patch aneurysms and are the basis for the recommendation to use separate side branches to these arteries at the initial aortic operation.

Aortic coarctation is the most common congenital lesion of the descending aorta and can present in adulthood with restenosis or false aneurysm formation. Open surgical repair remains the gold standard for primary coarctation, but regardless of the surgical technique used and despite excellent initial results, 3–38% of patients develop long-term anastomotic pseudoaneurysms with a rupture-related mortality of 7%. Reintervention is necessary since conservative management is associated with a 100% rate of rupture.

Infection of the prosthetic graft after surgery of the thoracic aortic is a devastating complication and occurs in 1–3% of descending or thoracoabdominal aneurysm repairs. The source of the infection is usually from either seeding of the graft by way of septic emboli or contiguous spread from an empyema. Occasionally, a graft infection results from an inadvertent esophageal injury at the initial aortic surgery.

Natural History

Aortic aneurysms follow a predictable course of continued enlargement and eventual rupture. The incidence of aortic aneurysms is estimated at 5.9 cases per 100,000 person-years and is increasing with over 40,000 people dying of aortic disease yearly in the United States. This increasing prevalence is likely the result of improved imaging techniques and awareness.

Descending and thoracoabdominal aortic aneurysms remain a surgical disease with survival rates for patients with untreated aneurysms of 13–39% at 5 years. Patients typically die from rupture, with the lifetime probability of rupture in untreated aneurysms nearing 80%. The size of the aneurysm remains the most important predictor of rupture. Aneurysms over 5 cm have a significantly higher risk of rupture, which exponentially increases as the aneurysm enlarges. Growth rates of aneurysms are variable, but have been estimated at 0.10–0.42 cm/year, and for aneurysms over 5 cm, the rate of expansion is exponential. Aortic rupture is clearly also influenced by comorbidities, including age, tobacco use, hypertension, and emphysema. Thus, control of these modifiable risk factors is paramount to prevent rapid expansion of aneurysms. Smoking cessation should be a cornerstone of managing patients with aneurysms as well as those who have had a repair to protect nonoperated segments from further growth since both smoking and chronic obstructive pulmonary disease have been implicated as risk factors for aortic rupture. Patients should have strict blood pressure control with beta-adrenergic blockers to decrease the pulse pressure (dp/dt), which has been shown by Wheat and Palmer to influence rupture.

Aortic aneurysmal disease does not cease after aortic repair since other segments of the aorta remain at risk. Bavaria et al. found that the mean time from initial aortic surgery to the need for additional aortic replacement was 6.2 years with some patients requiring reintervention within the first 2 years. For this reason, we advocate yearly radiographic surveillance after descending and thoracoabdominal aneurysm repairs.

Preoperative Evaluation

All patients with descending or thoracoabdominal aortic aneurysms undergo a complete imaging study to define their aortic anatomy from the proximal carotid arteries to the distal femoral arteries. Currently, multiple imaging modalities are available, but spiral CT is by far the most common method. Patients should undergo chest, abdomen, and pelvis CT angiography with a pre-stent protocol technique. Multiplanar reconstructions with centerline of flow analysis are performed on a workstation (TeraRecon Inc., San Francisco, CA) to accurately delineate aortic anatomy, size, calcification, and the location and topography of any related dissection flaps. Careful review of these studies is important in patients with previous aortic repairs because knowing the exact extent of planned reconstruction is necessary. Angiography is rarely, if ever, used for preoperative planning. In patients with marginal renal function, magnetic resonance imaging (MRI) with or without gadolinium can be used so long as the patient does not have any implanted magnetic devices.

All patients who undergo descending or thoracoabdominal aortic aneurysm repair undergo cardiac catheterization and echocardiography. If coronary artery disease is found, a decision must be made regarding medical management, percutaneous coronary intervention (angioplasty or stenting), or surgical revascularization. If a non-critical coronary vessel is involved, medical management will typically suffice. However, when a larger vessel with a critical area of myocardium is stenosed, then bare-metal stenting with an obligate 30-day course of clopidogrel before elective aneurysm repair is the best course. If severe or triple-vessel disease is encountered, the patient should undergo coronary artery bypass surgery prior to aneurysm repair. If the proximal descending aorta is involved, consideration should be given to using the left internal thoracic artery as a free graft in case the left subclavian artery is clamped during aortic repair. Finally, if a patient is found to have aortic insufficiency graded higher than 2+, the aortic valve should be replaced before elective aneurysm surgery.

All patients should be screened for severe chronic obstructive pulmonary disease with formal spirometry and an arterial blood gas sample. A forced expiratory volume in 1 s (FEV1) <1.2 L/min, or home oxygen use predicts an increased risk of postoperative respiratory failure. Pulmonary risk stratification is extremely important in reoperative descending and thoracoabdominal aneurysms since the left lung will likely incur more injury during dissection.

Operative Techniques

The surgical approach for each patient who requires redo descending or thoracoabdominal aortic aneurysm surgery should be individualized. The extent of the previous aortic repair, the previous incision and access, and prior complications should be taken into account when planning a reoperation. Strategic operative planning should involve a consideration of (1) operative approach (redo thoracotomy or thoracoabdominal incision vs. an extra-anatomic approach vs. an endovascular or hybrid approach), (2) method of visceral and lower extremity perfusion, and (3) technique of spinal cord protection. We will review our general strategy for redo descending and thoracoabdominal aneurysm surgery (Fig. 19.2) and then focus on specific surgical situations. Importantly, optimal results for reoperative aortic surgery can only be achieved with careful attention to preoperative planning, operative technique, and postoperative management.

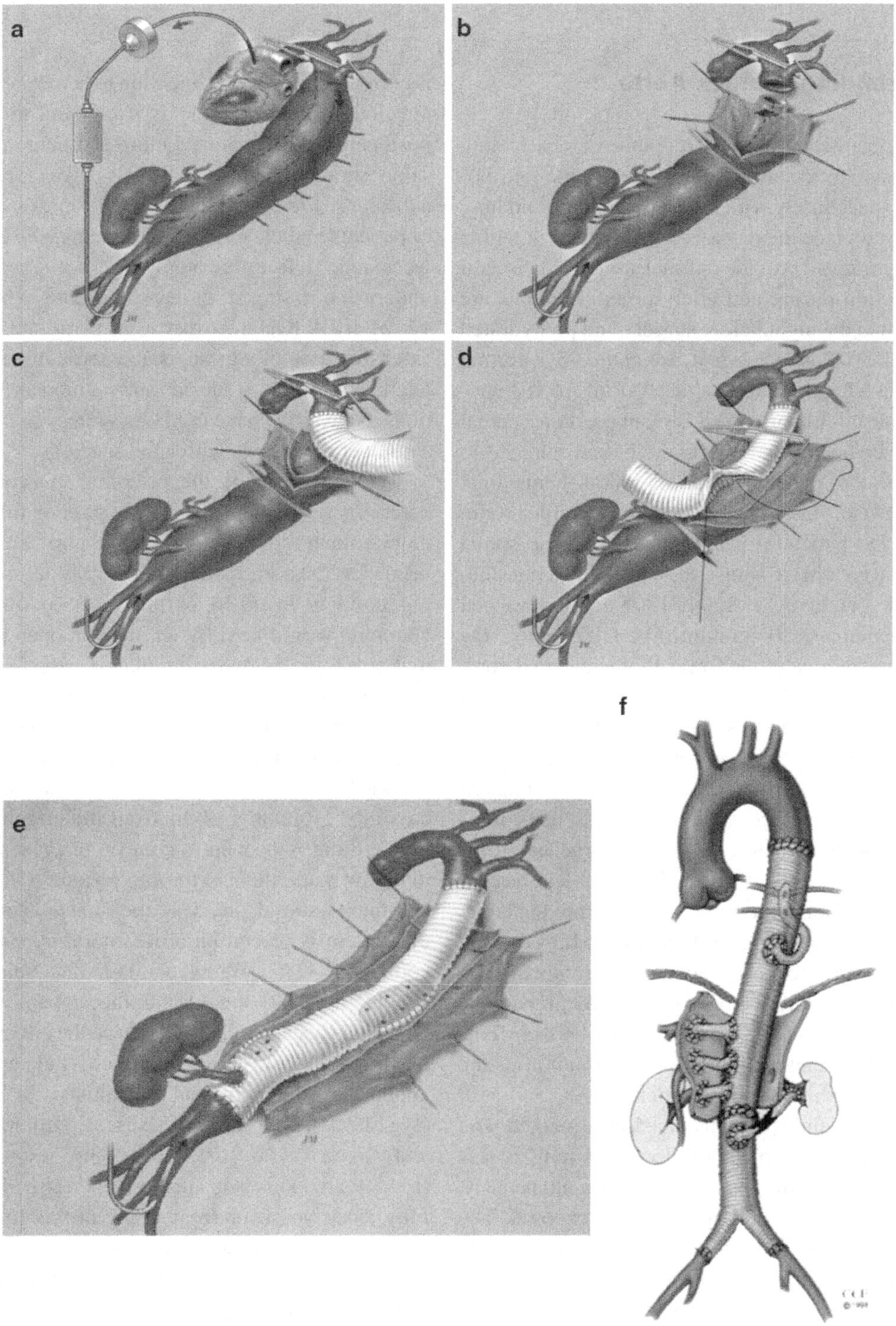

Fig. 19.2 Operative steps in the repair of a thoracoabdominal aortic aneurysm. (**a**) Insertion of an atriofemoral bypass circuit with heat exchanger and cooling the patient to 32°C followed by proximal cross-clamp application. (**b**) Complete transection of the aorta beyond the subclavian artery after clamping the mid-descending thoracic aorta. (**c**) Completion of the proximal anastomosis and oversewing of the upper intercostal arteries above T6. (**d**) Sequential movement of the proximal cross-clamp onto the graft and the lower cross-clamp to just above the celiac artery to allow intercostal artery reattachment. (**e**) Completion of repair by reattachment of the visceral segment and distal anastomosis. (**f**) Separate branched grafts to each intercostal and visceral artery are used in patients with Marfan's syndrome and other connective tissue disorders to avoid future patch aneurysm formation

Descending Thoracic Aorta

The operative goals of reoperative descending thoracic aortic surgery are to reenter the left thoracic space safely with minimal bleeding and lung injury, replace the diseased aortic segment with a tube graft, and provide optimal spinal and visceral protection during and after surgery. Patients are admitted the night before surgery and prehydrated with D5 1/2 NS (5% dextrose and 0.45% normal saline) + 1 amp $NaHCO_3$ at 100 mL/h. If hypothermic circulatory arrest is planned, then a spinal catheter is inserted the night before surgery to lessen the chance of an epidural hematoma. Otherwise, this is performed in operating room with the patient still awake. The silastic spinal drainage catheter is inserted under local anesthesia at the level of L3/4, L4/5, and advanced approximately 20–25 cm to the L1/2 region, the vulnerable area of the lower thoracic spinal cord. Cerebrospinal fluid (CSF) pressure is monitored and maintained at less than 10 mmHg throughout the procedure. Right upper and lower extremity arterial lines are placed in addition to standard central venous access, and the patient is intubated with a double-lumen endotracheal tube. Positioning for adequate left thoracic access involves placing the shoulders 70° from the table, which allows for a 45° rotation at the hips for safe left femoral access. In patients who require hypothermic circulatory arrest, we sterilely prepare the left arm so that access can be gained for right axillary artery cannulation with easy rotation of the left arm within the surgical field.

The patient's previous incision is marked, and this incision is typically followed as long as it is not too far from the planned access. Simultaneously, the left femoral artery and vein are exposed. The decision as to which interspace to enter is based on the anatomic region of most complexity (arch vs. distal descending thoracic aorta) and the previous entry point. All attempts are made to avoid access through a previously entered interspace because this is the site of most dense pleural adhesions, which can lead to lung injury. Typically, the fifth or sixth rib is removed, and dissection of the lung is commenced. Careful attention to hemostatis and prevention of lung injury is paramount to avoid postoperative respiratory failure and hemorrhage. Time should be taken carefully dissect pleural adhesions. Etz and colleagues [7] report that 7% of patients in their series of 60 patients who underwent redo left thoracotomy for aortic surgery underwent a staged, 2-day procedure whereby 12–24 h of ICU recovery was permitted, after extensive lysis of adhesions and aortic dissection, to allow bleeding to subside and pulmonary secretions to clear. We have used this strategy as well in a number of patients with good success.

The condition of the proximal anastomosis determines whether left heart bypass or full cardiopulmonary bypass with circulatory arrest is needed. If the aortic arch or very proximal ascending aorta is involved or proximal control and clamping would be difficult, then an open proximal anastomosis under circulatory arrest should be planned. For left heart bypass, the patient is heparinized with 1 mg/kg i.v. heparin. The pericardium is opened below the left phrenic nerve, and the left inferior pulmonary vein is cannulated, carefully excluding all air from the circuit. The pericardium is opened to confirm placement and to allow surveillance for tamponade. The left common femoral artery is then cannulated and the patient is placed on atriofemoral bypass and cooled to 32°C. While cooling, the patient is slowly given 30 mg of intrathecal papaverine, which has been kept at 37°C. Once the patient has reached the target temperature, cross-clamps are applied and the proximal anastomosis is begun (Fig. 19.2a). The aorta is transected completely and freed from the underlying esophagus (Fig. 19.2b). This step should be performed carefully since an esophageal injury at this location with a nearby aortic graft can be devastating. When tissue planes around the distal aortic arch or proximal descending thoracic aorta have been previously violated, identification and preservation of the recurrent laryngeal nerve can be difficult. The proximal anastomosis is sewn with continuous 4–0 prolene suture using a strip of bovine pericardium as a washer to aid in hemostasis

(Fig. 19.2c,d); this method works much better than felt reinforcement for aortic anastomoses and is more infection resistant. Once the proximal anastomosis is complete, the distal anastomosis is completed (Fig. 19.2e). If the graft does not go beyond T7 or T8, then the intervening intercostal vessels are rapidly oversewn to avoid steal phenomenon, and no intercostal reimplantation is necessary. However, if the graft extends to the diaphragm, then a long beveled anastomosis is typically created, so as to include the intercostal vessels from T7 down to T11 or T12. In patients with Marfan's syndrome or another defined connective tissue disease, one or two separate 8-mm grafts should be used to reattach intercostal vessels to avoid the late possibility of intercostal artery patch aneurysms (Fig. 19.2f).

Once the distal anastomosis is complete, the graft is de-aired, the patient is placed in a head-down position, and the graft is unclamped. The perfusionist must be attentive to keep the lower extremity pressure lower than the upper body pressure so as to avoid brain embolization. The patient is then rewarmed to 35°C, cannulas are removed, and protamine is administered.

Certain patients will have unfavorable anatomy that threatens safe application of a cross-clamp to the distal arch or proximal descending thoracic aorta. Hypothermic circulatory arrest has proven very valuable in these patients. In fact, Etz and colleagues reported a 30% use of hypothermic circulatory arrest for redo left thoracoabdominal surgery in their series. Preoperative dialog with the perfusionist is necessary to ensure a safe operation. We typically utilize an 8-mm graft sewn to the right axillary artery as arterial inflow, and then left femoral venous and arterial cannulation. This dual arterial cannulation affords complete control of upper and lower body perfusion during the case. Once on bypass, the patient is cooled to 18°C for a minimum of 30 min; cerebral oximetry is used to monitor cerebral blood flow. Transesophageal echocardiography is employed to be certain that no left ventricular distention occurs when the heart fibrillates. During circulatory arrest, 100–500 mL/min flow is maintained via the right axillary artery so as to prevent air entrainment in the arch and head vessels. Once the open proximal anastomosis has been completed, upper and lower body perfusion can be restarted independently.

Patients who have undergone a previous coarctation repair can present with stenosis or pseudoaneurysm and represent a significant surgical challenge. In adults who develop restenosis following a childhood coarctation repair, we advocate a bypass from the distal arch to the descending thoracic aorta (20 mm graft for females and 22 mm for males). This approach lessens the risk of recurrent laryngeal nerve injury and paraplegia since important collateral blood flow to the spinal cord is not interrupted. In patients who have had multiple left thoracotomies, an extra-anatomical graft can be performed via a median sternotomy. The patient is placed on cardiopulmonary bypass, the heart is arrested, and a graft is placed from the ascending aorta to the descending aorta. The distal anastomosis is performed by reflecting the heart up and approaching the distal descending thoracic aorta via the posterior pericardium. The graft is routed to the right side of the heart.

Graft infection in the descending aorta can be a challenging surgical problem. The classic approach to aortic graft infection involves complete excision of the graft material with remote reconstruction of the distal circulation. Treatment of aortic graft infection with graft excision and axillofemoral bypass may carry an increased risk of limb loss, aortic stump blowout, and pelvic ischemia. Studies by Kieffer et al. suggest that insertion of a homograft is useful in this situation. In most patients, we advocate resection of the graft, careful debridement of surrounding tissue, replacement with a new antibiotic-soaked tube graft, and omental flap coverage. Gel-impregnated grafts are soaked in 600 mg of rifampin or amphotericin B prior to insertion. In addition, we position a percutaneous irrigation catheter in the area of infection and place surrounding drainage tubes of the Blake variety to prevent suction of omentum into the holes of conventional chest tubes.

Thoracoabdominal Aorta

Reoperations on the thoracoabdominal aorta employ the same anesthesia set-up and spinal drainage protocols as descending thoracic reoperations. Patients are positioned slightly differently: the chest and shoulders should be positioned approximately 60° to the table, and the right groin should be accessible in case an aortic bifurcated graft is required. The incision is taken from behind the scapula across the costal margin and is curved to the umbilicus; for type II aneurysms, the incision is carried down to the pubic bone. The sixth rib is resected, and the dissection of the lung and retroperitoneum is begun. If the previous repair involved a retroperitoneal approach, it is often easier to approach the abdominal aorta through the peritoneum after mobilizing the left colon but without medial rotation of the left kidney. If the diaphragm was previously mobilized, leaving it intact on reoperation may improve postoperative respiratory function. Atriofemoral bypass is established as previously described. A segmental sequential repair is then performed. The sequence of repair involves (1) the proximal anastomosis and oversewing of intercostals above T6; (2) intercostal segment revascularization with either a Carrell patch or separate grafts (in patients with Marfan's or another defined connective tissue disorder) to two or more selected intercostal arteries; (3) visceral and renal segment revascularization; and (4) distal anastomosis. During visceral reattachment, cold crystalloid is instilled into each renal artery; Pruitt catheters are inserted into the celiac and superior mesenteric arteries to provide 300–600 mL/min active perfusion derived from a separate line from the atriofemoral bypass circuit. Distal control of the aorta during performance of the distal anastomosis can be difficult in patients who have had a previous retroperitoneal dissection. Here, we either perform this anastomosis open with lower extremity flow minimized or insert a Coda (Cook Medical, Bloomington, IN) endovascular occlusion balloon for endoluminal control. In patients who have had high aortic segments replaced and require completion replacement to their iliac bifurcation or beyond, we attempt to bevel our distal anastomosis so as to include lumbar arteries as the lumbar arteries are usually critical in maintaining spinal collateral flow in such extensive aortic replacements.

Postoperative Management

Prior to leaving the operating room, the double-lumen endotracheal tube is changed to a single-lumen tube, provided there is no vocal cord edema. Mean arterial blood pressure is maintained at 80–100 mmHg; volume and vasopressors are used, if needed, for blood pressure support. Cerebrospinal drainage is continued for 48 h. Upon returning from the operating room, the patient is awoken and neurologic status is assessed. Neurologic status is continually reevaluated in case delayed neurologic deficits develop. In patients who develop delayed neurologic deficits, a rapid action plan is commenced involving induced hypertension and aggressive spinal drainage. We typically keep patients intubated for 48 h to clear pulmonary secretions from the left lung and maintain adequate oxygenation as this has been shown to reduce the risk of delayed neurologic deficit. Patients typically have their spinal drains removed on postoperative day 2, and are subsequently extubated and transferred to the step-down floor on postoperative day 4.

Spinal Cord Protection

The incidence of neurologic deficit (either paraplegia or paraparesis) in descending, and thoracoabdominal aneurysm surgery has slowly declined over the past decade due to a greater awareness of the etiologic factors. The three major events that contribute to spinal cord injury are as follows: (1) the degree and duration of spinal cord ischemia during the period of aortic cross-clamping; (2) failure to re-establish spinal cord blood flow during aortic cross-clamping; and (3) postoperative damage to the spinal cord from ischemia/reperfusion injury.

The degree of spinal cord ischemia is dependent on both the extent of aortic repair and the available collateral blood flow [8]. Multiple studies have correlated the extent of aortic replacement with the risk of neurologic injury in both open and endovascular aortic repair, with type II thoracoabdominal aneurysm repair posing the greatest risk. Additionally, the duration of aortic cross-clamping has been repeatedly shown to correlate with spinal cord ischemia and eventual neurologic dysfunction. A useful approach for reducing the degree of spinal cord ischemia entails maintaining adequate blood flow with the use of distal aortic perfusion and decreasing spinal cord metabolic demands with moderate hypothermia (Fig. 19.3). In fact, studies looking at deep hypothermia and circulatory arrest for thoracoabdominal aneurysm repair have reported very low rates of paraplegia, emphasizing the importance of hypothermia in the overall protection strategy.

An additional adjunct that lessens spinal cord ischemia is CSF drainage. Two prospective randomized trials, one by Svensson and colleagues [9] and one by Coselli and colleagues [1], have shown that for extent I and II thoracoabdominal aortic aneurysms, CSF drainage significantly reduces the incidence of neurologic deficits. Paraplegia rates in both studies utilizing CSF drainage were approximately 3%. We use intrathecal papaverine in addition to continuous CSF drainage to improve collateral blood flow down the longitudinal vessels of the spinal cord. The optimal protective strategy utilizes all three adjunctive measures: (1) distal aortic perfusion, (2) moderate hypothermia, and (3) CSF drainage.

Re-establishment of spinal blood flow relies on both intercostal and collateral blood flow. Many studies have shown a higher risk of paraplegia in patients whose collateral network (importantly, the left subclavian and internal iliac arteries) has been compromised. To preserve as much spinal blood flow as possible, we advocate

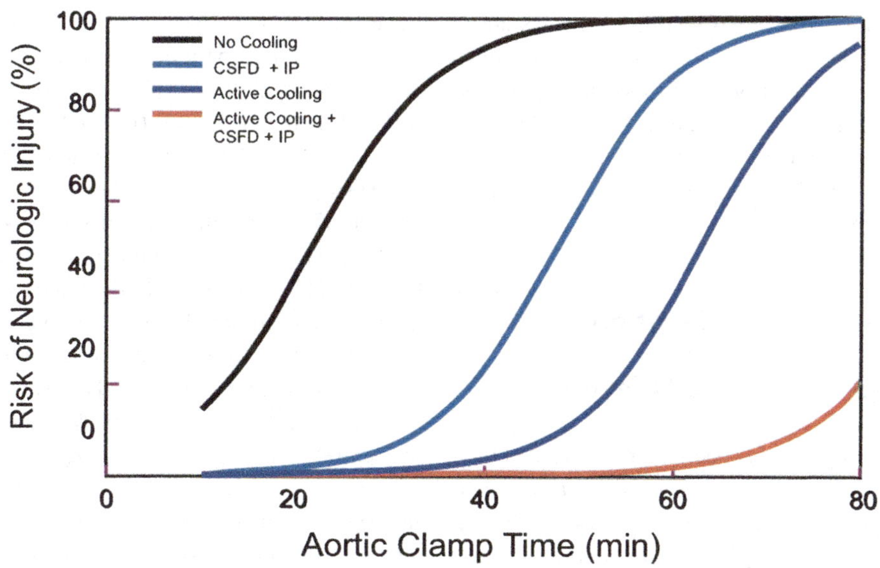

Fig. 19.3 The relationship between aortic cross-clamp time and risk of neurologic injury based on a prospective randomized study showing the risk according to increasing use of adjunctive measures (CSF drainage with intrathecal papaverine and moderate hypothermia) (Reprinted from Svensson et al. [11]. Copyright (1998), with permission from Elsevier)

reimplantation of selective patent intercostal arteries from T6 down to L2. Intraoperative attention to steal phenomenon is also important; intercostals arteries that are not being reimplanted should be rapidly oversewn. With the increasing success of intraoperative spinal cord protection, we have begun to see a greater proportion of delayed deficits after surgery. Hypotension, hypoxia, the need for reintubation, and bleeding are all related to delayed neurologic deficits. For this reason, we keep patients intubated for 48 h.

Renal and Visceral Protection

Postoperative renal failure remains a significant comorbidity in thoracoabdominal aneurysm repair. Reports cite incidences between 4 and 29%, and patients who incur renal failure have a greater 30-day mortality and poorer overall recovery and survival. Risk factors associated with renal failure include preoperative renal insufficiency (creatinine (Cr) >2.0 mg/dL) and the use of the clamp-and-sew technique [10]. No renal protection strategy has yet proven superior. We have used 180 mL of 4°C cold crystalloid infusion for renal protection; this has consistently maintained the kidneys at 15°C in our early studies. Visceral protection is important to prevent liver ischemia and resultant coagulopathy. We routinely use direct visceral perfusion through Pruitt catheters during type II thoracoabdominal aneurysm repair.

Alternative Surgical Options

Branched–Fenestrated Stent grafts

Standard surgical approach to redo descending and thoracoabdominal aneurysms is considerably demanding, and outcomes correlate with the number and severity of associated comorbidities. Many large studies have reported mortality rates ranging from 7 to 17% with the mortality in most series of reoperations exceeding 10%. Cardiac, neurologic, respiratory, and renal complications limit the number of patients who are eligible for open reoperative surgery. We have been actively involved with the development of fenestrated and branched stent grafts to target this high-risk patient population (Figs. 19.4 and 19.5). The branched thoracoabdominal stent graft is a modular system based on the Zenith stent graft (Cook Inc., Bloomington, IN). The main body component is a custom-designed straight or tapered device with reinforced fenestrations or directional helical branches precisely constructed to correlate with the patient's target vessels. Reinforced fenestrations are mated to balloon-expandable covered stents (Jomed, Abbot Labs, Abbott Park, IL), and the directional branches are mated to self-expanding covered stents (Fluency, Bard Inc., Tempe, AZ). Greenberg et al. [11] reported the first, 50 patient series of branched endografts used to treat thoracoabdominal aortic aneurysms. Despite the high-risk patient cohort, there was only one perioperative death (2%) and two cases of spinal cord ischemia (4%). The largest series to date of endovascular thoracoabdominal repair using stent grafts has been reported by our group at the Cleveland Clinic. Roselli et al. [12] described 73 patients who underwent fenestrated–branched endograft repair for thoracoabdominal aortic aneurysms (type I, II, or III, $n=28$; type IV, $n=45$) between 2004 and 2006. Mean aneurysm size was 7.1 cm. Thirty-day mortality was only 5.5%; mean length of stay was 8.6 days. Major perioperative complications occurred in 11 patients (14%) and included paraplegia (2.7%), renal failure (1.4%), prolonged ventilator support (6.8%), myocardial infarction (5.5%), and minor hemorrhagic stroke (1.4%). Target branch vessel patency was 100%. These results are extremely encouraging for the high-risk reoperative patient with a thoracoabdominal aneurysm. Because of these data, we routinely screen reoperative descending or thoracoabdominal aneurysm patients for their anatomic suitability for branched–fenestrated stent graft repair.

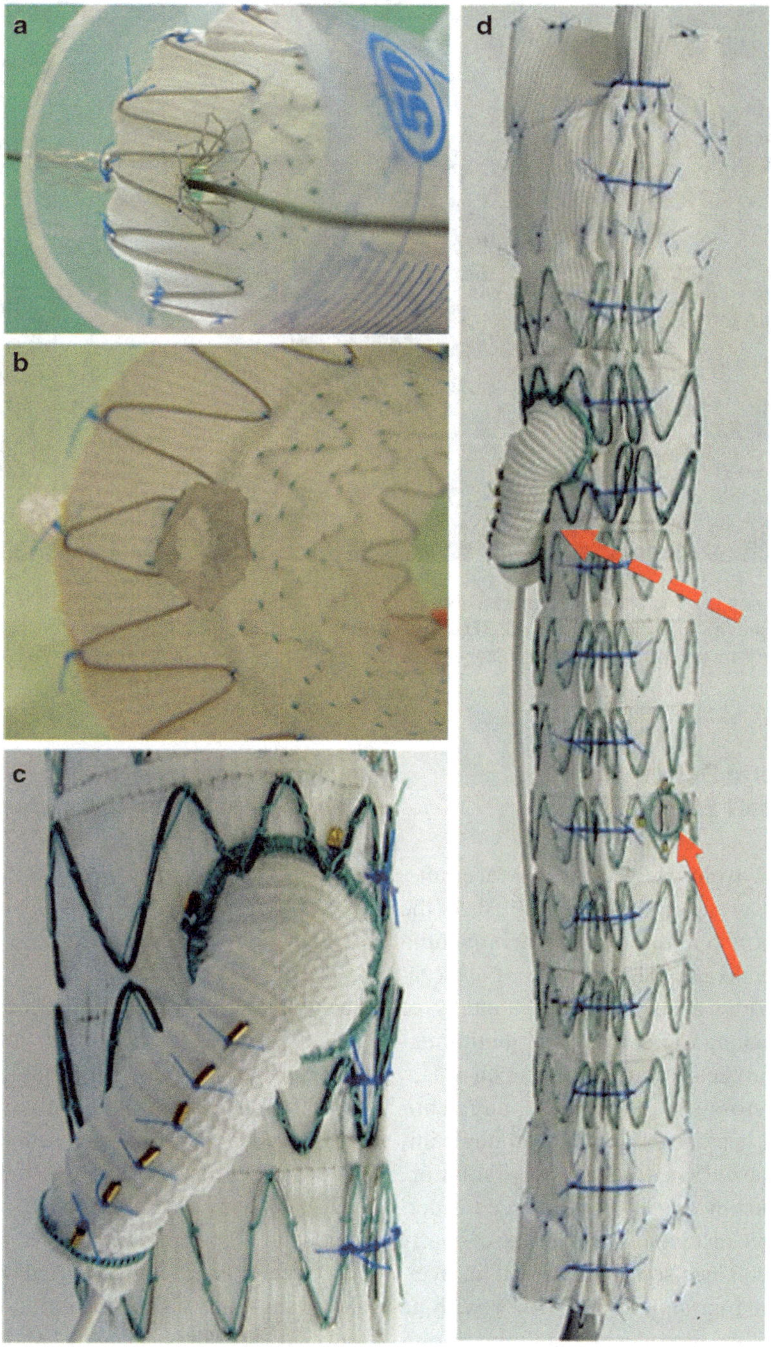

Fig. 19.4 Fenestrated-branched stent graft for thoracoabdominal aortic aneurysm repair. (**a**) Circumferentially reinforced fenestration is shown with wire access into a target visceral and deployment of a balloon-expandable stent graft partially extending within the aortic stent graft lumen. (**b**) Flaring of the aortic segment of the balloon-expandable stent graft to abut the stent graft to the aortic graft, achieving a seal around the fenestration. (**c**) A helical branch (*directional branch*) consisting of an 8-mm polyester graft sewn to the aortic prosthesis above the target vessel. (**d**) The entire main body device showing both a fenestration (*solid arrow*) and a helical branch (*dashed arrow*). (Reprinted from Soltesz et al. [15]. Copyright (2010), with permission from Elsevier)

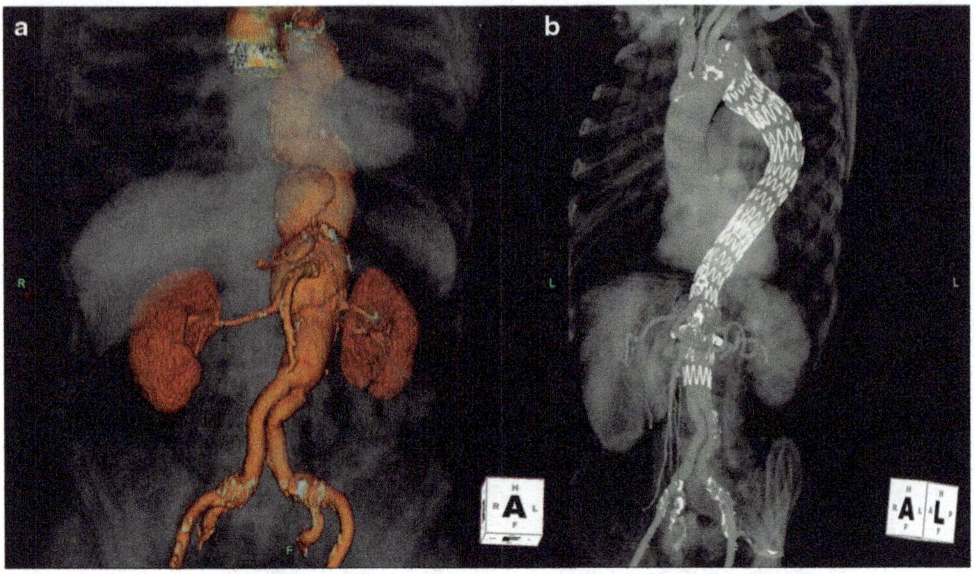

Fig. 19.5 Endovascular repair of a type III thoracoabdominal aortic aneurysm. (**a**) Arterial contrast phase 3D reconstruction of aneurysm preoperatively. (**b**) Postoperative 3D reconstruction after repair with a composite design four-branch reinforced fenestrated device

Hybrid Visceral Debranching and Stent Graft Exclusion

Soon after the advent of abdominal stent grafts, the St. Mary's group in London published the first large series of complete visceral debranching followed by endovascular exclusion of thoracoabdominal aortic aneurysms. The strategy of visceral debranching is predicated upon minimizing the morbid aspects of a traditional open repair, namely, aortic cross-clamping, single lung ventilation, and left heart bypass [13]. Although initially conceptualized as a straightforward solution, visceral debranching procedures can be considerably morbid and involved. Donas et al. recently reviewed 13 published series and found an overall perioperative mortality rate of 10.7% with no paraplegia or other procedure-related neurological deficits. Subsequent reports have showed disparate outcomes with paraplegia rates exceeding 15% and perioperative mortality above 14%. We have abandoned this approach for primary thoracoabdominal aortic aneurysm repairs but continue to use this method in carefully selected patients on a case-by-case basis for reoperative thoracoabdominal repairs (Fig. 19.6).

Results

The reported outcomes of reoperative descending and thoracoabdominal aneurysms repair vary widely. Some reports include patients with previous infrarenal aneurysm repairs and aortic arch repairs and do not truly represent the patient population described herein. A recent report by Etz and colleagues sought to clarify these issues by reviewing 60 patients who underwent reoperative descending ($n=22$) or thoracoabdominal ($n=38$) aneurysm surgery through a redo lateral thoracotomy. Nine patients (15%) had Marfan's syndrome and 27 patients (45%) had previous dissections. Hospital mortality was 13.3%; paraplegia occurred in one patient (1.6%), respiratory insufficiency occurred in 13 (21.6%), and renal failure in two (3.3%). Lombardi et al. [14] reviewed 76 patients

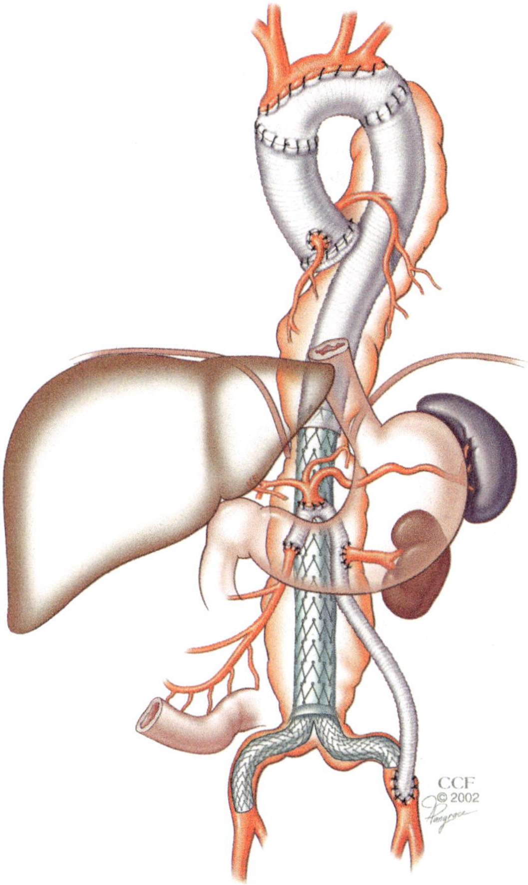

Fig. 19.6 Hybrid visceral debranching and completion stent graft treatment of a thoracoabdominal aortic aneurysm. Shown is a bypass graft placed from the left iliac artery to the left kidney, celiac artery, and the superior mesenteric artery. The remaining part of the aorta is lined with stent grafts. Reprinted with permission, Cleveland Clinic Center for Medical Art and Photography c 2009–2011. All Rights Reserved

with previous aortic surgery who underwent reoperative thoracoabdominal aortic repair. Overall 30-day mortality was 11.4%, and paraplegia occurred in 7.6%.

Overall, these and other scant reports suggest that reoperative aneurysm surgery is safe and efficacious, especially since there is no real alternative to surgery to prevent inevitable aneurysm rupture in patients with descending and thoracoabdominal aortic aneurysms. A careful individualized treatment plan for each patient is paramount to determining the best method of repair (open, branched–fenestrated stent graft, or hybrid visceral debranching). Careful attention to preoperative imaging and risk stratification will result in acceptable outcomes for this growing cohort of patients.

References

1. Coselli JS, Lemaire SA, Köksoy C, Schmittling ZC, Curling PE. Cerebrospinal fluid drainage reduces paraplegia after thoracoabdominal aortic aneurysm repair: results of a randomized clinical trial. J Vasc Surg. 2002 Apr;35(4):631–9.
2. Crawford ES, Crawford JL, Safi HJ, Coselli JS, Hess KR, Brooks B, Norton HJ, Glaeser DH. Thoracoabdominal aortic aneurysms: preoperative and intraoperative factors determining immediate and long-term results of operations in 605 patients. J Vasc Surg. 1986 Mar;3(3):389–404.
3. Crawford ES, Cohen ES. Aortic aneurysm: a multifocal disease. Presidential address. Arch Surg. 1982; 117:1393–400.
4. Carrel T, Pasic M, Jenni R, Tkebuchava T, Turina MI. Reoperations after operation on the thoracic aorta: etiology, surgical techniques, and prevention. Ann Thorac Surg. 1993;56:259–68; discussion 269.
5. Svensson LG, Crawford ES, Hess KR, Coselli JS, Safi HJ. Experience with 1509 patients undergoing thoracoabdominal aortic operations. J Vasc Surg. 1993; 17:357–68; discussion 368–70.
6. Kulik A, Allen BT, Kouchoukos NT. Incidence and management of intercostal patch aneurysms after repair of thoracoabdominal aortic aneurysms. J Thorac Cardiovasc Surg. 2009;138:352–8.
7. Etz CD, Zoli S, Kari FA, Mueller CS, Bodian CA, Di Luozzo G, et al. Redo lateral thoracotomy for reoperative descending and thoracoabdominal aortic repair: a consecutive series of 60 patients. Ann Thorac Surg. 2009;88:758–66; discussion 767.
8. Svensson LG, Hess KR, Coselli JS, Safi HJ. Influence of segmental arteries, extent, and atriofemoral bypass on postoperative paraplegia after thoracoabdominal aortic operations. J Vasc Surg. 1994;20:255–62.
9. Svensson LG, Hess KR, D'Agostino RS, Entrup MH, Hreib K, Kimmel WA, et al. Reduction of neurologic injury after high-risk thoracoabdominal aortic operation. Ann Thorac Surg. 1998;66:132–8.
10. Svensson LG, Coselli JS, Safi HJ, Hess KR, Crawford ES. Appraisal of adjuncts to prevent acute renal failure after surgery on the thoracic or thoracoabdominal aorta. J Vasc Surg. 1989;10:230–9.
11. Greenberg RK, West K, Pfaff K, Foster J, Skender D, Haulon S, Sereika J, Geiger L, Lyden SP, Clair D, Svensson L, Lytle B. Beyond the aortic bifurcation: branched endovascular grafts for thoracoabdominal and aortoiliac aneurysms. J Vasc Surg. 2006 May;43(5):879–86; discussion 886–7.

12. Roselli EE, Greenberg RK, Pfaff K, Francis C, Svensson LG, Lytle BW. Endovascular treatment of thoracoabdominal aortic aneurysms. J Thorac Cardiovasc Surg. 2007;133(6):1474–82.
13. Farber MA, Ford PF. Hybrid procedures for thoracoabdominal aortic aneurysms. Semin Vasc Surg. 2009;22:140–4.
14. Lombardi JV, Carpenter JP, Pochettino A, Sonnad SS, Bavaria JE. Thoracoabdominal aortic aneurysm repair after prior aortic surgery. J Vasc Surg. 2003; 38:1185–90.
15. Soltesz EG, Greenberg RK. Endovascular repair of thoracoabdominal aortic aneurysms with fenestrated-branched stent-grafts. Oper Tech Thorac Cardiovasc Surg 2010;15:86–99.

20 Reoperations Following Endovascular Aortic Repair

Eric E. Roselli

Introduction

Endovascular repair has become the preferred treatment option for descending thoracic aortic disease because of the reduced morbidity associated with this approach compared with the open operation [1]. Since they became commercially available in 2005, the use of endovascular devices has expanded rapidly. However, the current generation of thoracic stent grafts cannot be used in all patients due to the anatomic requirements for a durable repair. Specifically, secure fixation of a stent graft within the aorta requires 2 cm of normal-caliber, parallel aorta at both the proximal and distal seal zones. The aorta should be a healthy substrate without severe calcification or thrombus to tolerate the radial forces applied by the devices. In long-segment disease, the endovascular devices should be placed with maximum overlap to compensate for later aortic remodeling. The delivery system needs to accommodate the tortuosity of the aorta and the caliber of the iliofemoral system during the manipulation required to gain access and deploy the stent grafts.

In their current iterations, thoracic stent grafts simply do not fit all patients and all pathologies [2]. Nonetheless, so many patients with complex thoracic aortic disease present at high risk for death without intervention; it is not uncommon for patients to be treated with stent grafts, even though they do not meet the recommended instructions for use. This has been especially true in the last few years because stent grafts have become commercially available, and surgeons have become more familiar with their use.

As a consequence of the widespread use of endovascular devices in a broader population of patients and pathologies, we are seeing more patients with life-threatening complications from thoracic endovascular aortic repair (TEVAR) who require reoperations. These complications can occur during the acute perioperative period or later in the course of follow-up and may require additional endovascular or open treatment. Indications for reoperation include endoleaks, device migration, stent collapse, proximal aortic dissection, infection, persistent aortic growth, or access site injury. This chapter will review the methods to prevent a reoperation, indications for doing a reoperation, and operative techniques of performing reoperations after TEVAR using a case-based approach.

Endoleaks

The term endoleak refers to the presence of blood flow and pressure in the excluded portion of the aorta outside of the stent graft. Endoleaks are classified by source in relation to the stent graft [3]. Type I endoleaks are defined as those which occur at the proximal (Ia) or distal (Ib) seal zones of the

E.E. Roselli, MD (✉)
Department of Thoracic and Cardiovascular Surgery, Cleveland Clinic, Cleveland, OH, USA
e-mail: roselle@ccf.org

V.R. Machiraju et al. (eds.), *Redo Cardiac Surgery in Adults*,
DOI 10.1007/978-1-4614-1326-4_20, © Springer Science+Business Media, LLC 2012

aortic stent graft. Type II endoleaks originate from branch arteries arising from the excluded segment, which continue to pressurize the aneurysmal sac in a retrograde fashion, and Type III endoleaks occur when blood leaks between the overlap zones of sequential stent graft devices.

Type Ia Proximal Endoleaks

Case 1: An 84-year-old female underwent thoracic aortic stent grafting involving coverage of the left subclavian artery with a TAG endoprosthesis (Gore Medical, Flagstaff, AZ) via a transfemoral approach for a 7-cm distal arch and descending aortic aneurysm. The proximal landing zone was limited to 1.5 cm. Although she tolerated the procedure well, an adequate seal was not achieved. Over the several months that followed, she underwent multiple additional endovascular procedures including placement of additional uncovered stents (Palmaz stent; Cordis, Miami Lakes, FL) and attempts at coil embolization of the aneurysm without success. Approximately 1 year following the initial procedure, she developed severe chest pain and presented to the emergency room, where a repeat computed tomography (CT) scan demonstrated a Type Ia endoleak with associated expansion of the aneurysm and a contained leak (Fig. 20.1).

Case 2: A 69-year-old female involved in a high-speed motor vehicle collision sustained multiple blunt traumatic injuries including splenic laceration, tibia and fibula fractures, pulmonary contusion with multiple rib fractures, and traumatic aortic transaction. She was transferred to a trauma center and underwent splenectomy, open reduction and internal fixation of her fractures, and thoracic aortic stent grafting with a TAG device. She recovered well from her acute injuries but, in 1-month follow-up imaging of her aorta, was found to have a persistent Type Ia endoleak with a large pseudoaneurysm extending into the mediastinum (Fig. 20.2).

Case 3: A 62-year-old female presented with acute chest and back pain associated with oliguria and diminished peripheral pulses. CT at the presenting hospital demonstrated a distal aortic dissection with the entry tear beyond the left subclavian artery and a compressed true lumen (Fig. 20.3). She was transferred to our center and, because of the acute complications of end-organ malperfusion, was taken for emergency stent grafting. She tolerated this procedure well with improved distal pulses and increased urine output as a result of true lumen re-expansion. There was concern, however, during the procedure as to the adequacy of her proximal landing zone due to the proximity

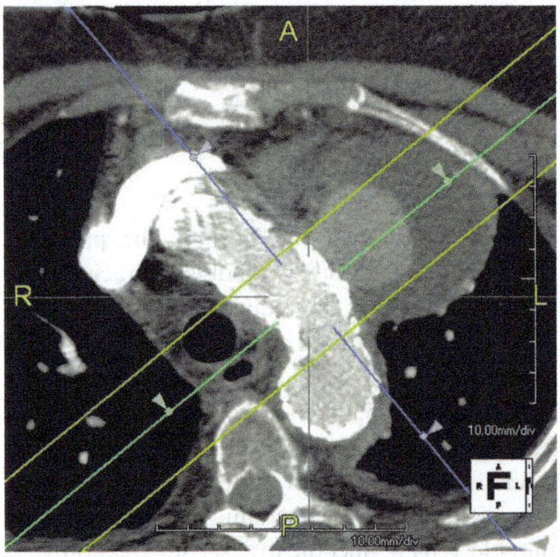

Fig. 20.1 Multiplanar (MPR) CT reconstruction of Type Ia endoleak into an arch aneurysm

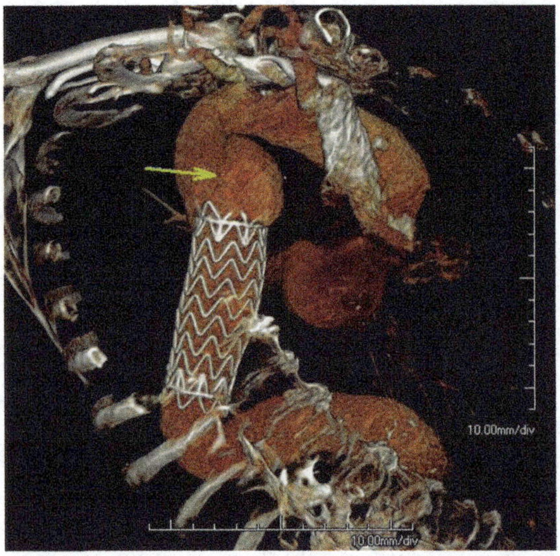

Fig. 20.2 Volume-rendered reconstruction (VRE) CT depicting proximal endoleak and persistent pseudoaneurysm (*arrow*)

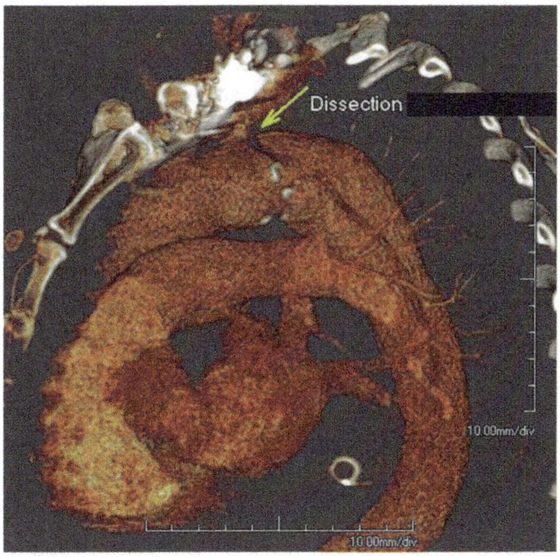

Fig. 20.3 VRE CT of acute Type B dissection adjacent to the left subclavian artery

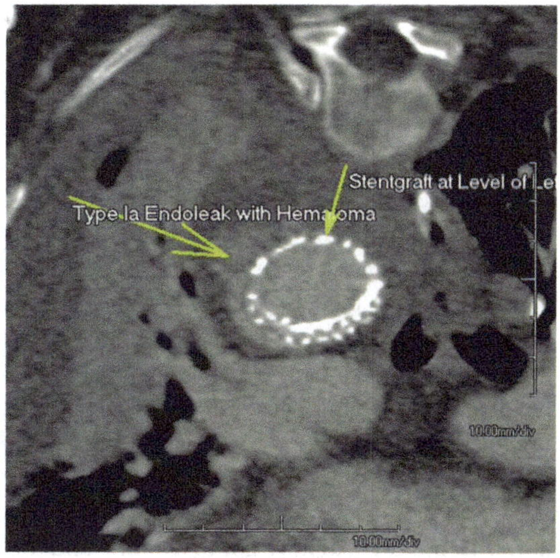

Fig. 20.4 MPR CT demonstrating endoleak and expanding hematoma after TEVAR of a Type B dissection

of the entry tear to the aortic arch. Follow-up CT scan on postoperative day 1 demonstrated a Type Ia endoleak with persistent flow around the device, raising concern for its stability (Fig. 20.4).

Case 4: A 70-year-old male with moderate chronic obstructive pulmonary disease (COPD), large penetrating ulcerations with two large, associated saccular aneurysms of the arch, and descending aorta and multivessel coronary artery disease presented with chest pain. He underwent coronary artery bypass grafting (with four grafts placed) and single-stage repair of his aortic arch and proximal descending aorta through a sternotomy using deep hypothermic circulatory arrest and frozen elephant trunk repair with direct placement of a TX2 stent graft (Cook, Bloomington, IN) sutured to the proximal aortic arch. On a predischarge CT scan, he was noted to have a Type Ia endoleak (Fig. 20.5).

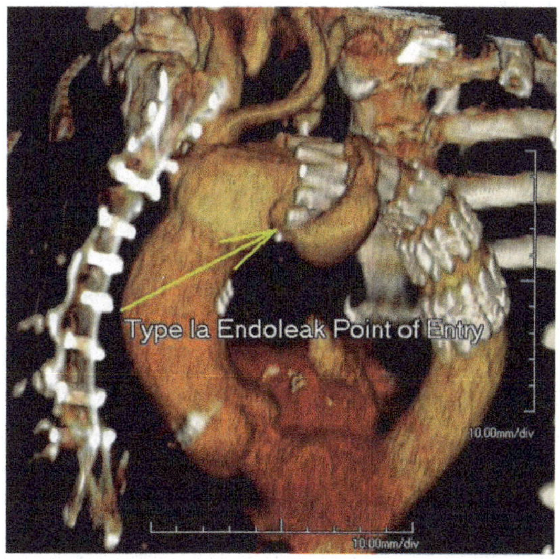

Fig. 20.5 VRE CT of endoleak after frozen elephant trunk repair

Prevention

Cases 1–4 demonstrate common indications for thoracic stent grafting. Cases 1 and 4 are elderly patients with severe degenerative thoracic aneurysmal disease. Case 2 is a patient with a traumatic transection, and Case 3 is a patient with a complicated distal aortic dissection. The indications to operate were clear in all these patients. The results of conventional open surgery in each of these patients were sufficient to warrant consideration of endovascular repair.

The most critical issue, after assuring that the intervention is warranted, relates to the adequacy of the proximal seal zone. This assessment can only be performed accurately with proper imaging, which includes CT with three-dimensional reconstruction techniques or the use of intravascular ultrasound. Degenerative aneurysms in elderly patients often involve or encroach on the aortic arch, and aortic transections and acute distal dissections most commonly occur near the left subclavian artery. When assessing the seal zone in elderly patients requiring reoperation, the distance from the left common carotid artery to the leading edge of the aneurysm must be greater than 15 mm, at a minimum, on both the greater and lesser curves of the arch. In patients with a large degenerative aneurysm where only the proximal most stent is sealing within the aorta, 15 mm of seal may not be enough and this zone may need to be expanded to as much as 30 mm. This is especially true if the sealing zone segment of aorta has a significant atherosclerotic burden resulting in a patient–device interface that is not ideal. Similarly, if the device has to extend around a tight curve, the landing zone must be within a parallel segment of aorta so as to optimize circumferential sealing of the device and, therefore, a longer distance between the left carotid and the aneurysm may be necessary.

The error in Case 1 was due to either miscalculation or intentional compromise on the length of the sealing zone for the device in this patient, and she was, therefore, left with a persistent Type Ia endoleak. As described earlier, the patient was rescued from this error but may have fared better if the inadequate seal zone was properly assessed at the time of elective repair. Theoretically, this patient has a partially treated aorta, in which the Type Ia endoleak continued to pressurize the aneurysm and the distal landing zone was adequately sealed, may be more dangerous than the untreated aneurysm since there was no outflow. This is not necessarily the case with Type Ia endoleaks in the infrarenal aorta, however, based on some elegant studies performed in dogs [4].

In patients with traumatic aortic transection or acute dissection, the arch may be very angulated at the point of injury. In this situation, 15 mm of aorta beyond the left carotid artery may not be good enough, despite the aorta otherwise being normal in caliber and morphology. There must be a 15 mm segment of aorta within which the device will lie flat and parallel with circumferential seal. In Case 2, the implanting surgeons were rightfully concerned about having the device lie within the angulated segment of the proximal descending aorta. However, in their decision to avoid this so-called no-man's zone, they compromised the proximal landing zone and did not provide enough coverage of the injured segment. It is unclear whether this proximal endoleak was present immediately after the intervention since the predischarge CT scans were not available. However, patients with traumatic aortic transection or acute dissection often have associated hematoma in the more proximal aorta. As this treated aorta heals, it must be imaged at regular intervals to assess morphologic changes within the seal zone. Predischarge and 1-month postprocedure CT scans are very important in these patients.

In Case 3, the implanting surgeon was fully aware of the potential for an inadequate proximal seal with the device but the initial objectives of the procedure were to optimize true lumen flow and reperfuse the compromised end organs. This understanding of the compromise that was being made allowed for prompt diagnosis and intervention of the endoleak. Similarly, in Case 4, the inadequacy of the seal zone prompted the decision to perform the repair using a hybrid, frozen elephant trunk technique. The error here was a technical one either of sizing or of misplacement of the proximal fixation sutures into the frozen elephant trunk graft.

Indications

Intervention is recommended in all patients with a Type 1a endoleak [3]. Type Ia endoleaks occur in 10% of patients whose stent graft is landed in zones 0 or 1 (the distal ascending aorta or more proximal aortic arch) [5]. This is emphasized in Cases 1 and 2, both of whom returned with emergencies. In patients with acute distal dissections, like the patient in Case 3, it is sometimes difficult to differentiate a proximal, Type II endoleak originating from bronchial arteries from a true Type I endoleak. If the suspicion for a Type I leak is low and the risk of surgical intervention is inordinately high, then some of these patients may be closely monitored with frequent, early CT scans. Intravascular ultrasound can also help to differentiate some of these endoleaks but is an invasive procedure. Patient 4, with the Type Ia endoleak in the setting of a sutured device, is less at risk for device migration than the others but may be at high risk of rupture due to increased pressurization of the aneurysm sac.

Operative Approach

Open Surgical Repair: Reverse Frozen Elephant Trunk: The patient in Case 3 was taken for emergency sternotomy, ascending and transverse arch replacement, and reverse elephant trunk repair. This was performed under deep hypothermic circulatory arrest with arterial cannulation via the right axillary artery and antegrade brain perfusion. The arch was reconstructed using the Griepp technique; first, sewing a graft to the brachiocephalic vessels to allow for antegrade brain perfusion. The distal anastomosis was performed to the proximal end of the stent graft and included the native aorta as well as felt Teflon strips within the media and on the outside of the aorta.

Endovascular Device Extension: The patient in Case 2 was taken for emergency stent grafting of her more proximal aorta with planned coverage of the left subclavian artery. Careful assessment of the cervical portion of the CT scan demonstrated a nondominant left vertebral artery, and so left subclavian revascularization was not performed before the procedure [6]. The device was delivered via common femoral cut-down and, because of the very short margin for error in this tight sealing zone, the device was deployed using rapid ventricular pacing to reduce the pulsatile displacement forces on the device [7].

Endovascular Embolization: The patient in Case 4 was returned to the hybrid operating suite for endovascular repair. Access was obtained via the right brachiocephalic artery and using a 6 Fr by 55-cm sheath delivered in the proximal aortic arch, access was obtained into the aneurysm sac across the point of leak. After first gaining access with a hydrophilic wire and catheter, exchange was made for a stiffer wire into the aneurysm sac. The long sheath was then delivered into the aneurysm and multiple coils were delivered into the aneurysm sac. Finally, an 8-mm vascular plug (Amplatzer, AGA Medical, Plymouth, MN) was placed across the orifice and deployed. Completion arch angiography and follow-up CTs confirmed adequate sealing of the endoleak and shrinking of the aneurysm (Fig. 20.6). In situations where the stability of the device is in question, this embolization technique for Type Ia endoleaks should be avoided, as there may be risk of dislodging the device in the attempts to access the aneurysm sac. The durability of such a repair is also unknown, and it should be reserved for patients considered too high risk for open repair.

Hybrid Debranching and Stent Grafting: The patient in Case 1 was taken for emergency surgery to undergo a more proximal repair of her aorta. In this particular case, the patient's more proximal aorta was relatively spared of disease, and because of her age, she was felt to be at particularly high

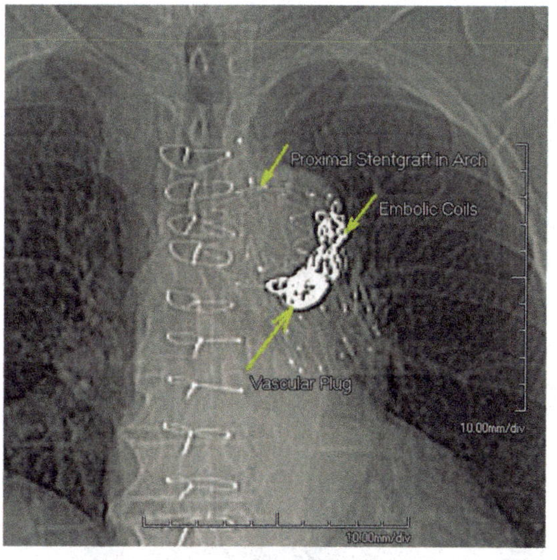

Fig. 20.6 Postprocedure chest X-ray of the patient in Case 4 demonstrating the stent graft device, vascular plug, and embolization coils into the endoleak sac

risk for circulatory arrest, especially in the setting of a contained rupture. Through a sternotomy, she underwent ascending to innominate and left carotid bypass followed by antegrade delivery of an additional thoracic stent graft to achieve seal within a favorable landing zone (Fig. 20.7). This was performed successfully in combination with off-pump coronary bypass grafting of the right coronary artery. These procedures can be performed in a single-stage approach, as was performed here because the aneurysm was leaking, or in a two-stage approach. Device delivery may either be performed in a standard retrograde fashion from the iliofemoral arteries or antegrade from the subclavian artery or ascending aorta [2].

Type Ib Distal Endoleaks and Chronic Distal Dissections

Case 5: An 84-year-old woman with a large thoracoabdominal aortic aneurysm was treated with a Talent thoracic stent graft (Medtronic, Minneapolis, MN) 5 years earlier, extending from the left subclavian artery to the visceral segment including coverage of the celiac artery, which subsequently thrombosed. In routine follow-up, she was noticed to develop aneurysmal degeneration of her thoracoabdominal aorta with associated Type Ib endoleak and was referred to our outpatient clinic. On evaluation, she complained of severe upper abdominal and mid- to lower back pain, and the CT scan revealed an 8-cm thoracoabdominal aneurysm with a large distal endoleak and considerable aneurysmal growth since the last CT (Fig. 20.8).

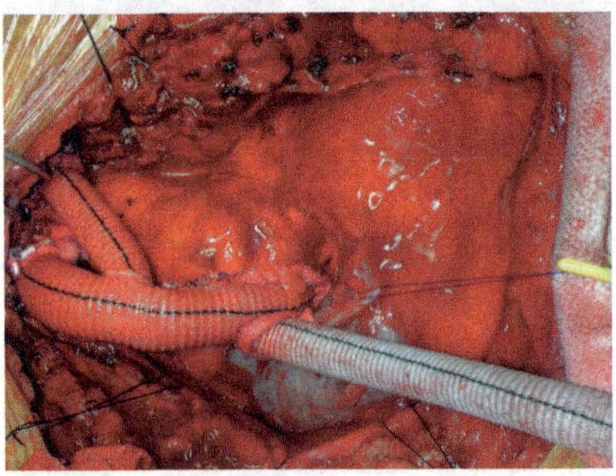

Fig. 20.7 Intraoperative photograph from the patient in Case 1 demonstrating arch debranching and conduit for antegrade device delivery

Case 6: A 72-year-old woman underwent endovascular thoracoabdominal aortic aneurysm repair with a TAG device 2 years earlier for a 5.5 cm aneurysm via retroperitoneal access from the infrarenal aorta due to severe iliofemoral occlusive disease. She was initially lost to follow-up but later presented with lower back pain and was found to have growth of her aneurysm to over 7 cm with a distal Type Ib endoleak (Fig. 20.9). Her celiac artery was also occluded. Because of her poor access and the need for a significant operation to achieve access, she underwent a full cardiac workup, which revealed ischemic myocardium and multivessel disease involving all territories.

Case 7: A 75-year-old man with a history of uncomplicated Type B aortic dissection was followed with serial cross-sectional imaging studies and found to have rapid expansion of his thoracoabdominal aorta with maximum diameter of 58 mm in the most proximal descending aorta. He was obese and had marginal pulmonary function. He quit smoking and underwent thoracic endovascular repair just beyond the left subclavian artery to the level of the celiac. His distal

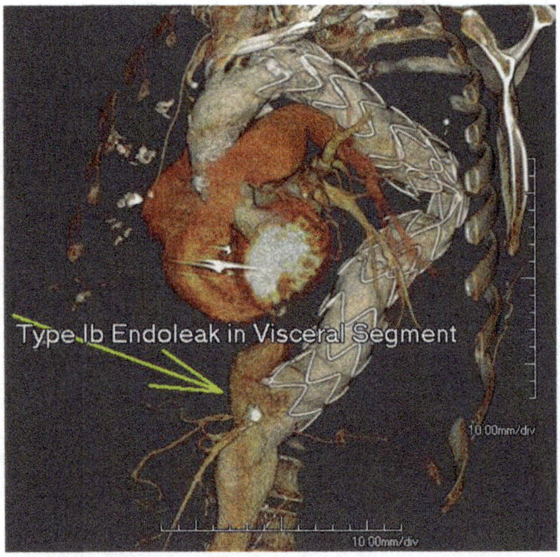

Fig. 20.8 VRE CT demonstrating distal endoleak at the level of the visceral segment and a compromised distal landing zone

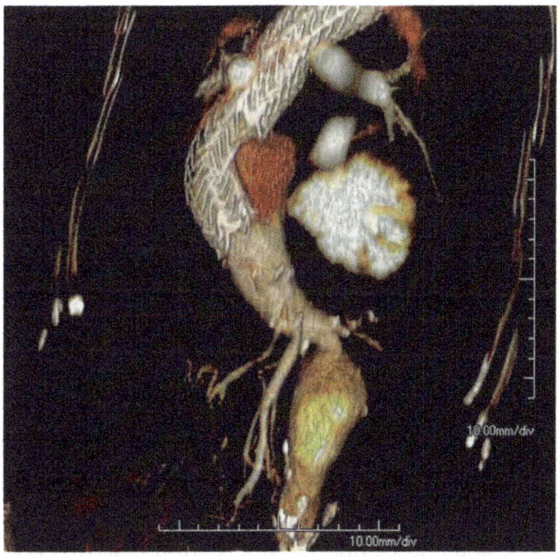

Fig. 20.9 VRE CT demonstrating distal endoleak after thoracic stent graft with acceptable distal landing zone

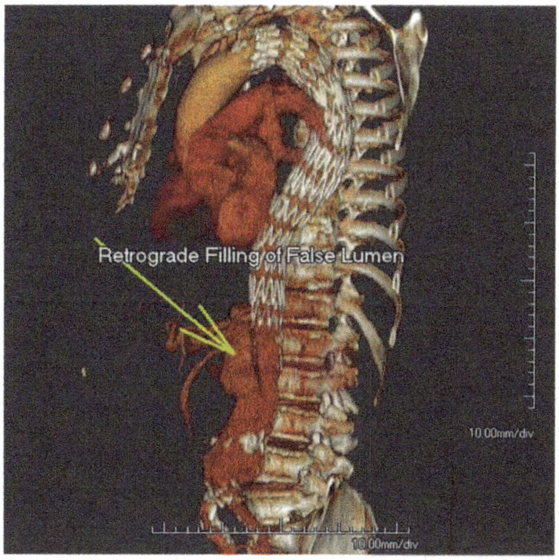

Fig. 20.10 VRE CT after descending TEVAR for chronic dissection with retrograde filling of false lumen in abdominal aorta

descending aorta was over 4 cm, and his infrarenal aorta was aneurysmal to 5.5 cm. After the initial phase of recovery from his thoracic stent graft, he dedicated himself to cardiac rehab and lost 30 lb. On follow-up imaging, his abdominal aneurysm was stable in size, and the false lumen in the upper half of his thoracic aorta was partially thrombosed but he had persistent false-lumen flow and pressurization (Fig. 20.10).

Prevention

Since all the currently available thoracic stent grafts are held in place by the radial force of their Z-shaped stents, their durability is dependent upon the aorta to which they are secured. More specifically, long-term durability of endovascular aortic repair is most closely correlated with the stability of the proximal and distal aortic seal zones. Although the patient described in Case 5 came to our attention several years after her initial repair, it is clear that the distal landing zone was compromised from the beginning because the decision was made to cover her otherwise patent celiac artery. Similarly, the patient in Case 6 had an occluded celiac artery due to severe atherosclerotic disease in the visceral and distal descending aortic segments. The tapered neck of this aneurysm likely indicated an aneurysm in evolution at the time of initial repair. Understanding the limitations of the distal seal zone is critical to the preoperative planning and discussions about durability with the patient before endovascular repair. Although coverage of the celiac artery can be performed safely in some patients, there is a significant risk of foregut ischemia associated with this strategy and it should only be utilized in emergency situations [8].

The use of thoracic stent grafts to treat distal chronic aortic dissections, like that in patient 7, represents a unique type of case and is included here with Type Ib endoleaks because of similarities in the approaches to treatment. It is quite common for these patients to have retrograde filling of the false lumen from distal fenestrations, but this is not necessarily a Type Ib endoleak. The dissection flap in the chronic state is thickened and stiff, and once the adventitial layer of the dilated false lumen dilates, it is unlikely that the morphology of these degenerated aortas will change much. There is a growing body of evidence, however, that the use of stent grafts in the chronically dissected aorta can promote healing and reduce the risk of rupture in approximately 75% of patients [9]. This occurs as a result of thromboexclusion with radial expansion of the true lumen and the promotion of thrombosis within the false lumen in treated segments of aorta. Unfortunately, the success with the endovascular technique in these patients is not consistent. This is especially true of patients in whom the dissection extends more distally into the infrarenal aorta and pelvic vessels and in those who develop aneurysmal degeneration in these more distal segments of the aorta.

Indications

Like patients with Type Ia endoleak, all patients with Type Ib endoleak require intervention. If the proximal fixation is secure; however, treatment for Type Ib endoleaks is not necessarily an emergency as it often is with Type Ia endoleaks where there is concern for device migration, collapse, and aortic occlusion. With distal Type Ib endoleaks, the timing of treatment can be determined by the growth rate of the aneurysm.

The patient described in Case 5, unfortunately, developed rapid growth of her aneurysm and impending rupture with severe symptoms requiring urgent intervention. The patient described in Case 6 was not directly symptomatic from her aorta but had significant interval growth and a large associated endoleak. The findings of ischemia and associated multivessel coronary occlusive disease added another indication for intervention. Patients like the patient described in Case 7 are becoming increasingly common as more people are surviving the acute phases of aortic dissection [9]. The challenge in patients with chronic aortic dissection and extensive aneurysmal degeneration is that simply stent grafting the descending aorta is less likely to lead to thrombosis of the more distal false lumen. The patient in Case 7 had a large abdominal aneurysm and the visceral segment was dilated as well, so his repair was planned in a staged fashion.

Operative Technique

Open repair: The patients in Cases 5 and 7 underwent conversion to open repair, but Case 5 was performed as an emergency and Case 7 was performed as an electively planned procedure. If the proximal seal and proximal fixation are stable, then repair can be performed by focusing on the distal repair and converting it to a sutured anastomosis. All the available stent grafts may be safely clamped with standard aortic cross-clamps but the native aorta needs to be included in both the clamp and the anastomosis. Depending on how dilated the native aorta is, the surgeon may wish to first secure the stent graft to the aorta by transecting it and running a suture around the end of the stent graft and the native aorta. A standard polyester graft can then be anastomosed to this composite aorta with the stent graft acting as a neointima (Fig. 20.11).

The need for urgent intervention with involvement of the visceral segment relegated the patient described in Case 5 to a direct open conversion. The combination of extensive aortic aneurysm and chronic dissection dictated that the patient in Case 7 has an open completion of the first stage of endovascular repair.

These operations are performed through a left thoracoabdominal incision with the use of partial left heart bypass with left atrial-to-femoral bypass with cerebrospinal fluid drainage and active cooling. Because the stent graft is left in situ, the incision can be relatively low depending on the site of distal leak. The operation is much like an elephant trunk completion procedure, with or without visceral reimplantation (Fig. 20.12).

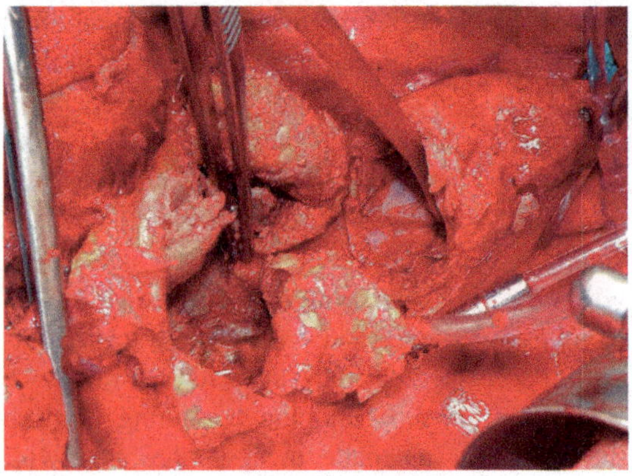

Fig. 20.11 Intraoperative photograph of stent graft within lumen of thoracic aorta clamped and transected to facilitate conversion to open repair

Endovascular Device Extension: Because of the morbidity associated with open repairs on the descending or thoracoabdominal aorta, an endovascular repair strategy is preferred. For most of these patients with Type Ib endoleak, however, the landing zone is suboptimal. The diseased segments of aorta encroach upon the visceral segment of the aorta. Like Type Ia endoleaks and their usual involvement with the aortic arch, the branch vessels present additional difficulty for an endovascular repair. If time permits construction of a custom-designed device, patients with suboptimal landing zone may be treated with a branched graft device (Fig. 20.13) [10]. The patient in Case 5 was not offered this luxury and underwent open repair. The patient in Case 6 had a less urgent indication for repair of the endoleak, and the celiac artery was already chronically occluded allowing for additional stent grafting with a commercially available device. An additional consideration for in the patient in Case 6 was pre-existing severe iliofemoral disease, which necessitated initial placement through an open exposure of the infrarenal aorta, and multivessel coronary disease. The difficulty imposed by her access issues and the need for coronary revascularization led us to pursue an antegrade delivery approach for the stent graft through a conduit on the ascending aorta, concurrent with three-vessel coronary artery bypass grafting. This approach has been used in many situations at our institution, as well as by others, with very good results [2, 5].

Endovascular embolization: The use of prothrombotic materials to treat Type I endoleaks in either the proximal or distal seal zone is a compromised approach with questionable durability and is not generally recommended except in the most desperate of situations. In the setting of a chronic dissection with retrograde filling of the false lumen, however, this may prove to be a reasonable approach. There has been little written with regard to this technique, but the intentional placement of a collapsed stent graft or iliac occluder device into the distal inflow portion of the false lumen can promote thrombosis in the aneurysmal false lumen and is worthy of further investigation (Fig. 20.14).

Hybrid Debranching and Stent Grafting Another alternative to direct open repair or the use of custom-branched endografts for patients in whom the

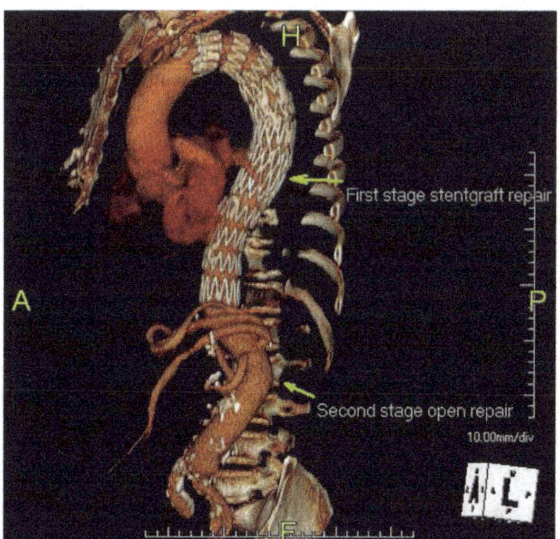

Fig. 20.12 VRE CT after hybrid repair of a Type II thoracoabdominal aneurysm and chronic dissection with stent graft in descending and open branch grafting of the abdominal aorta

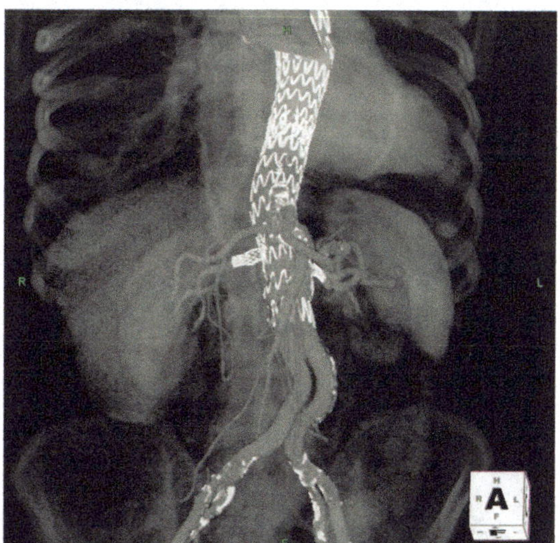

Fig. 20.13 Maximum intensity projection (MIP) CT of thoracoabdominal branched graft repair

distal landing zone abuts the visceral arteries is the hybrid approach of debranching followed by stent grafting. This approach is not new, and many have described their experiences in small series of patients, generally using a retrograde revascularization approach in which a multibranched graft is constructed from the iliac artery to the visceral and renal arteries in the first stage of the operation. The stent graft can then be placed within the visceral segment of aorta without end-organ compromise. In most of the published reports on this technique, the mortality and morbidity are still moderate to high [11–13]. In some patients with combined severe cardiac disease and thoracoabdominal aneurysms, we have utilized an antegrade approach to debranching by constructing the visceral bypasses off the ascending aorta with good early success (Fig. 20.15).

Type II Endoleaks

Type II endoleaks are those that originate from branch arteries arising from the excluded segment that continue to pressurize the aneurysm sac in a retrograde fashion.

Case 8: A 59-year-old man with aneurysmal degeneration of a chronic residual dissection after emergent Type A dissection repair with a supracoronary graft underwent a staged thoracic aortic repair. This was performed as a reverse frozen elephant trunk technique because the true lumen was so compressed distally. The stent graft was placed in the descending aorta as the first stage. Subsequent to this, a redo sternotomy and arch replacement, including the stent graft into the distal anastomosis, was performed. On follow-up imaging, he was noted to have a Type II endoleak that was filling the false lumen aneurysm in a retrograde fashion from the persistently dissected left subclavian artery.

Prevention

With precise preoperative imaging and the use of 3D reconstruction techniques, issues with persistent retrograde flow from the left subclavian artery can be predicted. Specifically, when the origin of the left subclavian artery is within an aneurysmal or diseased segment of aorta, it is more likely to lead to Type II endoleak. If it is simply covered within the otherwise normal landing zone, the left subclavian artery is less likely to be involved in a

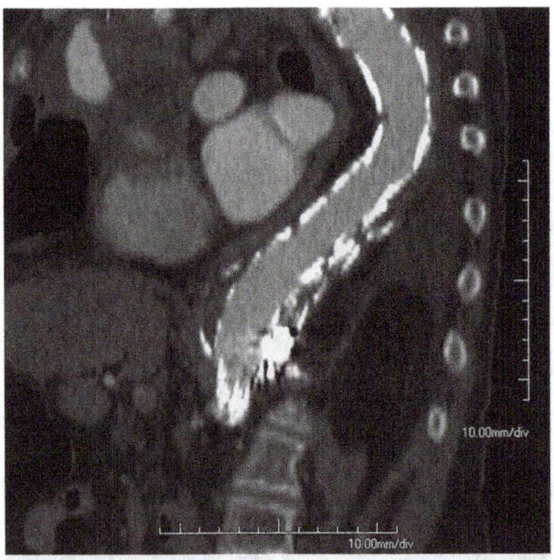

Fig. 20.14 Postoperative VRE CT with standard TEVAR in true lumen and collapsed stent graft with embolization coils in false lumen to prevent retrograde filling of the false lumen

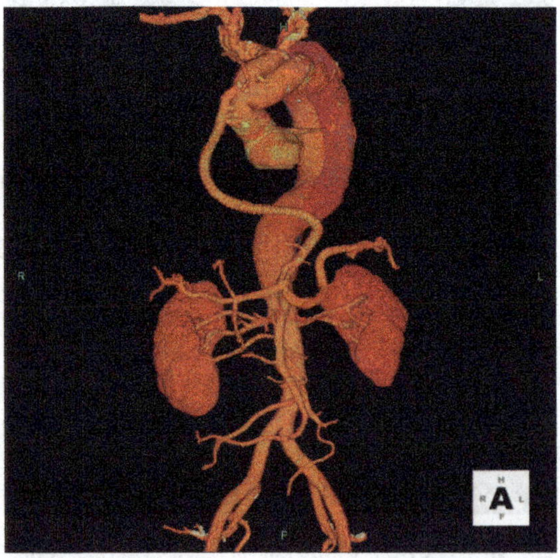

Fig. 20.15 VRE CT after ascending to celiac artery bypass to facilitate endovascular elephant trunk completion with the distal landing zone in the upper abdominal aorta

Type II endoleak. In elective cases, the left subclavian should be revascularized first and can then be occluded proximally, either at the time of the arterial transposition or endovascularly during the stent graft procedure, with vascular plugs or coils [6].

Indications

Type II endoleaks are mostly benign because they are most often characterized by low flow and low pressure. With watchful waiting, the majority of Type II endoleaks resolve spontaneously as the branch vessels thrombose over a period of months. The exception is when the source of the Type II endoleak is a larger vessel, such as the left subclavian artery or a covered visceral artery. Type II endoleaks are rarely associated with aneurysm growth, which warrants intervention.

Operative Techniques

Open repair: If an important endoleak from the left subclavian artery is anticipated, we prefer to revascularize it preemptively. This is especially true in the case of a patent left internal thoracic artery-to-coronary bypass, when the left vertebral artery is dominant and when there will be extensive aneurysmal coverage and the loss of cervical spinal cord collaterals may increase the risk of spinal cord ischemia. An additional advantage to left subclavian revascularization is that it provides access into the left common carotid origin via percutaneous brachial puncture at the time of stent grafting to assist with accurate device placement or troubleshooting within the arch, if needed. This revascularization can be performed by means of carotid subclavian bypass or left subclavian transposition. In the case of a bypass, the proximal left subclavian artery can either be ligated proximal to the vertebral artery during the cervical operation or occluded endovascularly with coils or a vascular plug at the time of the endovascular portion of the operation. Our preference is for carotid to subclavian bypass with later coil embolization as this is a simpler neck dissection with less risk of vertebral artery injury.

The use of video-assisted thoracoscopic techniques have also been described to ligate segmental arteries causing a Type II endoleak but this is very rarely indicated as these vessels almost always thrombose and the endoleaks resolve within months.

Endovascular embolization: This can be performed quite readily via 6 Fr access to the left subclavian artery via a percutaneous brachial artery approach with the use of prothrombotic coils (Nestor, Cook Inc., Bloomington, IN) or vascular plugs (Amplatzer, Plymouth, MN). In the event that a patient has an aneurysmal left subclavian artery, preemptive placement of the larger caliber iliac occluder device has been described [14].

Type III Endoleaks

Type III endoleaks are those that occur when blood leaks between the overlap zones of sequential stent graft devices.

Case 9: An 81-year-old man had undergone descending aortic stent grafting with the placement of two devices extending from just beyond the left subclavian artery to the level of the diaphragm 1-year earlier. He presented to an outside emergency room with back pain and hemoptysis. A CT scan was performed and demonstrated separation of two endografts in the overlap zone with a rapidly expanding, descending aneurysm and a possible contained rupture into the mediastinum (Fig. 20.16).

Prevention

During the preoperative planning phase, assessing the diameters and length are not enough but the morphology of the entire segment of aorta within which the device will lie must be evaluated. The displacement forces on the thoracic stent graft in the region of the aortic isthmus are directed cephalad and laterally (Fig. 20.17) [15]. These force vectors should be understood by the implanting surgeon and taken into consideration when assessing the lie of the device within the aneurysm and at the proximal seal zone. After assessing the adequacy of the landing zones and making diameter determinations, one has to decide upon device length and the number of devices to use. In a patient with a large proximal aneurysm, it is important to understand that the forces on the device are going to be directed at the greater curve and outer wall of the aorta. These forces will push the device toward the outer wall of the descending thoracic aorta. If the overlap between two devices is not maximized in a patient with a particularly large aneurysm, the two devices can slide completely apart from each other creating a Type III endoleak, which can be as deadly as a Type I endoleak.

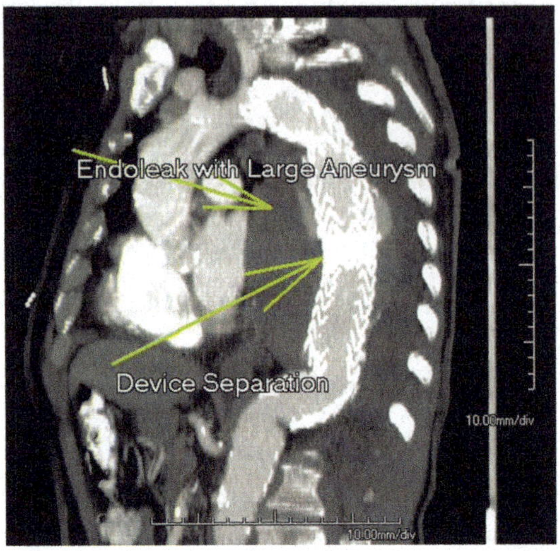

Fig. 20.16 MIP CT demonstrating minimal overlap between devices with an endoleak pressurizing a contained aortic rupture extending into the mediastinum

Each of the manufacturers describes a minimum length of overlap in their instructions for use. The TAG device recommends 5 cm of overlap for two devices of the same caliber and 3 cm of overlap when placing a larger device within a smaller one with no more than two steps up in sizing between components. The Talent device has markers on the grafts to guide minimum overlap, which is generally about 5 cm. The TX2 device is recommended to have a minimum overlap zone of two stent lengths (5 cm) between successive components. These recommendations are only guidelines, and the important point to remember is that it is best to optimize the amount of overlap between successive devices so as to avoid Type III endoleaks. This is especially important in patients with a very large and long

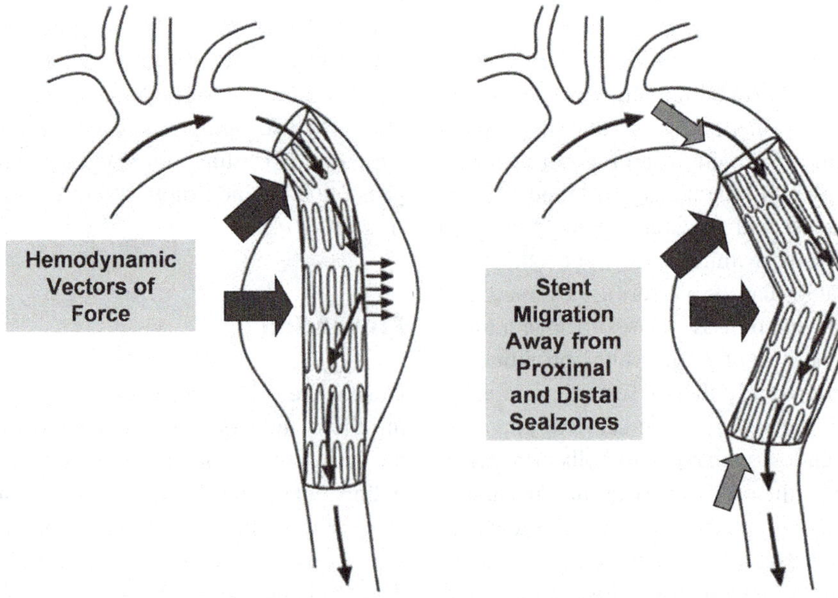

Fig. 20.17 Migration forces within the descending thoracic aorta after stent graft repair. Dark *gray arrows* depict force vectors, and light gray arrows depict direction of migration

aneurysm where the device between sealing zones will be prone to shift within the aneurysm sac.

Indications

The high flow and high pressure associated with this type of endoleak can quickly lead to aneurysmal growth as well as instability in the proximal and distal fixation of the devices. The presence of a Type III endoleak is an absolute indication for intervention.

Operative Techniques

Type III endoleaks should always be amenable to endovascular repair techniques with the placement of additional stent grafts to bridge the gap between devices. This was the approach taken in the patient described in Case 9. When doing so, it is critical to reassess the access vessels beforehand as patients may have had progression of occlusive disease or sustained focal injury to the access vessels in the interim between the operations. Gaining wire access across the separated devices may require a dual approach from both above and below with possible use of a snare to achieve through-and-through access. The overlap device is generally oversized by approximately 10% and the longest piece possible, to achieve maximum overlap, is selected. In patients who present with rupture or contained leak after developing a Type III endoleak, it may be necessary to evacuate the hemothorax or hemomediastinum after first treating the aortic hemorrhage endovascularly.

Migration

Case 10: A 62-year-old man with an aneurysm involving the distal aortic arch and proximal descending thoracic aorta demonstrated rapid aneurismal growth from 4.5 to 5.4 cm on CT scans 6 months apart. He underwent left common carotid–left subclavian artery bypass followed by TEVAR. A Type I endoleak was noted on completion angiography, and the decision was made to balloon-expand the proximal portion of the stent graft. Despite pharmacologically lowering the systolic blood pressure to 60 mmHg, the device migrated distally during brief inflation of a conforming balloon. A second device was delivered just distal to the left common carotid artery and, again, required balloon-expansion. During the second round of balloon-expansion, rapid right ventricular pacing was used, and an excellent angiographic result was obtained. Coils were inserted in the left subclavian artery origin to treat a Type II endoleak. The patient tolerated the procedure well and follow-up CT imaging demonstrated no evidence of an endoleak.

Case 11: A 77-year-old man with COPD and a large distal arch and proximal descending aortic aneurysm underwent attempted endovascular repair. Although the initial device deployment was uncomplicated, he did have a persistent endoleak. A CT scan performed in-hospital demonstrated that the device had migrated distally into the arch aneurysm sac but was well seated distally in the normal-caliber mid-descending aorta (Fig. 20.18).

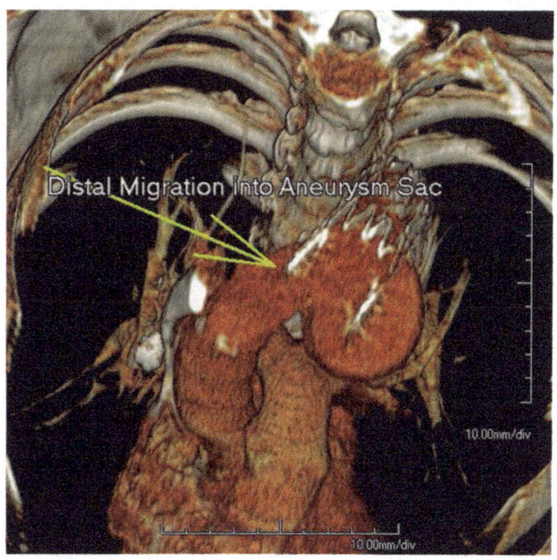

Fig. 20.18 VRE CT cephalad view over arch depicting proximal device migration into the aneurysm sac

Prevention

As described earlier, the displacement forces in the thoracic aorta are directed upward and laterally toward the greater curve. A patient with a particularly large aneurysm at the level of the aortic isthmus has a large space within which the device can be displaced and, in patients with a large aneurysm at this level, a longer proximal landing zone, in the range of 25–30 mm, may be desirable. Just as was seen in Case 9, an understanding of the displacement forces on the implanted devices helps during the preoperative planning phase. If a single long device is chosen to span a particularly large (in diameter) aneurysm in this location, these displacement forces will be directed at displacing the device from the proximal and distal landing zones. However, if two devices are chosen to span the distance across the diseased segment, the displacement forces will be directed to the overlapping segment of the two devices. This trombone mechanism between the two overlapping devices acts to unload the more critical proximal and distal landing zones and can reduce the risk of migration [16].

To optimize the seal zone in the arch, precise placement of the endovascular device against the origin of the left carotid artery is often necessary. Because of the inherent tortuosity of the arch, achieving a good seal often requires the use of a conforming balloon after deployment. This maneuver can be complicated by the very high hemodynamic forces in the proximal aorta, and balloon-expanding the device within a short proximal landing zone can sometimes lead to migration of the whole endovascular device into the aneurysm sac as the heart ejects against the inflated balloon and device. To facilitate this balloon-expansion process and reduce the displacement forces, it is helpful to reduce the blood pressure and cardiac output by pharmacologic manipulation with beta-blockers or the use of adenosine. The reproducibility of this effect is not ideal, and another fine option is the use of rapid ventricular pacing [7].

Indications

If migration happens acutely during the procedure, it must be addressed immediately, as was seen in Case 10. The indications to intervene upon a delayed device migration are less clear than with acute migrations or Type I and III endoleaks. In fact, the determination of whether or not thoracic migration has actually occurred can be confused with less pathologic aortic growth in the longitudinal plane and requires the use of 3D CT techniques. During this analysis, focus is directed on the device in relation to stable landmarks as reference points because the aorta itself may grow and elongate over time giving the appearance of migration [16]. The determination of migration requires close inspection and any uncertainty about the stability of the seal zones requires intervention before an endoleak develops that may threaten the stability of the device.

Treatment

Open repair: Since migration often occurs as a result of aortic growth in the landing zone, there may not be adequate aortic length available for additional stent grafting. When the arch is involved, migration is best treated with conversion to open repair. This can be addressed with open arch and thoracic aortic repair using conventional techniques through a left thoracotomy with the use of deep hypothermic circulatory arrest, but this is a morbid operation and many patients have significant comorbidities, which led them to undergo endovascular repair initially.

Hybrid techniques: The two most feasible alternative options are hybrid techniques that are performed through a median sternotomy approach [2, 5]. The debranching technique can be performed with or without the use of cardiopulmonary bypass depending on the state of the ascending aorta and the need for other cardiovascular interventions. The reverse frozen elephant trunk technique is performed with the use of deep hypothermic circulatory arrest, and the previously placed stent graft is included in the open proximal repair with direct placement of sutures through both the device and the surrounding aortic wall. Further descriptions of both of these hybrid techniques is included in the section on Type Ia endoleaks earlier.

Endovascular repair: Endovascular repair can be achieved with the placement of an additional device that acts as a proximal extension when there is adequate aortic length for sealing. An accurate assessment of the aortic diameter with precise sizing is critical as the landing zone may have grown since the initial procedure. When endovascular repair requires placement within the proximal aortic segments, rapid ventricular pacing is a useful adjunct.

In patients with migration and a limited proximal landing zone who are at high risk for conversion to an open repair, some have suggested the use of additional endovascular techniques to allow for extension into the more proximal aortic arch. The so-called chimney technique involves the placement of additional stent grafts within the supra-aortic branches alongside the thoracic stent grafts to extend the thoracic repair more proximally while maintaining the patency of the branch arteries (Fig. 20.19). This represents a feasible approach but there is no long-term data to support the durability of this technique, and it should only be used as a salvage procedure in the highest-risk patients [17].

Stent Collapse

Case 12: A 30-year-old male sustained multiorgan trauma after a fall caused by partial opening of his parachute during a skydive. He was resuscitated and stabilized but part of his treatment included endovascular stent grafting of a traumatic aortic transection. This initially went well, but he later developed distal malperfusion and was found to have complete stent graft collapse on CT.

Case 13: The woman in Case 2 underwent additional stent grafting for a Type Ia endoleak due to inadequate coverage during the initial repair, as described earlier. A follow-up surveillance CT scan 1 year later demonstrated partial collapse of the mid-descending aortic stent graft (Fig. 20.20).

Prevention

This is a complication that has been most commonly described with the Gore TAG stent graft device. Of the commercially available devices, it has the lowest radial force. Geometrically speak-

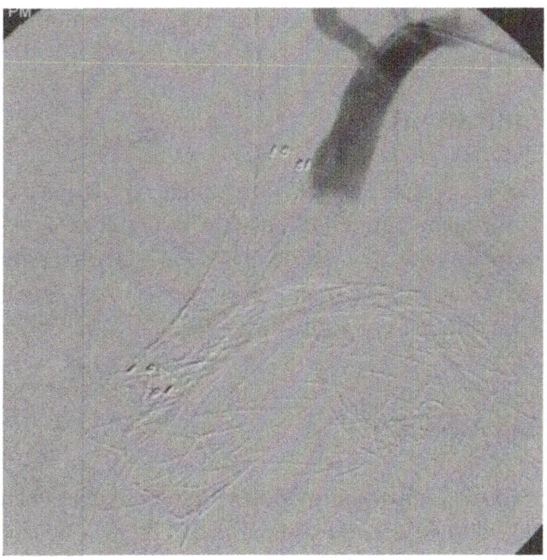

Fig. 20.19 Fluoroscopic still of a covered stent in left carotid artery adjacent to a thoracic stent graft allowing for extension of the seal into zone 1 – "chimney technique"

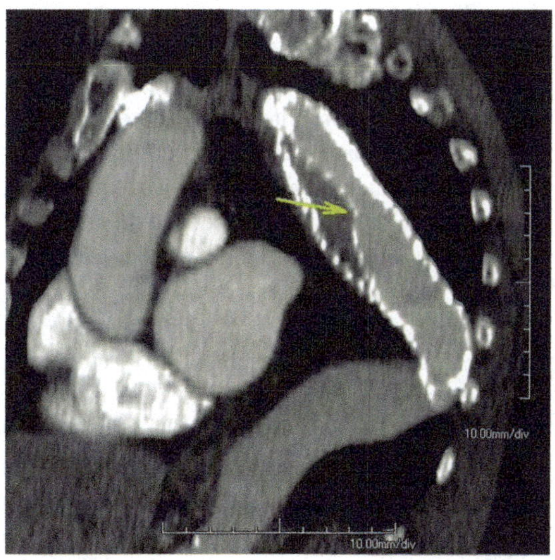

Fig. 20.20 MPR CT demonstrating collapsed stent graft in the descending aorta within a previously placed device. Note the thrombus between devices as this collapse was chronic

ing, the preferred shape of the stent in its expanded state is a circle but if it is not fully expanded, it tends to sit in a crescent configuration. When the device collapses into the crescent shape, it can obstruct blood flow through the aorta with complete acute aortic obstruction or pseudocoarctation, and the resulting distal malperfusion can be life-threatening. The device is also prone to migration when collapse occurs. The most important way to keep device collapse from occurring is by accurate sizing and device selection. A sizing chart is provided with each of the commercially available devices with to assist with device selection but, as a general rule, the devices are oversized by 10–20% in relation to the native aortic diameter. Most of the cases where device collapse has occurred have been patients who present with traumatic aortic injury and who have an otherwise normal-caliber aorta. Since the smallest diameter TAG device is 26 mm, if it is placed in an aorta that is less than 20 mm in diameter, it will not be able to fully expand and is at risk for collapse. The smallest diameter TX2 device is 28 mm and the smallest diameter Talent device is 22 mm. Abdominal stent graft device cuffs, as well as iliac extension limbs, have been used as alternatives to treat the aorta in patients who present with acute traumatic aortic transection and a small-caliber aorta. The issue with many of these alternative devices is that their delivery systems are often too short to reach the proximal most descending aorta, and they may require alternative routes of delivery, like the axillary artery or ascending aorta [2].

The other situation in which device collapse can occur is when the device is placed at an angulated segment of the aorta in such a way that leaves the leading edge incompletely opposed to the aortic wall. This most commonly occurs at the distal aortic arch in patients with a tight angle of curvature, and this region is sometimes referred to as "no-man's land." The hemodynamic forces directed behind the leading edge of the device can push upon the outer side of the stent graft and lead to device collapse (Fig. 20.21). The best approach to avoid this cause of collapse is to either place the device distally, beyond the angle of curvature, or more proximally within the aortic arch. The problem with placing the device distally is that the extent of coverage of the diseased aorta is often

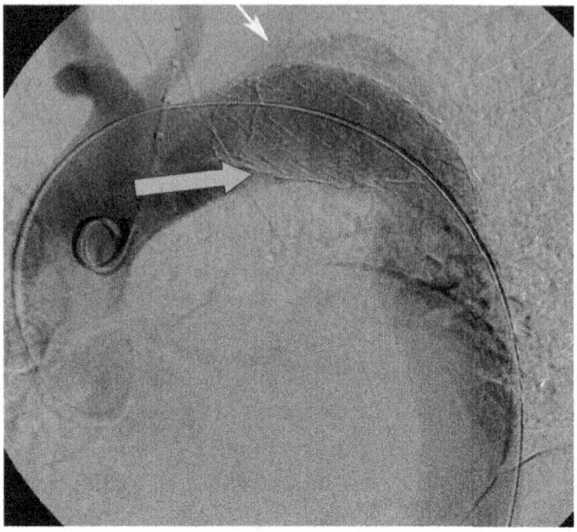

Fig. 20.21 Fluoroscopic image of a stent graft with proximal end in "no-man's land." The large arrow is directed at the area of malposition within the arch, and the smaller arrow shows an associated endoleak

compromised, and the patient may end up with persistent Type Ia endoleak. The issue with placing the device more proximally is that it most often requires coverage of the left subclavian artery, which may require additional revascularization. The risk of revascularization is significantly lower than the risk of an inadequate proximal seal, and so the seal zone should never be compromised, especially in the setting of acute dissection or traumatic transection.

Indications

Device collapse requires treatment, if the patient is fortunate enough to have the collapse detected before a complete aortic occlusion leads to death or by surveillance imaging, as was seen in Case 13 with only partial aortic occlusion.

Treatment

Endovascular repair: Most collapsed devices can be addressed endovascularly. If collapse occurs during the initial device deployment, it can be treated with the use of a conforming balloon to initially open the collapsed stent. However, additional stenting should also be performed to extend the seal of the device into a more parallel segment of the aorta and to optimize the radial force of the stents so as to avoid collapse. Sometimes additional radial force can be provided with the use of an additional balloon-expandable stent (10×40 mm Palmaz stent, Cordis, Miami Lakes, FL). With a delayed presentation, the endovascular treatment options are the same but the additional stent graft should be placed first and needs to extend beyond the area of collapse because in the chronic setting, a thrombus can accumulate within the collapsed portion of the stent graft, and simple balloon-expansion may force that thrombus into the bloodstream leading to embolization.

Open repair: Depending on the location of the device and the adequacy of the proximal landing zone, device collapse may require open repair. As described for many of the other complications earlier, this may be approached through a left thoracotomy and will most likely require the use of deep hypothermic circulatory arrest. Preferably, device collapse is treatable through a sternotomy and the use of hybrid techniques. The options are either an arch debranching procedure with subsequent endovascular stent graft proximal extension or the frozen elephant trunk approach, which is performed with deep hypothermic circulatory arrest. The issue that may arise when using either of the approaches with circulatory arrest is that the occlusive, collapsed device may compromise distal perfusion. A good option in this situation is to "Y" the arterial inflow and cannulate both the right axillary artery and the common femoral artery to assure good perfusion both proximally and distally.

Proximal Dissection

Case 14: A 58-year-old presented with severe ripping chest and back pain, and was found to have a Type B intramural hematoma with a false lumen of greater than 15 mm and persistent pain despite blood pressure control. She successfully underwent descending thoracic stent grafting and on postoperative day 5 began complaining of severe abdominal pain without other complaints. A CT scan was ordered and demonstrated a significant retrograde dissections and small pericardial effusion (Fig. 20.22).

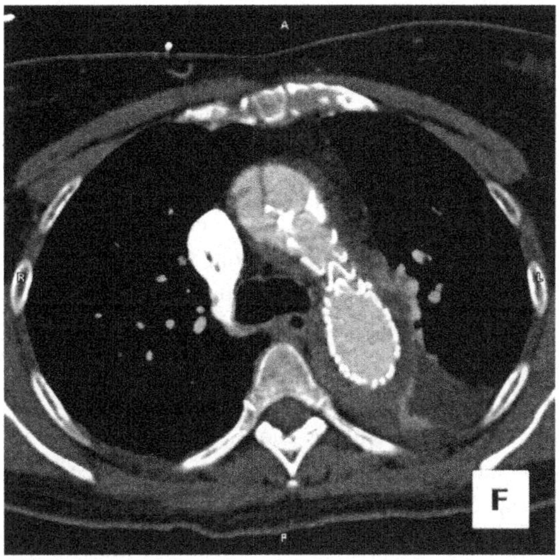

Fig. 20.22 Axial CT demonstrating proximal aortic dissection after TEVAR

Prevention

Stent grafting of Type B aortic dissections has become the treatment of choice for patients with complicated acute presentations and is playing an increasingly important role in high-risk patients with uncomplicated presentations and patients with complicated chronic dissections [9]. In the acute setting, the aorta is fragile and endovascular interventions can lead to worsening of the initial aortic injury. Patient selection is crucial and the results of the INSTEAD trial, which compared best medical therapy with early stent grafting, demonstrated no benefit to endovascular repair because of some of the associated complications. Younger patients (<60 years old) with aortic dissection are more likely to have a connective tissue disorder, which may make their more proximal aorta prone to retrograde dissection. In patients with acute complicated dissections, it is important to avoid balloon-expansion so as to minimize aortic trauma. Also, during the planning phases of these procedures, the device is sized based on the aorta in the proximal landing zone. It is important to avoid oversizing as it may lead to excessive force on the already vulnerable aortic wall. In the acute setting, the CT scan may not have been acquired in the usual manner for aortic imaging as many of these patients undergo CT to rule out pulmonary embolism or for other differential diagnoses; therefore, the sizing based on the CT scan may not be accurate. If there is suspicion about the accuracy of aortic sizing, then intravascular ultrasound can be very helpful to confirm the proper device selection. When choosing a device, it is also advisable to avoid stent grafts with bare metal stents at their proximal end as these can be more traumatic to the more proximal aorta. Finally, as described earlier in the discussion on stent graft collapse, it is critical to avoid placement of the sealing stent upon the distal angle of aortic arch. The motion and orientation of the device in this setting can lead to focal intimal trauma from the leading edge of the device. This is especially in the patients with a "Gothic" arch.

Because these retrograde dissections can occur in a delayed fashion, it is important to have a high index of suspicion, and all patients undergoing stent grafting of acute Type B dissections need to undergo predischarge CT scan or during their hospital stay should undergo reimaging of the aorta if they develop new symptoms of chest pain. The incidence of retrograde dissection is estimated to be ~2.5% after stent grafting of Type B dissections and is a life-threatening event with a mortality of 27%, which is probably underrecognized [18].

Indications

As is the case for any other etiology of Type A dissection, the presence of proximal dissection is an indication for surgical intervention.

Treatment

Open repair: The initial objective is to get the patient out of the operating room alive and the key is cardiac and brain protection. At Cleveland Clinic, these operations are performed using deep hypothermic circulatory arrest with right axillary arterial return via a vascular graft conduit. Brain protection is achieved either via retrograde brain perfusion alone or as a combination of both retrograde brain perfusion and antegrade brain perfusion depending on the extent of repair required. Most likely, however, the patient will require a complete arch repair with suture anastomosis to the proximal end of the stent graft including the aortic wall with the additional use of felt between dissected layers as a reverse elephant trunk procedure. If there is a reasonable segment of healthy aortic arch, the procedure could be performed as a single anastomosis by tacking the stent graft to the aorta adjacent to the brachiocephalic vessels from the inside and also including a portion of the device in the distal aortic anastomosis, much like a long beveled arch anastomosis. The aortic root is almost always salvagaeable with valve resuspension as long as the diagnosis is not delayed for very long and the patient did not have pre-existing serious valve pathology.

Endovascular repair: There have been no published reports of stent grafting the ascending aorta after retrograde dissection associated with stent grafting of the descending aorta, but stent grafts have been used to treat spontaneous dissection of the ascending aorta in a few selected patients with limited success. As devices specially designed for the ascending aorta evolve, it is likely that endovascular repair may become an option if retrograde dissection occurs [19].

Infection

Case 15: A 46-year-old woman who underwent stent graft repair 3 years earlier for a complicated Type B aortic dissection presented with fevers and back pain. CT scan revealed a fluid collection around the descending aorta and a stent graft suspicious for graft infection. After a full course of antibiotics, the bacteremia returned and repeat imaging confirmed the stent graft as the source. She underwent a stage repair with extra-anatomic bypass based on the ascending aorta followed by complete device removal (Fig. 20.23).

Case 16: A 34-year-old man was involved in a motor vehicle collision and sustained multiple vertebral fractures. The fractures were treated with open reduction and fixation through an anterior approach via thoracotomy. The devices were later found to be unstable and he underwent additional posterior fixation but this was complicated by deep wound infection. He returned 5 months

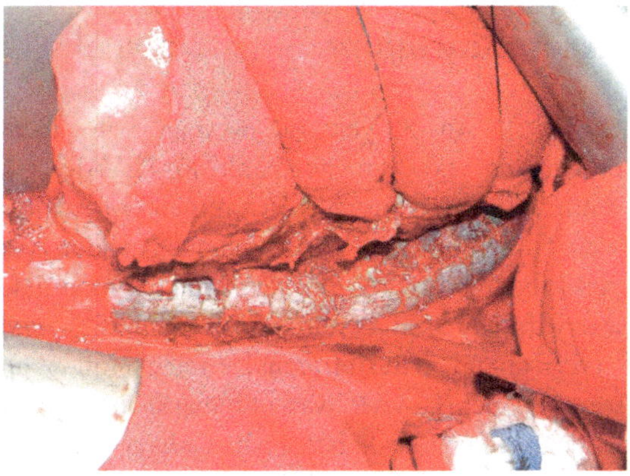

Fig. 20.23 Intraoperative photograph of an infected stent grafts in situ after extra-anatomic bypass from the ascending to arch and bilateral femoral arteries

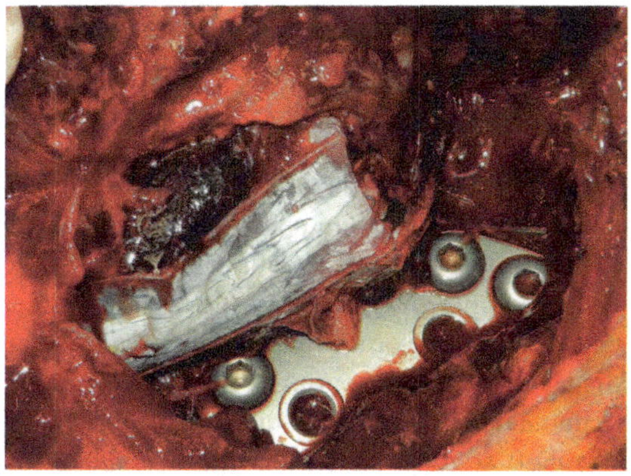

Fig. 20.24 Intraoperative photograph of infected spine hardware after posttraumatic transaction TEVAR and an additional proximal extension for proximal endoleak with contained rupture

after the initial operation with severe back pain and contrast-enhanced CT demonstrated a focal dissection of the descending aorta in the region of the hardware. This was treated with a single thoracic stent graft. He later returned complaining of severe pain and was found on CT to have a contained rupture of the descending aorta with loose anterior vertebral hardware, and he was bacteremic. He underwent immediate stent grafting with the placement of proximal extension devices and had symptomatic relief. He then returned to the operating room 1 week later for definitive removal of the infected spinal hardware and flap coverage of the stent graft (Fig. 20.24).

Prevention

Infection of an aortic graft, whether it was placed through and open or endovascular approach, carries a very high operative risk and is one of the most dreaded cardiovascular complications. Currently, no recommendations exist regarding the use of prophylactic antibiotics for patients with aortic grafts but it may be prudent to treat patients with a long segment of stent grafts with antibiotic prophylaxis as if the patient had a prosthetic valve. When stent grafts were examined in autopsy patients late after initial placement, the devices were not totally endothelialized by gross examination.

Indications

Although surgical principles dictate that an infected prosthetic device needs to be removed for eradication of the infection, the risks of the surgery must always be weighed against the risks of best medical therapy including a lifetime of antibiotics for some patients. The risk of complications related to the aorta increases when there is concern for aortic stability (i.e., inflammatory aneurysm, expanding aneurysm, pseudoaneurysm, anaerobic infections suggestive of enteric or bronchial fistula, and contained rupture), and in these situations, even high-risk surgery may be a patient's only option for treatment. In patients with persistent bacteremia, all other sources must be ruled out. In younger patients who can better tolerate multiple, staged operations, surgical objectives may change between phases of treatment but a more aggressive approach is usually the rule.

Treatment

Open repair: The most complete operative treatment requires removing all the prosthetic graft materials without leaving any prosthetic in its stead. This is usually accomplished as a staged approach first consisting of extra-anatomic bypass followed by stent graft removal and oversewing of the residual aortic stump. The extra-anatomic bypass can either be based off the axillary arteries or the ascending aorta. To avoid using diseased aortic tissue in the stump closure, bypasses to the supra-aortic vessels can also be performed simultaneous with the abdominal aortic bypass from the ascending aorta. This debranching procedure is then combined with oversewing of the healthier distal ascending aorta while avoiding the infected distal arch. It is important, when creating the extra-anatomic bypass, to understand the extent of runoff so as to match the inflow conduit and the outflow to the end-organ demands. For most patients, the axillary arteries are inadequate and the conduit must be greater than 16 mm in diameter. After a successful first stage, the patient is later returned to the operating room for complete removal of the endovascular device, debridement, and oversewing of the distal aortic stump. The infected field and the aortic stumps are then covered with an omental or other fatty or muscular flap. This approach was utilized in the patient described in Case 15, but is an extensive series of trauma for an already sick patient and the recovery can be very difficult.

For patients in whom the risk of a staged approach is too high, the option to remove the infected stent graft and replace the aorta with either a homograft or a rifampin-soaked vascular graft is reasonable. It is always wise to cover these grafts with an omental flap. Depending on the infecting organism, these patients sometimes require lifelong antibiotic treatment.

Endovascular repair: Stent grafts have a role in patients with device infection; they provide stability to an unstable aorta. Even if the devices are to be removed later, they play an important role in acute salvage procedures [20]. It is likely that most stent grafts placed into an already infected aorta will require removal, but this is not always true. The patient described in Case 16 kept his stent graft devices after removal and debridement of the associated spinal hardware infection. A pericardial fat flap and a bovine pericardial patch were used to cover the stent grafts. This was performed in two stages after initial stabilization of his aorta was achieved by the placement of an additional proximal stent graft.

Access Site Injury

Case 17: An 82-year-old woman with focal descending aneurysm amenable to TEVAR presented for elective repair. Her iliofemoral vessels were 5 mm in diameter, and a planned conduit was performed at the origin of the right common iliac artery through a small retroperitoneal incision with a cross-clamp on the infrarenal aorta. On follow-up imaging, her TEVAR was unremarkable without evidence of endoleak, but she had a large pseudoaneurysm of the infrarenal aorta that required additional stent grafting to repair (Fig. 20.25).

Prevention

Precise and complete vascular-enhanced CT imaging of the entire aorta and pelvic vessels with 3D reconstruction analysis is the best way to determine whether a patient has safe access from the femoral artery or requires the use of an abdominal aortic or iliac conduit. One should have a low threshold for conduit use as this procedure is very well tolerated [21].

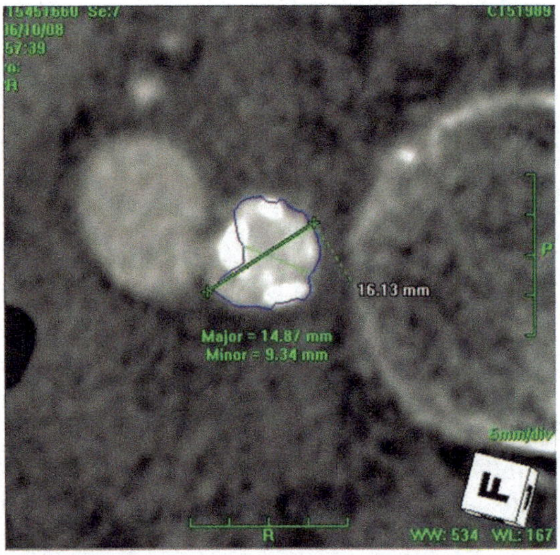

Fig. 20.25 Axial CT image of infrarenal aorta with a focal pseudoaneurysm secondary to cross-clamp for construction of the access conduit

Indications

Vascular access injuries occur as a spectrum from focal stable dissection of the iliofemoral arteries to complete disruption with hemodynamic instability. The decision to intervene is based on the extent of injury and the presence of active bleeding.

Treatment

If an artery has only focal dissection with no compromise in distal perfusion or evidence of extravasation, it may be left alone. All arterial access sites need to be included in the surveillance imaging studies, especially if there has been an injury. In the event that there is dissection in an access vessel without bleeding, it should be assessed with angiography and, possibly, intravascular ultrasound. If there is concern about compromised flow, it can be further assessed by direct measurement of a pressure gradient. These lesions can usually be treated quite easily with the placement of a self-expanding or balloon-expandable stent. In the event that there is extravasation, the situation becomes an emergency and the first matter of business is to gain vascular control. This is best achieved either through the working side or the contralateral side with an occlusive balloon in the more proximal aorta or iliac vessels. Once the patient is resuscitated, the injured vessel can be repaired either endovascularly using a repaving technique with covered stents or by direct retroperitoneal repair through an open incision.

It is important to remember that all segments of the vasculature that are traversed or manipulated during endovascular intervention may be vulnerable to injury, and these injuries may present later. The pseudoaneurysm in the previous case was only found incidentally by complete imaging during the early follow-up, averting an emergency surgery or potentially mortal complication.

Miscellaneous Failed Endovascular Procedures

Case 18: A 22-year-old woman with a history of Takayasu disease previously underwent a modified Bentall procedure that was later complicated by a large pseudoaneurysm with maximum diameter of 8 cm. Initial attempts to treat this were performed endovascularly with the placement of atrial septal defect closure devices across the defects in the suture line. She later presented to the Cleveland Clinic with persistent flow into the pseudoaneurysm with continued growth.

Case 19: A 37-year-old woman with long-segment coarctation complicated by claudication underwent endovascular stenting with the placement of several stents extending from just beyond the left subclavian artery to the level of the diaphragm. She had little change in her symptoms and was referred to cardiovascular surgery. The maximum diameter of her descending thoracic aorta was 10 mm on CT angiography but her supraceliac aorta was larger, ~16 mm. She underwent median sternotomy and ascending-to-abdominal aortic bypass without complications and had significant improvement in her symptoms, and the gradient was less than 10 mmHg.

Prevention

The most important thing when performing a procedure using a device outside of its intended indication is to understand the limitations of its engineering. The patient in Case 18 had too large of an anastomotic defect to safely secure it with the use of the septal defect closure device. The patient in Case 19 had too long of a narrow lumen within her descending aorta to benefit from dilatation to only 10 mm. Nonetheless, these procedures were performed, and their failures did not preclude either patient from undergoing a successful reoperation.

Indications

Neither of these patients had the intended outcome of their endovascular procedures: obliteration of flow into the pseudoaneurysm and optimal distal arterial perfusion, respectively. The indications that prompted the endovascular attempts still apply for the reoperation.

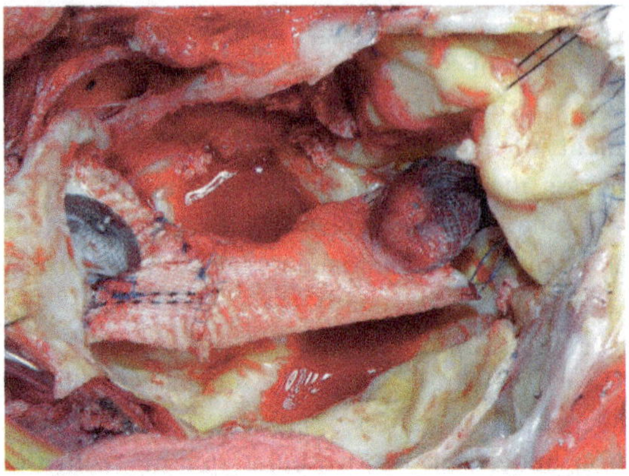

Fig. 20.26 Intraoperative photograph from Case 18 of ascending graft and failed septal closure devices for ascending pseudoaneurysm

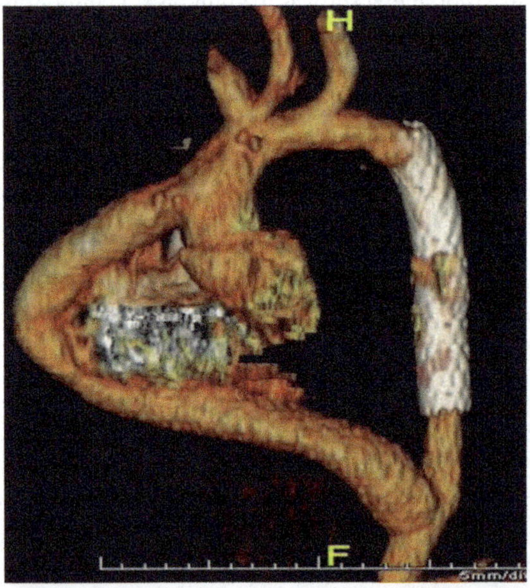

Fig. 20.27 Postoperative VRE CT from Case 19 demonstrating the ascending to supraceliac aortic bypass for inadequate stenting of a long-segment coarctation

Treatment

Open repair was the only feasible option in both of these patients. The first underwent standard open repair under deep hypothermic circulatory arrest. Great care must be taken when performing reoperations on a patient with aortic pseudoaneurysm [22]. The chest was opened with the patient already heparinized and cannulated in preparation for early institution of cardiopulmonary bypass with cooling. The pseudoaneurysm was safely controlled, and the devices and old graft removed and replaced with reconstruction of the proximal and distal anastomoses (Fig. 20.26). The second patient with the long coarctation and failed stenting underwent an extra-anatomic ascending-to-abdominal aortic bypass with very good success (Fig. 20.27). The old endovascular devices were removed in the first patient and left in situ in the second patient.

Conclusions

Increasing availability and comfort with the use of endovascular devices will lead to expanded usage of the devices. The first step in performing a reoperation in these patients is to avoid it by selecting the patient and devices that will fit best for a particular problem. The user of endovascular devices has to understand the limits of each device and the tolerances of the diseased aorta. Most complications after endovascular repairs can be addressed with additional endovascular reoperations, but the fundamental principles of what makes an endovascular repair durable should not be compromised if the patient can tolerate an open operation. Converting an endovascular repair to an open repair requires precise imaging to facilitate the planning stage of what can be a creative series of procedures. These are difficult problems that are best handled in a center with experience and the resources of a multidisciplinary aortic team.

References

1. Svensson LG, Kouchoukos NT, Miller DC, et al. Expert consensus document on the treatment of descending thoracic aortic disease using endovascular stent-grafts. Ann Thorac Surg. 2008;85(Suppl):1–41.
2. Roselli EE, Soltesz EG, Mastracci T, Svensson LG, Lytle BW. Antegrade delivery of stent grafts to treat complex thoracic aortic disease. Ann Thorac Surg. 2010;90(2):539–46.
3. Veith FJ, Baum RA, Ohki T, et al. Nature and significance of endoleaks and endo-tension: summary of opinions expressed at an international conference. J Vasc Surg. 2002;35:1029–35.

4. Soulez G, Lerouge S, Salazkin I, Darsaut T, Oliva VL, Raymond J. Type I and collateral flow in experimental aneurysm models treated with stent-grafts. J Vasc Interv Radiol. 2007;18:265–72.
5. Schoder M, Lammer J, Czerny M. Endovascular aortic arch repair: hopes and certainties. Eur J Vasc Endovasc Surg. 2009;38:255–61.
6. Matsumura JS, Lee WA, Mitchell RS, et al. The Society for Vascular Surgery Practice Guidelines: management of the left subclavian artery with thoracic endovascular aortic repair. J Vasc Surg. 2009;50:1155–8.
7. Moon MC, Dowdall J, Roselli EE. The use of right ventricular pacing to facilitate stent graft deployment in the distal aortic arch. J Vasc Surg. 2008;47:629–31.
8. Rao AS, Rhee RY. Coverage of the celiac artery during TEVAR: is it ever appropriate? Semin Vasc Surg. 2009;22:152–8.
9. Subramanian S, Roselli EE. Thoracic aortic dissection: long-term results of endovascular and open repair. Semin Vasc Surg. 2009;22:61–8.
10. Roselli EE, Greenberg RK, Pfaff K, et al. Endovascular treatment of thoracoabdominal aortic aneurysms. J Thorac Cardiovasc Surg. 2007;133:1474–82.
11. Resch TA, Greenberg RK, Lyden SP, Clair DG, Krajewski L, Kashyap VS, et al. Combined staged procedures for the treatment of thoracoabdominal aneurysms. J Endovasc Ther. 2006;13:481–9.
12. Patel R, Conrad MF, Paruchuri V, Kwolek CJ, Chung TK, Cambria RP. Thoracoabdominal aneurysm repair: hybrid versus open repair. J Vasc Surg. 2009;50:15–22.
13. Hughes GC, Nienaber JJ, Bush EL, Daneshmand MA, McCann RL. Use of custom Dacron branch grafts for "hybrid" aortic debranching during endovascular repair of thoracic and thoracoabdominal aortic aneurysms. J Thorac Cardiovasc Surg. 2008;136:21–8, 28.e1–6.
14. Roselli EE, Ganapathi A. The use of an Zenith iliac plug device to treatment left subclavian artery aneurysm at the time of thoracic endovascular repair of a chronic distal dissection. Ann Thor Surg. 2010 (submitted for publication).
15. Figueroa CA, Taylor CA, Chiou AJ, Yeh V, Zarins CK. Magnitude and direction of pulsatile displacement forces acting on thoracic aortic endografts. J Endovasc Ther. 2009;16:350–8.
16. O'Neill S, Greenberg RK, Resch T, Bathurst S, Fleming D, Kashyap V, et al. An evaluation of centerline of flow measurement techniques to assess migration after thoracic endovascular aneurysm repair. J Vasc Surg. 2006;43:1103–10.
17. Ohrlander T, Sonesson B, Ivancev K, et al. The Chimney graft: a technique for preserving or rescuing aortic branch vessels in stent-graft sealing zones. J Endovasc Ther. 2008;15:427–32.
18. Dong ZH, Fu WG, Wang YQ, et al. Retrograde type A aortic dissection after endovascular stent graft placement for treatment of type B dissection. Circulation. 2009;119:735–41.
19. Moon MC, Morales JP, Greenberg RK. The aortic arch and ascending aorta: are they within the endovascular realm? Semin Vasc Surg. 2007;20:97–107.
20. Topel I, Stehr A, Steinbauer MG, et al. Surgical strategy in aortoesophageal fistulae: endovascular stent grafts and in situ repair of the aorta with cryopreserved homografts. Ann Surg. 2007;246:853–9.
21. Abu-Ghaida AM, Clair DG, Greenberg RK, et al. Broadening the applicability of endovascular aneurysm repair: the use of iliac conduits. J Vasc Surg. 2002;36:111–7.
22. Roselli EE, Pettersson GB, Blackstone EH, et al. Adverse events during reoperative cardiac surgery: frequency, characterization, and rescue. J Thorac Cardiovasc Surg. 2008; 135: 316–23, 323.e1-6.

Percutaneous Approaches to Valvular Heart Disease After Previous Cardiac Surgery

21

John M. Stulak and Hartzell V. Schaff

Introduction

While open surgical correction is the best treatment for most patients with valvular heart disease, there have been recent technical advances that permit percutaneous approaches to valve replacement and valve repair in selected circumstances. The most widely accepted catheter-based therapy for valvular heart disease is percutaneous balloon dilatation for rheumatic mitral valve stenosis, and this might be applicable to some patients who require relief of mitral valve stenosis after previous aortic or tricuspid valve surgery. As discussed earlier, degenerative mitral valve disease is the most common mitral valve etiology in Western populations, and considerable effort has been extended toward catheter-based methods for repair of mitral valve prolapse. Patients with aortic valve stenosis constitute the largest population of patients who might be considered for transcatheter therapy. Percutaneous and transapical insertion of collapsible bioprostheses has been used widely in elderly high-risk patients, and many of these patients have had previous cardiac surgery [1, 2].

Transcatheter techniques are a valuable alternative in circumstances where patients are too frail to undergo conventional operation, and these methods offer hope to patients who would otherwise not be candidates for treatment. In addition, transcatheter aortic valve implantation (TAVI) has also been used as an alternative to open prosthetic replacement in patients who have degeneration of bioprostheses [3]. Another novel application of catheter-based therapy is repair of paravalvular leaks with Amplatzer occlusion devices (AGA Medical, Plymouth, MN) [4].

J.M. Stulak, MD (✉) • H.V. Schaff, MD
Division of Cardiovascular Surgery, Mayo Clinic, Rochester, MN, USA
e-mail: schaff@mayo.edu

Aortic Valve

In the last half decade, two systems have been introduced for sutureless TAVI, the CoreValve (Medtronic, Minneapolis, MN), and the Edwards SAPIEN valve (Edwards Lifesciences, Irvine, CA). Both utilize pericardium for leaflet cusps; however, the CoreValve is self-expanding and is deployed with some of the mesh frame extending below the aortic valve annulus. The SAPIEN valve is balloon expandable and is deployed in an intra-annular, subcoronary position. The first valve was implanted using a TAVI procedure in 2002 [5], and it is now estimated that over 10,000 patients have received either the CoreValve or the SAPIEN prosthesis [6]. In the early series, TAVI was utilized in high-risk patients, many of whom had undergone previous coronary artery bypass operations (17–34%) [7–13].

Early results of TAVI have been encouraging with procedural success in 80–90% of patients and 30-day mortality ranging from 10 to 22%. In a more recent series with 646 patients, the

V.R. Machiraju et al. (eds.), *Redo Cardiac Surgery in Adults*,
DOI 10.1007/978-1-4614-1326-4_21, © Springer Science+Business Media, LLC 2012

procedure was successful in 97% of patients and mortality was 8% [14].

Outcomes of TAVI in patients who had previous cardiac surgery were described by Walther et al., who reported their experience with 25 patients who underwent TAVI after prior cardiac surgery [15]. Mean preoperative logistic EuroSCORE was 40% and mean preoperative STS risk score was 17%. Consistent with prior studies, the most common previously performed operation was coronary bypass grafting (72%); 12% of patients had undergone prior mitral valve operations and 8% had prior aortic valve surgery. The rate of in-hospital or 30-day mortality was 12%, and there were no new-onset strokes in any patient. There were four additional deaths during follow-up (mean approximately 1 year) for a 72% actuarial 1-year survival; none of the early or late deaths were thought to be directly related to the valve. In the face of significantly elevated operative risk, these data suggest that TAVI may represent an attractive therapeutic option.

Ensuring antegrade blood flow through the coronary ostia is critical after TAVI; however, prior coronary bypass grafting may offer "protection" from this potentially lethal complication. When utilizing the transapical approach for TAVI in patients with prior surgery, access to the apex of the left ventricle is usually uncomplicated. Pericardial adhesions rarely interfere with identification of the apical puncture site, which can be performed directly through the pericardium. The potential disadvantage is limited visualization of the left anterior descending coronary artery, but, in general, other technical aspects of TAVI are similar to those in patients who have not had prior surgery.

A potential disadvantage to TAVI is the risk of neurological injury. In a report by Smith et al. [34] on cohort A in the Placement of Aortic Transcatheter Valves (PARTNER) trial, the risk of stroke or transient ischemic attack within 30 days after transcatheter replacement was 5.5%, and this risk increased to 8.3% after 1 year. In comparison, the early and late risks of neurologic injury were 2.4 and 4.3%, respectively, in patients who had surgical aortic valve replacement. The early risk of stroke or transient ischemic attack in the PARTNER trial is consistent with previous studies and is similar to the 6.7% risk in patients who were not candidates for surgery. For patients who are not surgical candidates, this increased risk of neurological complications may be acceptable, but for patients who are candidates for surgery, the risk must be balanced against the benefits of avoiding sternotomy and cardiopulmonary bypass.

TAVI has been evaluated in clinical protocols that enrolled high-risk patients in the United States. FDA approval is imminent, but guidelines need to be developed for patient selection and certification of hospitals, surgeons, and interventionalists. It seems clear, however, that TAVI will be an important alternative treatment for many patients who would otherwise be candidates for aortic valve reoperation, and this approach should be considered when reoperation is necessary.

Pulmonary Valve

Isolated pulmonary valve disease is rare, but pulmonary valve regurgitation is a common consequence of repair of congenital heart diseases that involve the right ventricular outflow tract (RVOT) reconstruction, including tetralogy of Fallot with or without pulmonary atresia, transposition of the great arteries with pulmonary stenosis, and truncus arteriosus. Reconstruction of the RVOT is an integral part of the repair of these lesions, and repair is usually undertaken at an early age. Consequently, late reoperation is often necessary as a result of somatic growth or failure of the initial procedure. Indeed, reoperation on the RVOT is one of the most common indications for surgery in adult congenital heart disease [16].

The timing of reoperation for correction of pulmonary valve regurgitation has been debated, but, in general, surgery is indicated to reduce the deleterious effects of right ventricular enlargement due to volume overload [17]. Furthermore, reintervention is also indicated for patients with severe stenosis of right ventricle-to-pulmonary artery conduits (peak gradient greater than 50 mmHg). Reoperation should be considered in patients who have pulmonary regurgitation or stenosis and who exhibit decreased exercise capacity, reduced right ventricular function, increased right ventricular end-diastolic dimension, or moderate or severe tricuspid valve regurgitation. [18]. Because all the current options for RVOT reconstruction degenerate over time, many patients may require several reoperations over their lifetime.

Percutaneous approaches are a particularly attractive treatment option in patients with RVOT reconstruction. Bonhoeffer et al. described the first percutaneous pulmonary valve implantation in humans [19, 20]. This device consisted of a bovine jugular venous valve sutured to the wall of a balloon expandable stent. Due to the large caliber of the sheath required for delivery, the experience was initially limited to patients older than 5 years or heavier than 20 kg, and all patients treated in these studies had prior cardiac surgery (extracardiac conduits).

The Melody valve (Medtronic Inc), a modified version of the initial device, was approved by the US Food and Drug Administration in January 2010, and in an update from the multicenter trial evaluating the Melody valve, there was significant relief of the RVOT gradient (postprocedure mean gradient, 13 mmHg) and successful correction of pulmonary valve regurgitation (trivial or absent in all patients) [21]. Similar to the previously discussed studies, all patients in this report had undergone prior cardiac surgery with an extracardiac right ventricle-to-pulmonary artery conduit, and approximately half of the patients had undergone more than one previous repair. In addition, a significant number also had undergone prior interventional procedures including a single prior stent placement in 17% and multiple stent placements in 9% of patients. Procedural mortality for insertion of the Melody pulmonary valve was very low, and 94% of patients were free of valve dysfunction or reintervention 1 year after percutaneous pulmonary valve insertion. As more durable valve substitutes are developed, this approach will undoubtedly decrease the need for reoperation in these complex patients.

Mitral Valve

Several percutaneous devices have been developed to reduce mitral valve regurgitation, but direct attempts at annuloplasty have not been successful. The most advanced percutaneous method is the MitraClip device (Abbott, Abbott Park, IL) that is intended to mimic the surgical edge-to-edge repair first described by Alfieri [22]. This technology was initially evaluated in the EVEREST (Endovascular Valve Edge-to-Edge REpair STudy) phase I feasibility trial (55 patients) and roll-in phase of the EVEREST II trial (52 patients). These trials demonstrated procedural/in-hospital mortality of <1%, and 66% of patients had mild or no mitral regurgitation at 1 year of follow-up [23]. Previous mediastinal surgery was an exclusion criterion for the first 27 patients. The EVEREST II trial was the first randomized trial of a percutaneous mitral valve repair device compared with conventional surgical therapy and demonstrated a lower incidence of major adverse events, but at the expense of a a lower incidence of efficacy even after 2-year follow-up [24]. In this trial, 38 of the 184 patients (21%) in the percutaneous cohort had undergone prior coronary artery bypass grafting.

Since receiving CE Mark approval in 2008, the majority of MitraClip implants have been performed in Europe. In the German experience, 51 patients with a mean logistic EuroSCORE of 29% and STS risk score of 15% underwent correction of mitral regurgitation with the MitraClip. There were no procedure-related major adverse events and no in-hospital mortality [25]. Five of the fifty-one patients had undergone prior cardiac surgery, including prior bypass grafting in four and aortic valve replacement in one. In the Italian experience, 31 patients had MitraClip implantation with acute device success in 97% [26]. Only two of these patients had undergone prior coronary bypass grafting. It is important to note that in these studies the use of the MitraClip device did not preclude future mitral valve surgery when required.

While most of the patients in these studies examining the early experience with the MitraClip device underwent prior bypass grafting or aortic valve replacement, there are very few studies reporting use of the MitraClip after prior mitral valve surgery. One case report described its successful use in two patients after prior partial band annuloplasty [27]. Important technical considerations in this clinical setting include the following (1) the need for transthoracic echocardiography for device postioning due to excessive interference from the annuloplasty band when using transesophageal imaging, and (2) the awareness that in the setting of prior annuloplasty, there is a higher risk of creating mitral stenosis after deployment compared to use in patients who have not had prior mitral valve surgery.

In addition to addressing leaflet pathology, a percutaneous mitral annuloplasty device (PMAD; Cardiac Dimensions, Inc., Kirkland, WA) was developed for deployment in the coronary sinus to address functional mitral regurgitation with a dilated annulus [28]. Early experience in five patients demonstrated shortening of the septal–lateral mitral annular dimension and a resultant decrease in the amount of mitral valve regurgitation; one of these five patients (20%) had undergone prior coronary bypass grafting.

Tricuspid Valve

Only case reports have been published on the use of percutaneous access to address tricuspid valve disease. The first publication reports the off-label use of the Edwards SAPIEN transcutaneous aortic valve in an 8-year-old child with bioprosthetic degeneration 5 years after tricuspid valve replacement [29]. This case report demonstrated the ability to percutaneously implant a valved stent virtually "anywhere" in the heart provided that a stiff anchoring site is present. Examples of this could be a valve ring in any location, a rigid conduit in the pulmonary position, or a calcified annuloplasty band in the mitral or tricuspid position. Another case report described the use of the MitraClip device to address significant tricuspid regurgitation in a patient with corrected congenital transposition of the great arteries [30]. Three months after device deployment, the patient was asymptomatic with mild residual tricuspid valve regurgitation.

Paravalvular Leak

Leakage around a previously placed valve prosthesis is a well-recognized complication after valve replacement, and reoperation in this setting carries a significantly increased risk of operative morbidity and mortality, especially when the mitral valve is involved [31, 32]. Catheter-based attempts at closure of paravalvular leaks are particularly attractive in this clinical setting. Sorajja et al. reported their experience in 16 patients who underwent prior valve replacement (14 mitral and 2 aortic) and developed heart failure or hemolytic anemia [31]. Under echocardiographic and fluoroscopic imaging, implantation of either the Amplatzer Septal Occluder or Duct Occluder was attempted in all 16 patients (19 defects, 21 separate percutaneous attempts). Procedural success was obtained in 17/21 attempts (81%) without periprocedural death, stroke, or myocardial infarction. Furthermore, there was no obstruction of the existing valve prosthesis, and New York Heart Association function class improved significantly during follow-up. Although challenging, percutaneous repair of paravalvular regurgitation is feasible; however, careful patient selection is necessary.

Future Directions

The therapies discussed represent a diverse array of options to problems that were previously only amenable to open surgical repair. These techniques are in different stages of development, but it is clear that this field is evolving from experimental concepts to potentially viable long-term solutions to a growing burden of degenerative valvular heart disease. Future devices and approaches will need to be rigorously evaluated for sound proof-of-principle, positive long-term outcomes in animal models, and benefits in humans as demonstrated by randomized trials. New percutaneous approaches should be compared with the contemporary standard of care, conventional open cardiac surgery [33].

References

1. Iung B. Management of the elderly patient with aortic stenosis. Heart. 2008;94:519–24.
2. Block PC. Percutaneous transcatheter repair for mitral regurgitation. J Interv Cardiol. 2006;19:547–51.
3. Klaabarg K-E, Egeblad H, Jakobsen C-J, et al. Transapical transcatheter treatment of a stenosed aortic

valve bioprosthesis using the Edwards SAPIEN transcatheter heart valve. Ann Thorac Surg. 2009;87: 1934–6.
4. Hoffmayer KS, Zellner C, Kwan DM, et al. Closure of a para-valvular aortic leak: with the use of 2 AMPLATZER devices and real-time 2- and 3-dimensional transesophageal echocardiography. Tex Heart Inst J. 2011;38(1):81–4.
5. Cribier A, Eltchaninoff H, Bash A, et al. Percutaneous transcatheter implantation of an aortic valve prosthesis for calcific aortic stenosis. Circulation. 2002;106: 3006–8.
6. Walther T, Chu MWA, Mohr W. Transcatheter aortic valve implantation: time to expand? Curr Opin Cardiol. 2008;23:111–6.
7. Cribier A, Eltchaninoff H, Tron C, et al. Treatment of calcific aortic stenosis with the percutaneous heart valve: mid-term follow-up from the initial feasibility studies: the French experience. J Am Coll Cardiol. 2066;47:1214–23.
8. Grube E, Laborde JC, Gerckens U, et al. Percutaneous implantation of the CoreValve self-expanding valve prosthesis in high risk patients with aortic valve disease. The Siegburg first-in-man study. Circulation. 2006;114:1616–24.
9. Lichtenstein SV, Cheung A, Ye J, Thompson CR, Carere RG, Pasupati S, et al. Transapical transcatheter aortic valve implantation in humans: initial clinical experience. Circulation. 2006;114(6):591–6.
10. Gruge E, Schuler G, Buellesfeld L, et al. Percutaneous aortic valve replacement for severe aortic stenosis in high risk patients using the second- and current third-generation self-expanding CoreValve prosthesis. Device success and 30-day clinical outcome. J Am Coll Cardiol. 2007;50:69–76.
11. Webb JG, Pasupati S, Humphries K, et al. Percutaneous transarterial aortic valve replacement in selected high-risk patients with aortic stenosis. Circulation. 2007; 116:755–63.
12. Walther T, Falk V, Borger MA, et al. Minimally invasive transapical beating heart aortic valve implantation – proof of concept. Eur J Cardiothorac Surg. 2007;31:9–15.
13. Walter T, Simon P, Dewey T, et al. Transapical minimally invasive aortic valve implantation: multicenter experience. Circulation. 2007;116(11 Suppl):I240–5.
14. Piazza N, Grube E, Gerckens U, et al. Procedural and 30-day outcomes following transcatheter aortic valve implantation using the third generation (18 Fr) CoreValve ReValving system: results from the multicenter, expanded evaluation registry 1-year following CE mark approval. EuroIntervention. 2008;4:242–9.
15. Walther T, Falk V, Borger MA, et al. Transapical aortic valve implantation in patients requiring redo surgery. Eur J Cardiothorac Surg. 2009;36(2): 231–4.
16. Dore A, Glancy DL, Stone S, Menashe VD, Somerville J. Cardiac surgery for grown-up congenital heart patients: survey of 307 consecutive operations from 1991 to 1994. Am J Cardiol. 1997;80:906–13.
17. Perloff JK, Natterson PD. Atrial arrhythmias in adults after repair of tetralogy of Fallot. Ann Thorac Surg. 1995;91:2118–9.
18. Warnes CA, Williams RG, Bashore TM, Child JS, Connolly HM, Dearani JA, et al. ACC/AHA 2008 Guidelines for the management of adults with congenital heart disease: a report of the American College of Cardiology/American Heart Association Task Force on Practice Guidelines (writing committee to develop guidelines on the management of adults with congenital heart disease). Circulation. 2008;118:2395–451.
19. Bonhoeffer P, Boudjemline Y, Saliba Z, et al. Percutaneous replacement of pulmonary valve in a right ventricle to pulmonary artery prosthetic conduit with valve dysfunction. Lancet. 2000;356:1403–5.
20. Bonhoeffer P, Doudjemline Qureshi SA, et al. Percutaneous insertion of the pulmonary valve. J Am Coll Cardiol. 2002;39:1664–9.
21. McElhinney DB, Hellebrand WE, Zahn EM, et al. Short- and medium-term outcomes after transcatheter pulmonary valve placement in the expanded multicenter US Melody valve trial. Circulation. 2010;122:507–16.
22. Alfieri O, Maisano F, De Bonis M, et al. The double-orifice technique in mitral valve repair: a simple solution for complex problems. J Thorac Cardiovasc Surg. 2001;122:674–81.
23. Feldman T, Kar S, Rinaldi M, et al. Percutaneous mitral repair with the MitraClip system. Safety and Midterm Durability in the Initial EVEREST (Endovascular Valve Edge-to-Edge REpair STudy) cohort. J Am Coll Cardiol. 2009;54:686–94.
24. Feldman T, Foster E, Glower DG, et al. Percutaneous repair of surgery for mitral regurgitation. N Engl J Med. 2011;364:1395–406.
25. Franzen O, Baldus S, Rudolph V, et al. Acute outcomes of MitraClip therapy for mitral regurgitation in high-surgical-risk patients: emphasis on adverse valve morphology and severe left ventricular dysfunction. Eur Heart J. 2010;31:1373–81.
26. Tamburino C, Ussia GP, Maisano F, et al. Percutaneous mitral repair with the MitraClip system: acute results from a real world setting. Eur Heart J. 2010;31: 1382–9.
27. Lim DS, Kunjummen BJ, Smailing R. Mitral valve repair with the MitraClip device after prior surgical mitral annuloplasty. Catheter Cardiovasc Interv. 2010;76:455–9.
28. Duffy SJ, Federman J, Farrington C, Reuter DG, Richardson M, Kaye DM. Feasibility and short-term efficacy of percutaneous mitral annular reduction for the therapy of functional mitral regurgitation in patients with heart failure. Catheter Cardiovasc Interv. 2006;68(2):205–10.
29. Gewillig M, Dubois C. Percutaneous Re-Revalvulation of the tricuspid valve. Catheter Cardiovasc Interv. 2011;77:692–5.
30. Franzen O, von Samson P, Dodge-Khatami A, Geffert G, Baldus S. Percutaneous edge-to-edge repair of tricuspid regurgitation in congenitally corrected transposition of the great arteries. Congenit Heart Dis. 2011;6(1):57–9.

31. Sorajja P, Cabalka AK, Hagler DJ, et al. Successful percutaneous repair of perivalvular prosthetic regurgitation. Catheter Cardiovasc Interv. 2007;70:815–23.
32. De Cicco G, Russo C, Moreo AN, et al. Mitral valve periprosthetic leakage: anatomical observations in 135 patients from a multicentre study. Eur J Cardiothorac Surg. 2006;30:887–91.
33. Vassiliades Jr TA, Block PC, Cohn LH, et al. The clinical development of percutaneous heart valve technology: a position statement of the Society of Thoracic Surgeons (STS), the American Association for Thoracic Surgery (AATS), and the Society for Cardiovascular Angiography and Interventions (SCAI) endorsed by the American College of Cardiology Foundation (ACCF) and the American Heart Association (AHA). J Am Coll Cardiol. 2005;45:1554–60.
34. Smith CR, Leon MB, Mack MJ, et al. Transcatheter versus surgical aortic-valve replacement in high-risk patients. N Engl J Med 2011;364:2187–2198.

Index

A

Abiomed AB 5000, 68–70, 74
Abiomed BVS, 69, 70
Acar, C., 16
Acute kidney injury (AKI), 37–46
Acute renal failure, 37, 118
Acute tubular necrosis (ATN), 39
Ad, N., 114
AKI. *See* Acute kidney injury
Alfieri, O., 197
Allen, S.P., 15
Allograft, 134, 141, 142, 144–146, 148–150
Aminocaproic acid, 14, 60, 64, 83
Anesthesia, 29, 41, 42, 63–64, 86, 162, 164
Annuloplasty, 18, 33, 90, 92–95, 122, 123, 197, 198
ANP. *See* Atrial natriuretic peptide
Anterior leaflet, 90, 91, 93, 95, 96
Antibiotic prophylaxis, 189
Antibiotic therapy, 143, 149
Antifungal therapy, 150
Aortic aneurysm, 8, 159–161, 167, 168, 172, 176, 178, 183
Aortic arch, 11, 13, 30, 83, 128, 151–156, 162, 168, 173–175, 179, 183, 185, 186, 188
Aortic coarctation, 117, 159
Aortic cross-clamping, 11, 113, 134, 136, 164, 165, 168
Aortic dissection, 71, 128, 153, 155–157, 162, 171–173, 177, 178, 187, 188
Aortic transection, 174, 185, 186
Aortic valve
  repair, 125
  replacement, 18, 33, 81, 93, 117, 118, 125, 128, 133–139, 196–198
Arghami, A., 81–86
Artery stenosis, 30
Ascending aorta, 2, 11, 18, 23, 25, 27, 71, 73, 77, 82–86, 103, 112, 128, 134, 143, 147, 148, 151, 155, 162, 163, 174, 176, 179, 180, 184, 186, 188–190
Atelectasis, 54
ATN. *See* Acute tubular necrosis
Atrial fibrillation, 29, 90, 109–118, 122, 123
Atrial natriuretic peptide (ANP), 45, 115
Atriotomy, 101, 102, 105
Aviram, G., 82
Axial flow pumps, 67

B

Bacteremia, 100, 107, 141, 143, 147, 188, 189
Balloon-expansion, 183, 184, 187
Barnett, S.D., 114
Barratt-Boyes, B.G., 133
Bavaria, J.E., 160
Bermudez, C., 67–78
Biological valves, 106, 126
Bioprostheses, 141, 195
Biventricular support, 68, 73–76
Blood transfusion, 39, 57, 60
Bonhoeffer, P., 197
Brain imaging, 145
Brain perfusion, 31, 151, 154, 156, 175, 188
Branched-fenestrated stent grafts, 166–167
Brawley, R.F., 102

C

CABG. *See* Coronary artery bypass grafting
Cabrol graft, 138
CAD. *See* Coronary artery disease (CAD)
Calafiore, A.M., 122
Calcification, 126, 134, 136, 137, 171
Calcified ascending aorta, 2
Candidemia, 143
Cardiac catheterization, 76, 147, 160
Cardiac tamponade, 4
Cardiogenic shock, 1, 5, 23, 40, 67–78
Cardioplegic solution, 3, 5, 11–14
Cardiopulmonary bypass, 2, 4, 5, 8, 10–15, 20, 21, 29, 36, 39, 54, 56, 63, 67, 81, 83–85, 101, 102, 112, 114, 122, 125–127, 153, 155, 162, 163, 184, 191, 196
Carotid endarterectomy, 30

V.R. Machiraju et al. (eds.), *Redo Cardiac Surgery in Adults*,
DOI 10.1007/978-1-4614-1326-4, © Springer Science+Business Media, LLC 2012

Carotid Revascularization Endarterectomy *vs* Stent Trial (CREST), 30
Carrell, 158
Centrifugal flow pumps, 67, 69
CentriMag, 68–70, 72, 74–75
Chertow, G.M., 37
Chimney technique, 185
Chordal replacement, 96
Chronic aortic dissections, 177
Chronic obstructive pulmonary disease (COPD), 38, 53–55, 159, 160, 173, 183
Clonidine, 46
Clopidogrel, 14, 57, 58, 83, 160
Coagulopathy, 3, 42, 49, 57, 60, 64, 71, 81, 166
Cohen, E.S., 158
Cohn, L.H., 14
Comorbid conditions, 1, 5, 18, 63, 146
Computed tomography (CT), 31, 63, 135, 145, 157, 172
Congenital heart disease, 109–111, 114, 196
Conlon, P.J., 37
Cooley, D.A., 67
COPD. *See* Chronic obstructive pulmonary disease
Coronary angiography, 145
Coronary arteriography, 135
Coronary artery branches, 8, 10–12, 16–18
Coronary artery bypass grafting (CABG), 7–9, 13–18, 20–27, 29–33, 37–39, 54, 56, 59, 63, 82, 93, 117, 118, 125, 145, 173, 197
Coronary artery disease (CAD), 7, 12, 30, 53, 59, 63, 92, 128, 151, 160, 173
Coronary sinus perfusion, 3
Coselli, J.S., 165
Crawford classification, 158
Crawford, E.S., 157–159
Creatinine, 1, 37–40, 42, 44, 54, 83, 127, 166
Crooke, G.A., 84
Cryoablation, 113–117
Cryopreservation, 134
Custom-branched endografts, 180
Cytokines, 42, 43

D

David, T.E., 104
David, T.M., 126
De-airing of the heart, 3–4, 84
Debranching, 155–156, 168, 169, 176, 180, 184, 187, 189
Debridement, 102–103, 105, 135, 136, 138, 141, 142, 148–150, 163, 190
Decompensated heart failure, 67, 68
Deep hypothermia circulatory arrest, 152
Defibrillation, 63
Descending aorta, 26, 70, 151–157, 159, 160, 163, 173, 174, 177, 178, 180, 183, 185, 186, 188, 189, 191
Dexamethasone, 46
Diffuse microvascular hemorrhage, 60
Diltiazem, 16, 17, 46
Di Mauro, M., 27
Donas, 168
Dopamine, 45
Double-valve endocarditis, 149
Dumont, E., 94, 96
Duran, G., 133

E

Early postoperative stroke, 29, 30
Echocardiography, 22, 29, 63, 83, 84, 86, 89, 95, 99, 100, 121, 135, 139, 143–145, 147, 151, 160, 163, 198
ECMO. *See* Extracorporeal membrane oxygenation
Elderly patients, 15, 16, 46, 63, 64, 129, 173, 174
Elephant trunk procedure, 155, 156, 168
Emergency redo cardiac surgery, 5
Endocarditis, 1, 81, 83, 99–107, 121–124, 126, 128, 135, 138, 141–150
Endoleak, 171–186, 189, 190
Endovascular
  embolization, 175, 179, 181
  procedures, 159, 172, 191–192
  repair, 168, 171, 173, 175, 177–179, 183–188, 190, 192
  techniques, 178, 185
Enterococcus, 99, 143
Etz, C.D., 162, 168
Euko-reduced blood, 13
Extracorporeal membrane oxygenation (ECMO), 4, 69–73, 75, 78, 118

F

Factor VII, 14, 60
Fenoldopam, 45, 46
Fibrin sealant, 59
Fibrous trigone, 92, 94, 122
Fraser, T., 141–150
Free radicals, 42, 43, 45, 46
Frozen elephant trunk technique, 174, 180, 184
Fukuda, I., 32
Fungal pathogen(s), 101, 143

G

GFR. *See* Glomerular filtration rate
Gibbon, 67
Glomerular filtration rate (GFR), 41, 44, 45
Gold, J.P., 42
Graft, 2, 7, 21, 31, 46, 54, 57, 63, 71, 82, 93, 101, 117, 123, 125, 135, 143, 151, 159, 171, 196
Graft infection, 143, 145, 159, 163, 188
Greason, K.L., 99–107
Green, 8
Greenberg, R.K., 166
Griepp technique, 175
Griffin, B., 141–150
Guiraudon, G.M., 102
Gunning, A., 133

H

HACEK group, 99
Heartstring device, 2

Hemiarch, 136, 151
Hemodialysis, 1, 7, 17, 37, 38, 123, 143
Hemolysis, 39, 42, 72, 75, 93, 95, 96
Hemostasis, 10, 31, 57–60, 81, 83, 162
Heparin, 13, 16, 24, 58, 63, 72, 77, 83, 162
High-risk patients, 33, 44, 63, 130, 157, 187, 195, 200
High surgical risk, 1, 127
Homograft, 123, 126, 133–139, 145, 163, 190
Hybrid techniques, 157, 184, 187
Hybrid visceral debranching, 168, 169
Hypertension, 4, 5, 39, 42, 53, 63, 76, 81, 90, 121, 123, 135, 159, 164
Hypofibrinogenemia, 59

I

Iliofemoral disease, 179
Impella, 4, 68–70, 77
Indications, 17, 67, 70, 89–90, 93, 100, 106, 109–110, 115, 145, 146, 171, 173, 174, 178, 181, 183, 184, 186, 188–191, 196
Inflammatory response, 42, 43
Inotropic support, 11, 13, 40, 45, 64, 70, 78
Interagency Registry for Mechanically Assisted Circulatory support (INTERMACS), 69
Internal thoracic artery (ITA), 2, 8–11, 13, 15–17, 160, 181
Intra-aortic balloon pump (IABP), 23, 38, 40, 64, 68–71, 77, 78
Intra-arterial thrombolysis, 32, 33
Intraoperative preparation, 83
Intrapericardial dissection, 23
ITA. *See* Internal thoracic artery

K

Kamdar, A.R., 82
Katzan, I., 33
Kieffer, 163
Kobayashi, J., 112
Kormos, R.L., 67–78
Kulik, A., 159

L

Lam, B.K., 95
Lassnigg, A., 38
Lateral thoracotomy, 26, 84, 101, 168
Leacche, M., 38
Leaflet plication, 90
Leaflet tethering, 95
Left subclavian artery, 153, 155, 160, 172–177, 180, 181, 183, 186, 191
Left ventricular dysfunction, 7, 42, 44, 70, 75, 78, 109
Leuko-reduced blood, 13
Liano, F., 38
Li, J.S., 143
Limited surgical dissection, 3
Lok, C.E., 38
Lombardi, J.V., 168
Loop, F.D., 8
Low cardiac output syndrome, 4, 121, 122

M

Machiraju, V.R., 1–5, 7–18, 121–124
Malik, A.M., 29–33
Mannitol, 45, 46
Marfan's syndrome, 155, 158, 159, 161, 163, 164, 168
Maze procedure, 93, 109–115, 118
Mechanical cardiac support, 67
Mechanical prostheses, 99, 100, 141
Mechanical valves, 73, 105, 126, 133
Medically inoperable, 127, 128
Minakata, K., 67–78
Minimally invasive cardiac surgery, 129
Minimally invasive direct coronary artery bypass (MIDCAB), 22, 26
Minithoracotomy, 26, 86, 118
Mitral valve
  disease, 81–86, 114, 122, 195
  reconstruction, 101, 103–105, 142, 149
  regurgitation, 4, 89, 197, 198
  repair, 3, 18, 89–96, 122, 197
  replacement, 4, 92–95, 99, 100, 106, 107, 122
  surgery, 54, 64, 81, 89, 101, 111, 112, 116–118, 122, 123, 197, 198
Moon, M.R., 105
Murray, A.W., 63–64
Myocardial protection, 8, 11–14, 21, 27, 64, 69, 78, 82, 86, 127, 147
Myung, R.J., 21–27

N

N-acetylcysteine (N-AC), 46
Nephrotoxic medications, 41, 44
Nishi, H., 2
North American Symptomatic Carotid Endarterectomy trial (NASCET), 30

O

O'Brien, M.F., 85, 134
Off-pump coronary artery bypass grafting (OPCAB), 21–23, 25–27, 38, 39
Oxygen consumption in 1 minute (VO_2), 41

P

Padmanabhan, A., 57–60
Park, C.B., 2
Patient-related factors, 1, 53, 54
Pentoxifylline, 46
Percutaneous devices, 69, 77, 197
Percutaneous valve insertion, 127–130
Perioperative hemorrhage, 8, 14–15
Perioperative ischemic stroke, 29
Perioperative period, 57, 83, 171
Pettersson, G.B., 126, 141–151

Placement of Aortic Transcatheter Valve (PARTNERS trial), 127
Plasma transfusion, 54, 57–59
Platelet transfusion, 58–60, 83
Portner, P., 67
Postcardiotomy, 67–75, 77, 78
Posterior leaflet, 90–96
Postoperative care, 55
Postoperative management, 18, 115, 139, 149–150, 160, 164
Postoperative pleural effusions, 54
Preoperative examination, 81, 84
Prolonged ventilation, 14, 53, 54
Prophylactic nasal continuous positive airway pressure, 54
Prosthetic valve, 1, 3–5, 99–103, 105–107, 109, 122, 123, 138, 141–143, 147, 189
Protamine, 25, 58, 163
Pseudointima, 135, 136
Pulmonary complications, 53–55
Pulmonary hypertension, 4, 5, 53, 63, 76, 90, 121, 135
Pulmonary vein isolation (PVI), 109, 117
Puskas, J.D., 21–27

R

Radial artery, 15–17
Radiofrequency ablation, 109, 114
Radiographic contrast agents, 44
Ramankutty, R., 141–150
Redo coronary artery bypass grafting (Redo CABG), 7–9, 13–18, 21, 22, 27, 54, 57
Redo sternotomy, 2, 5, 8–9, 22, 109, 180
Redo thoracotomy, 81, 160
Renal tubular injury, 39
Restrictive pulmonary impairment, 53
Retrograde, 3, 5, 12, 14, 64, 84, 102, 125, 126, 147, 148, 151, 154–156, 172, 176, 177, 179–181, 187, 188
Revascularization, 1, 2, 4, 5, 7, 8, 10, 14, 15, 17, 18, 21–33, 53, 59, 64, 68, 69, 71, 73, 78, 82, 160, 164, 175, 179–181, 186
Right thoracotomy, 64, 84, 86, 101
Right ventricular dysfunction, 4, 12, 64, 76
Ring annuloplasty, 90, 92, 93, 95, 122, 123
Root replacement, 134–136, 138, 139, 148
Roselli, E.E., 166, 171–192
Rosner, M.H., 37–46
Ross, D.N., 133
Ross operation, 139, 149

S

Saphenous vein, 5, 8, 13–18
Savage, E.B., 14
Schaff, H.V., 81–86, 89–96, 99–107, 109–118, 195–198
Seal zone, 173, 174, 177, 179, 182, 184, 186
Smith, R.L., 11, 196
Sohail, M.R., 100
Soltesz, E.G., 157–169
Sorajja, P., 198
Spinal cord protection, 160, 164–166
Staphylococcus, 100, 123, 142
Stent
  collapse, 171, 185–186
  graft, 155, 166–169, 171–190
  migration, 171, 175, 178, 182–184
Sternotomy, 2, 5, 8, 9, 21, 22, 26, 27, 63, 64, 83, 84, 90, 101, 102, 109, 116, 125–127, 135, 163, 173, 175, 176, 180, 184, 187, 191, 196
Streptococcus, 99, 100
Stroke, 1, 8, 11, 14, 26, 29–33, 63, 64, 69, 73, 82, 84, 86, 101, 102, 109, 111, 127, 128, 130, 145, 151–154, 156, 166, 196, 198
Stulak, J.M., 109–118, 195–198
Subcoronary approach, 133
Sundt, T.M., 126, 151
Sundt, T.M. III, 133–139
Surgical techniques, 16, 69, 78, 112–113, 123, 124, 141
Suri, R.M., 89–96
Svensson, L.G., 151–156, 159, 165

T

Tachyarrhythmias, 109, 110, 115
TAG endoprosthesis, 172
TandemHeart, 68–70, 76–77
Technical failure, 93, 94, 96
Thakar, C.V., 38
Theophylline, 45, 115
Thoracic aneurysmal disease, 173
Thoracic endovascular aortic repair (TEVAR), 171, 173, 177, 180, 183, 187, 189, 190
Thoracoabdominal aneurysm, 158–160, 164–166, 176, 177
Thoracoabdominal aorta, 155–157, 160–161, 164, 176, 177, 179
Thoracoabdominal incision, 157, 160, 178
Thoratec PVAD, 68–70, 73
Thrombocytopenia, 59, 60
Tissue plasminogen activator (t-PA), 14, 31
Tranexamic acid, 14, 60, 64, 83
Transfusion, 15, 39, 54, 57–60, 63, 72, 83
Triangular leaflet resection, 90–91
Tricuspid valve regurgitation, 81, 112, 121, 123, 197, 198
Tricuspid valve stenosis, 121
Triulzi, D.J., 57–60
Tuttle, K.R., 44
TX2 stent graft, 173

U

Univentricular support, 75

V

Valvular heart disease, 89, 111–112, 121, 122, 195–198
Valvular surgery, 1, 4, 29, 37, 111
Vascular access injury, 190
Vasoplegic syndrome, 4–5
Vein graft atheroscelorosis, 13, 14
Vein graft failure, 8, 13–14

W

Walther, T., 196
Wechsler, L.R., 29–33
Wells, C.M., 63–64
Wilson, D.O., 53–55

Y

Yacoub, M.H., 133, 134, 136
Yoshioka, I., 82

Z

Zegdi, R., 95, 96

Made in the USA
Monee, IL
13 September 2026

62976345R00122